KU-784-549

Clinics in Developmental Medicine
LIFE QUALITY OUTCOMES IN CHILDREN
AND YOUNG PEOPLE WITH NEUROLOGICAL
AND DEVELOPMENTAL CONDITIONS:
CONCEPTS, EVIDENCE, AND PRACTICE

Clinics in Developmental Medicine

Life Quality Outcomes in Children and Young People with Neurological and Developmental Conditions: Concepts, Evidence, and Practice

Edited by

GABRIEL M. RONEN
McMaster University
Hamilton, ON
Canada

PETER L. ROSENBAUM
McMaster University
Hamilton, ON
Canada

2013
Mac Keith Press

© 2013 Mac Keith Press
6 Market Road, London, N7 9PW

Editor: Hilary M. Hart
Managing Director: Ann-Marie Halligan
Production Manager: Udoka Ohuonu
Project Management: Prepress Projects Ltd

The views and opinions expressed herein are those of the author and do not necessarily represent those of the publisher.

All rights reserved. No part of this publication may be reproduced, stored in a retrieval system, or transmitted in any form or by any means, electronic, mechanical, photocopying, recording or otherwise, without the prior written consent of the copyright holders or the publisher.

First published in this edition in 2013

British Library Cataloguing-in-Publication data
A catalogue record for this book is available from the British Library

ISBN: 978-1-908316-58-5

Typeset by Prepress Projects Ltd, Perth, UK
Printed by Henry Ling Limited, Dorchester, England

Mac Keith Press is supported by Scope

Dedication

As the editors of this volume we take great pleasure in dedicating the book to the people whose presence in our lives has had an overwhelming impact on our own life quality – to Michele, Lea and Raphael Ronen, and to Suzanne, Pauline, Joanna and Daniel Rosenbaum. We wish to express to them our love and affection, and to thank them for a lifetime of support as we have developed and pursued our interests as physicians, mentors, researchers and authors. We have tried to infuse the book with the life lessons we have learned together with our families, promoting themes of love, compassion, hope, resilience, and achievement that we believe are viable for people with neurological and developmental conditions.

GMR and PLR

CONTENTS

Contents

AUTHORS' APPOINTMENTS

Dana Anaby
Assistant Professor, School of Physical and Occupational Therapy, McGill University, Montreal, QC, Canada

Joan K. Austin
Distinguished Professor Emerita, Indiana University School of Nursing, Indiana University-Purdue University, IN, USA

Rachel Birnbaum
Childhood and Social Institutions and Social Work, King's University College, University of Western Ontario, London, ON, Canada

Christine Blain-Arcaro
Faculty of Education, University of Ottawa, ON, Canada

Bernard Dan
Professor of Paediatric Neurology and Neurophysiology, Queen Fabiola University Children's Hospital, Free University of Brussels, Belgium

Aileen M. Davis
Division of Health Care and Outcomes Research, Toronto Western Research Institute, Toronto, ON, Canada

Jenny Downs
Telethon Institute for Child Health Research, Centre for Child Health Research, The University of Western Australia, Perth, WA, Australia

David Dunn
Riley Child and Adolescent Psychiatry Clinic, Indianapolis, IN, USA

Nora Fayed
Health Care and Outcomes Research, Toronto Western Research Institute, University Health Network, Department of Pediatrics, McMaster Children's Hospital, Hamilton, ON, Canada

Gina Glidden
Outcome Trajectories Among Children with Epilepsy, Department of Pediatrics, McMaster Children's Hospital, Montreal, QC, Canada

Jan Willem Gorter
CanChild Centre for Childhood Disability Research, McMaster University, Hamilton, ON, Canada

Jennifer Hepditch
Department of Psychology, University of Ottawa, ON, Canada

Ann Jacoby
Department of Public Health and Policy, Institute for Psychology, Health and Society, University of Liverpool, Liverpool, UK

Sheila Jennings
Osgoode Hall Law School, Toronto, ON, Canada

Elizabeth N. Kerr	Department of Psychology, The Hospital for Sick Children, Toronto, ON, Canada
Marjolijn Ketelaar	Senior Researcher, Rudolf Magnus Institute of Neuroscience, Center of Excellence for Rehabilitation Medicine, University Medical Center Utrecht, Utrecht, the Netherlands
Olaf Kraus de Camargo	McMaster University, Chedoke Site, Evel 311, 1280 Main Street West, Hamilton, ON, Canada
Amanda Krygsman	Faculty of Education, The University of Ottawa, ON, Canada
Lucyna Lach	Associate Professor, School of Social Work, McGill University, Montreal, QC, Canada
Mary Law	School of Rehabilitation Science, *CanChild* Centre for Childhood Disability Research, McMaster University, Hamilton, ON, Canada
Helen Leonard	Telethon Institute for Child Health Research, Centre for Child Health Research, The University of Western Australia, Perth, WA, Australia
Patricia McDougall	Department of Psychology, College of Arts and Science, University of Saskatchewan, Saskatoon, SK, Canada
Christopher Morris	Senior Research Fellow in Child Health, Peninsula Cerebra Research Unit, Peninsula Medical School, University of Exeter, Exeter, UK
Iona Novak	Head of Research, Cerebral Palsy Institute, Darlinghurst, University of Notre Dame, Sydney, NSW, Australia
Scott Reeves	Center for Innovation in Interprofessional Education, University of California, San Francisco, CA, USA
Rebecca Renwick	Department of Occupational Science and Occupational Therapy, University of Toronto, Toronto, ON, Canada
Miriam Riches	Special Education Teacher, Toronto District School Board, Toronto, ON, Canada
Marij Roebroeck	Transition and Lifespan Research, Department of Rehabilitation Medicine, Erasmus MC University Medical Center, Rotterdam, the Netherlands
Gabriel M. Ronen	Faculty of Health Sciences, McMaster University, Hamilton, ON, Canada

Authors' appointments

Peter L. Rosenbaum
CanChild Centre for Childhood Disability Research, McMaster University Hamilton, ON, Canada

Dianne J. Russell
CanChild Centre for Childhood Disability Research, McMaster University, Hamilton, ON, Canada

Kim Schonert-Reichl
Department of Education and Counselling Psychology, University of British Columbia, Vancouver, BC, Canada

Val Shilling
Peninsula Cerebra Research Unit, Peninsula Medical School, University of Exeter, Exeter, UK

Veronica Smith
Department of Educational Psychology, University of Alberta, Edmonton, AB, Canada

Debra Stewart
School of Rehabilitation Science, McMaster University, Hamilton, ON, Canada

David L. Streiner
Department of Psychiatry and Behavioural Neurology, McMaster University, Hamilton, ON, Canada

Michele C. Thorne
Clinical Psychologist, Indiana Psychiatric Associates, Indianapolis, IN, USA

Tracy Vaillancourt
Faculty of Education and School of Psychlogy, Falculty of Social Sciences, University of Ottawa, ON, Canada

Irene Vitoroulis
Department of Psychology, University of Ottawa, ON, Canada

Diana Wiegerink
Transition and Lifespan Research Group, Erasmus MC University Medical Centre, Rotterdam and Rijndam Rehabilitation Center, Rotterdam, the Netherlands

FOREWORD

Maximizing the health and well-being of all members of society requires an integrated approach to healthcare provision, psychological issues, and social dimensions. In recent decades, the pendulum of public and professional opinion has swung, without real evidence, between the assumption that persons with disabilities lack meaningful quality of life and that, therefore, no intervention is worthwhile and the assumption that all available interventions should be implemented regardless of impact.

Discussion on healthcare reform in North America and elsewhere focuses on health disparities introduced by race, ethnicity, culture, sex, and sexual orientation but often ignores disability. There is ample experience and some data strongly indicating that disability is a major source of disparity. Disability in childhood is not going away and may be increasing. Most children with disabilities live well into adult life. It is time to assemble and make sense of what has been learned over the last 30 or 40 years about the concepts of quality of life and health status with special attention to disability.

This book, edited by Professors Ronen and Rosenbaum, admirably addresses these issues with a particular emphasis on how investigation and policy are evolving in Canada. A biopsychosocial model of health lies at the core of the book. The authors use the conceptual model of the International Classification of Function, Disability and Health (ICF), developed over the last 30 years under the auspices of the World Health Organization. Coupled with the International Classification of Disease (ICD), the ICF provides a framework for taking into account the contributions of biological, environmental, social, and personal characteristics to the functional status. The model allows aggregation of functional status across populations, which makes measurement tools based on the ICF model valuable for public health and policy. This bridge between individual and public health is no mean feat. The ICD is a reasonably complete system for specifying biological causes of illness. The ICF provides a system for specifying individual functional abilities which, from management and policy points of view, are often 'non-categorical' with respect to cause. This is particularly true of developmental disabilities. Failure to recognize the distinction between causes of disability and the consequences has impeded both research and public understanding. The authors do a great service by illuminating the confusing literature that has evolved regarding the related but distinct concepts of health status, health-related quality of life, and a personal view of quality of life. Intuitive thinking and knee jerk assumptions about quality of life are particularly vexing when applied to developmental disabilities. Healthcare professionals consistently overestimate the perceived 'burden' of impaired health status and tend to conflate health status with quality of life. Even parents and family members may make erroneously negative assumptions. The authors nicely illustrate this 'disability paradox' in which individuals with impaired, even severely impaired, health status have a much more positive view of their personal quality of life. The ICF encourages resolution of this paradox by focusing attention on activity and participation in life and on environmental and social factors that can be changed more easily than biological causes.

This book will serve the needs of several broad audiences. Students will find a lucid introduction to the current core concepts that will help them organize thinking about disabilities. Healthcare professionals with an interest in chronic conditions will find the chapters on measurement especially useful in devising ways of taking account of quality of life issues among the children and families they serve. Researchers will appreciate the excellent review and identification of areas that need much more investigation. Healthcare policy makers, administrators, and executives will find a great deal of information that should enable them to better organize health care on behalf of the increasing number of persons growing up with disabilities who will have ever-improving longevity and could be actively earning income and participating in all aspects of society. The use of case examples is especially helpful for illustrating several of the most important issues. Canadian legislative and judicial experience is emphasized in a constructive way and will stimulate review of similar experience in other countries.

The authors have done the rest of us a real service with this pioneering publication. Given that the field is young and dynamic, they will need to give us a second edition in the next few years.

John F. McLaughlin MD
Professor of Paediatrics
Seattle Children's Hospital
Seattle, WA, USA

PREFACE

Health care in the Western world is undergoing a major renaissance in the twenty-first century. Among the exciting developments is the recognition of the importance for healthcare providers to identify, understand, respect, and measure people's existential experience of their life with a chronic health condition. These perspectives – complementary to clinicians' and researchers' traditional biomedical focus on health – include an awareness of the life-course experiences of people who have these disparate conditions. There is an increasing recognition of the need to take account of these collective implications in the development and delivery of services for the people we are trusted to help.

This book takes a 'non-categorical' approach to health issues. There is abundant evidence that, despite huge variation in the underlying biomedical causes and features of various chronic health conditions, there is considerable common ground among these conditions with respect to their impact on the lives of the people who have them. The science of the measurement of patient-reported outcomes is being developed and applied in ways that allow health service professionals and researchers to gain a solid understanding of what people with chronic conditions experience in their lives as a consequence of these conditions, and how professionals can use these insights to engage with people to develop and deliver services that are responsive to these personal realities.

In this book the authors address current concepts, evidence, measurement science, challenges, and opportunities to study, understand, and apply what we are learning from people about their lives with chronic health conditions. The particular focus of this volume is the experience of children and young adults – people who are growing up with neurological and developmental conditions. Unfortunately there has often been pessimism and a feeling that nothing could be done to help them. We believe that this book illuminates three major themes: (1) that people's lives are rich and often satisfying 'despite' even significant biological imperfections; (2) that there are important lessons to be learned from people living those lives; and (3) that there are respectable scientific methods to be applied to move the field forwards.

This book is written for everyone who is interested in these important aspects of the health of children and young people with neurological and developmental conditions and their families. As the editors of this book, we hope that readers will find these ideas accessible and useful. If these perspectives and concepts enrich the quality of the work we do in our roles as service providers, researchers, advocates, and policy makers, this book will have served its purpose.

Gabriel M. Ronen
Peter L. Rosenbaum
McMaster University
Ontario, Canada
December 2012

ABOUT THE EDITORS

Gabriel M. Ronen is a Professor of Paediatrics at McMaster University and a Paediatric Neurologist at McMaster Children's Hospital in Hamilton, Ontario. He graduated from the University of Basel, Switzerland, where he also trained in paediatrics. He continued his training in Child Neurology in Canada. Dr Ronen founded the paediatric neurology and epilepsy services in the province of Newfoundland and Labrador during his first faculty position at Memorial University of Newfoundland.

Peter Rosenbaum is a Professor of Paediatrics at McMaster University, Ontario, Canada, where he holds a Canada Research Chair in Childhood Disability, Mentoring and Dissemination. He is co-founder of the *CanChild* Centre for Childhood Disability Research.

ACKNOWLEDGEMENTS

Rebecca Renwick (Chapter 3) gratefully acknowledges assistance with the literature search and appraisal for this chapter by University of Toronto student research assistants, Kali Jacobs, Saira Qadir, and Chloe Tudor.

Tracy Vaillancourt (Chapter 8) acknowledges funding from the Canadian Institutes of Health Research Canada Research Chair Program.

David L. Streiner (Chapter 18) thanks Paula Goering, Diego Silva, and Edward Wise for their extremely helpful comments on a previous version of this chapter.

COMMONLY USED ABBREVIATIONS

ADHD	attention-deficit–hyperactivity disorder
ALS	amyotrophic lateral sclerosis
ASD	autism spectrum disorder
CNS	central nervous system
CP	cerebral palsy
DSM-IV	Diagnostic and Statistical Manual of Mental Disorders, 4th edition
HRQL	health-related quality of life
ICF	International Classification of Functioning, Disability and Health
ICF-CY	International Classification of Functioning, Disability and Health for Children and Youth
IPC	interprofessional collaboration
IPE	interprofessional education
KT	knowledge translation
KTA	knowledge into action
PRO	patient-reported outcomes
QOL	quality of life
WHO	World Health Organization

1
SETTING THE STAGE: INTRODUCTION AND GENERAL OVERVIEW

Gabriel M. Ronen and Peter L. Rosenbaum

Neurological and developmental conditions are highly prevalent and cause biomedical and functional impairments that frequently lead to disabilities. Neurologically disabled people experience enormous challenges that have been identified as a global health priority by major international organizations (Janca et al 2006) and are now recognized as having social and public health impacts. Among these conditions, those associated with prenatal, perinatal, and neonatal onset are considered to be most prevalent (Bergen and Silberberg 2002, Mwaniki et al 2012) and are an important cause of interference with the typical developmental processes of childhood and early adulthood (hence 'neurodevelopmental' impairments and disabilities).

It will be apparent that people with neurological and developmental conditions are at high risk for a variety of predicaments involving diverse biomedical, behavioural, psychological, academic, social, and existential dimensions of their lives. Even major scientific breakthroughs in our understanding of the cause of a disease or the discovery of interventions to arrest the progression of an illness or its acute exacerbation are not likely to resolve the personal and social challenges related to the underlying conditions among the people who already have them.

Increasingly, healthcare providers have come to realize that in terms of the influences on the daily lives and long-term outcomes of individuals with lasting impairments people's perceptions of their conditions and a host of related social factors are as important as the biomedical conditions themselves. Developments that have contributed to this rising awareness include: (1) national and international recognition for the rights, dignity, and protection of people with disabilities; (2) advocacy and awareness campaigns by countless organizations around the world for people with neurological and developmental conditions; (3) the continuous refinements of relevant theories and the development of conceptual frameworks of outcomes, health, and health-related constructs such as functioning, participation, and quality of life; (4) improvements in the development of health measurement tools that today consist of most health-related aspects including patient-reported outcomes, making it possible to expand empirical research into the field of biopsychosocial constructs; and (5) the development of powerful statistical methods that enable researchers to study, both simultaneously and longitudinally, the complex interrelationships of a wide range of interconnecting health components. These statistical methods reduce the risk of oversimplifying life issues by reductionist methods, in which the inclusion of a limited number of factors, and univariate analyses, can too easily result in a narrow perspective of human problems with the danger of missing completely the true picture in all its complexity.

Focusing on these multifaceted realities, the aim of this book is to provide service providers and health services researchers with critically reviewed up-to-date information about life quality outcomes, relevant concepts, and methodological approaches to reflect the complexity of the life issues of both children and young adults with chronic conditions and of their families. We bring together scientifically grounded views and pertinent illustrative examples that we hope will enhance people's understanding of both the holistic outlook and the specific perspectives that are so important for the functioning of individuals with chronic conditions and the achievement of their personal goals. We also seek to convey how these individuals and their families view their own lives, our interventions, and the healthcare management they receive.

We chose to include the outcomes of 'emerging' adults in this volume because young people with neurological and developmental conditions may not yet, in their late teens and early adulthood, have reached their full cognitive, communicative, and social capacity for dealing with all the challenges they may face in an adult world (Arnett 2004) (Fig. 1.1). We have come to understand that the processes of brain maturation take longer in many people with neurological and developmental conditions. For example, researchers have identified that there is great variability in the maturation of different components of the brain among typically developed individuals, with considerable remodelling of grey and white matter continuing into the third decade of life (Lenroote et al 2006). Other empirical data suggest further delays in brain maturation in young people with developmental conditions, particularly with regard to cortical myelination, which lags behind that of controls by 3.2 years (Pujol et al 2004). Unfortunately the biopsychosocial impact of the delayed brain maturation in these emerging adults has not received the attention it deserves with regard to the research needed in order to understand the specific care they require during these years of transition and emerging adulthood.

The current text stresses the importance for healthcare professionals and researchers to be aware of the diversity of the outcomes of young people that should be considered; to take advantage of the tools and methods that are available to assess people's health, functioning, and quality of life outcomes; to recognize the determinants for each of these outcomes; to consider these outcomes in planning interventions; and to take opportunities to evaluate these various outcomes precisely as a basis for implementing evidence-based improvements in services. There is little doubt that it should be possible to intervene strategically to minimize

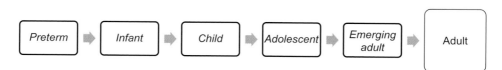

Fig. 1.1 The developmental stages included in the age range considered in this book.

threats to young disabled people's overall health and promote successful psychological, emotional, physical, and social development – even in the face of 'impairments' – in ways that will positively influence their health trajectories throughout their lifespan. We hope that this volume will inspire diverse opportunities to improve the life prospects of individuals with impairments, in order to help them achieve what they want to do and become who and what they want to become. We believe that this goal can be accomplished by promoting a variety of health-related interventions from various aspects of life that can be introduced at multiple points of entry in people's lives to any individual or population with impairments. Thus, this book should stimulate ideas for new approaches to study these outcomes in large populations and in different societies worldwide. We trust that by assembling these topics together in one book we are able to produce a reference work with significant impact beyond that achieved by the separate chapters.

It is expected nowadays that health professionals will be challenged to understand their patients' views about their conditions and the effects these conditions have on their patients' values, life goals, and welfare. With this objective in mind, Section A of this book covers an expanded range of relevant life quality outcomes that reflect the ways in which patients and families view their conditions and our interventions. We highly value the 'non-categorical' approach to our field, complementary to the 'categorical' or diagnostic approach, to reflect the extent to which the issues of interest in this text concern common matters that transcend specific diagnostic entities. We have tried to integrate advanced research-based knowledge from numerous biopsychosocial dimensions that are important to the life situations of young people with neurological and developmental conditions and their families.

Throughout this book we focus primarily on concepts that allow us to further develop and expand on current ideas, rather than concentrating on definitions with their set boundaries, which only limit such an approach. Chapters 2 to 5 in this section discuss in detail the World Health Organization (WHO) and others' concepts and definitions of 'health', 'functioning', 'participation', and 'quality of life'. We argue that although these ideas are related they are conceptually distinct. We have attempted to adhere to the terminology and organize the chapters in sequence according to the WHO biopsychosocial framework of the International Classification of Functioning, Disability and Health (ICF) (World Health Organization 2001). We see this way of thinking as a useful approach to 'rule in' relevant aspects of a young person's issues, create a dynamic structure of possible influences on outcomes, and foster an internationally accepted terminology.

We have tried to follow the ICF terminology throughout the entire book (World Health Organization 2001). Accordingly (see Chapters 2 and 4), disability and functioning are viewed as outcomes of interactions between *health conditions* (diseases, disorders, and injuries) and *contextual factors*. Therefore the term *impairment* is used for problems in body function or structure such as a significant deviation or loss, whereas *disability* is used as an umbrella term for impairments, limitations on activity, and restrictions on participation. Disability as used here is always meant to refer to an interaction between features of the person and features of the overall context in which the person lives. Note, however, that some aspects of disability are almost entirely internal to the person while other aspects are almost entirely external (World Health Organization 2001). At times the distinction between impairment and disability may not be as obvious. It is important to point out that legislation has not (yet) adapted to the ICF model. We have attempted in this book to use 'people or individuals with disabilities' when we refer to any substantive rights. For example, 'people with disabilities have the right to dignity.'

Chapters 6 to 9 focus on the developmental aspects of the lives of young people with neurodevelopmental conditions; the psychological impact of living with these conditions, using examples taken primarily from the authors' research on children with epilepsy; peer relationships; and developing sexual relationships, reporting details from studies of young people with cerebral palsy. Chapters 10 to 13 discuss a variety of potential contextual facilitators including resilience and the family; potential contextual barriers such as stigma (again using lessons learned from people with epilepsy); and what can be learned by examining legislation, drawing on examples from legal systems.

Section B (Chapters 14–18) is devoted to methods and measurement of life quality outcomes. This part of the book includes discussion of measurement concepts and standards and particular generic questions one should consider prior to selecting patient-reported outcome measures in clinical settings and research. For example, is the life quality problem clearly understood or is an initial exploratory qualitative research methodology required to identify the exact nature of the problem? And, when choosing a measure one needs to ask: 'What is the intended purpose for which any instrument is being considered?' (i.e. What is the question to be answered?), 'What information do I need this measure to capture?', 'Does the instrument selected cover the outcomes that are expected following the intervention?', 'Are the life quality outcomes that are an issue for my clinical group articulated by the measure?', 'Should I use self- or proxy informants?', 'What ethical issues need to be considered in this context?', and 'Are normative values relevant to this question and, if so, what norms should one consider as a point reference when measuring life quality issues in this population of interest?'.

Section C addresses questions that we believe will pose interesting challenges for healthcare providers, health administers, policy makers, and researchers regarding how we may positively influence life quality outcomes that are so important to the disabled individual and his or her family. Chapters in this section discuss generic innovative approaches, programming strategies, and recommendations. The chapters are organized in three subsections. Chapters 19 to 21 discuss topics on disability and education that include ideas on the introduction of interprofessional health education from the outset of professional school; recommendations for modifications to our practices to enhance the effective use of knowledge translation; and a re-evaluation of the impact of specialized education classes for specific individuals with disabilities related to academic impairments, with evidence from an experimental classroom for young people with complex epilepsy. Chapters 22 to 24 explore issues and programmes for people with childhood-onset conditions throughout their lifespan.

The final three chapters review social aspects of disability, emphasizing the palpable need to contribute to the work of parent organizations (mostly based on UK experience), and policy debates, and to understand and participate in court decisions in promoting better lives for our patients.

Finally, we continue to need to inform and enlighten the general public, the media, and policy makers that a person with an impairment should never be portrayed as having a tragic life without value. In the ICF concept of 'contextual factors' environment is usually thought of as referring to the physical and human elements of people's lives. We have deliberately invited chapters that remind us that the sociopolitical environment also exerts a powerful influence on the lives of the citizenry, including children and young people with developmental conditions and their families.

Readers will note that, while some chapters discuss broad issues without reference to specific biomedical conditions, at other times detailed data about a specific condition such as epilepsy or cerebral palsy are used to illustrate a complex generic issue relevant to many people with neurodevelopmental conditions. The editors deliberately sought authors on the basis of those researchers' extensive experience in their respective areas, expecting that readers will be able to glean the overarching concepts illustrated by particular examples. Most chapters are not meant to provide an exhaustive review of all the issues related to that topic; rather, authors were asked to illuminate the issues and concepts relevant to their assigned areas, and we hope that they will be seen to have done so.

Healthcare expertise should not remain static; rather, in a rapidly changing era we believe that health professionals must constantly build on our skills and sustain ourselves in a dynamic and relentless pursuit for improvement. Healthcare providers tend to devote little attention to fostering novel abilities and skills and show little willingness to accept innovative ideas. Moreover, we often tend to use intuitive thinking and be confident in the conclusions we reach – even when we are wrong. Daniel Kahneman, winner of the 2002 Nobel Prize in Economics, pointed out that '… questioning what we believe and want is difficult at the best of times, and especially difficult when we most need to do it, but we can benefit from the informed opinions of others' (2011). In a recent magazine article Gawande (2011) discussed approaches for overcoming some of these human susceptibilities by actively looking for coaching either by informed colleagues or others. Successful coaching would be more likely to help us detect our flaws, systematic biases, and errors in thinking, judgement, and decision making than we are generally able to do on our own, make us aware of things that we do not see from our vantage point, and help foster effective improvement and judgement, similar to the coaching that athletes and musicians seek for themselves.

Building on Kahneman's views (2011), we aim in this volume to improve people's ability to identify and understand the limitations of belief, judgement, and choice by providing a richer and more precise language with which to discuss them and by offering ideas and tools for evaluating our interventions.

In developing an unconventional text we cannot cover all relevant aspects, and errors of omission or emphasis may justifiably bring a variety of reactions from our readership. We would be grateful for any comments that will enhance the importance of this work for future editions.

REFERENCES

Arnett JJ (2004) *Emerging Adulthood. The Winding Road from the Late Teens through the Twenties*. Oxford, UK: Oxford University Press.

Bergen DC, Silberberg D (2002) Nervous system disorders: a global epidemic. *Arch Neurol* 59: 1194–1196. http://dx.doi.org/10.1001/archneur.59.7.1194

Gawande A. (2011) Personal best: top athletes and singers have coaches. Should you? *New Yorker*. Available at: www.newyorker.com/reporting/2011/10/03/111003fa_fact_gawande (accessed 27 August 2012).

Kahneman D (2011) *Thinking, Fast and Slow*. New York: Farrar, Straus, and Giroux.

Janca A, Aarli JA, Prilipko L, Dua T, Saxena S, Saraceno B (2006) WHO/WFN survey of neurological services: a worldwide perspective. *J Neurol Sci* 247: 29–34. http://dx.doi.org/10.1016/j.jns.2006.03.003

Lenroot RK, Giedd JN (2006) Brain development in children and adolescents: insights from anatomical magnetic resonance imaging. *Neurosci Biobehav Rev* 30: 718–729. http://dx.doi.org/10.1016/j.neubiorev.2006.06.001

Mwaniki MK, Atieno M, Lawn J, Newton CRJ (2012) Long-term neurodevelopmental outcomes after intrauterine and neonatal insults: a systematic review. *Lancet* 379: 445–452. http://dx.doi.org/10.1016/S0140-6736(11)61577-8

Pless IB, Pinkerton P (1975) *Chronic Childhood Disorders: Promoting Patterns of Adjustment*. Chicago, IL: Year Book Medical Publishers.

Pujol J, López-Sala A, Sebastián-Gallés N, Deus J, Cardoner N, Soriano-Mas C (2004) Delayed myelination in children with developmental delay detected by volumetric MRI. *NeuroImage* 22: 897–903. http://dx.doi.org/10.1016/j.neuroimage.2004.01.029

World Health Organization (2001) *International Classification of Functioning, Disability and Health*. Geneva: WHO Press.

Section A Concepts and Perspectives

2

CONCEPTS AND PERSPECTIVES OF 'HEALTH' AND 'LIFE QUALITY' OUTCOMES IN CHILDREN AND YOUNG PEOPLE WITH NEUROLOGICAL AND DEVELOPMENTAL CONDITIONS

Gabriel M. Ronen and Peter L. Rosenbaum

Overview

This chapter presents the framework and concepts of the 'non-categorical' approach to health and life quality outcomes – ideas that we believe help us to expand our professional approach to any clinical situation or health services research project. The chapter examines how we understand the health of an individual, and critically appraises the World Health Organization's definition of health. The text that follows reviews how one can conceptualize the term 'life quality outcomes' and discusses whose perspectives of outcomes are important. Next comes a discussion on the potential usefulness of the International Classification of Functioning, Disability and Health (ICF) framework, including the related concepts of impairment and disability. The following section reviews the meaning of the 'disability paradox', paving the way to conceptualize and define the life quality of an individual. We finish the chapter with a brief perspective of the term 'health-related quality of life' and its measurements.

Introduction

The distinguished microbiologist and philosopher René Dubos eloquently formulated one of the major theories of health, namely that:

> sickness and disability will, in varying degrees, always be with us and health care in all societies will always have to address the negative consequences of adaptation to existing and new social and environmental influences. Even under optimal arrangements, even where preventive care is integrated with curative care, the overwhelming concerns of healthcare providers will be providing not cure but care.
>
> (Dubos 1981, cited by Levine et al 1983: 401)

This quotation clarifies some of the challenges associated with how we need to understand health and life quality outcomes, specifically for children and young adults with neurological and developmental conditions. The citation challenges people to think about the exaggerated claims of the ability of science to eradicate neurological and developmental disorders; the urgent need for ongoing comprehensive scientific investigation and follow-up with empirical data to enrich our understanding of the essential issues for our patients and their families; the importance of facilitating not just evidence-based treatments but meaningful evidence-based care of patients; and indirectly the need to develop and apply proper measures that can be useful in describing people's daily life realities and planning life quality outcomes research. In this chapter we examine several key concepts, definitions, and perspectives of health and outcomes and assess their usefulness in the clinic and in research. To advance our understanding of these terms and concepts we will rely on theories that articulate the nature of the problems and provide us with the foundations for generating meaningful hypotheses that would enable specific theory-driven research. At the same time we aim to consider these concepts at a pragmatic and operational level as this volume is geared towards use by health professionals.

The non-categorical approach to health of patients
The non-categorical approach to chronic conditions emphasizes the commonalities in life experience across disease categories (diagnoses) while addressing the variation and diverse factors affecting health (Pless and Pinkerton 1975). The reason for highlighting this concept is in part because our biomedical traditions – so strongly rooted in disease-specific approaches to diagnosis and service delivery – have limited our ability to see common themes across conditions. In contrast, within a non-categorical perspective, limitations of daily functioning are seen as common manifestations of impaired health (whatever the reason for the impairment) rather than being specific to particular aetiologies.

A landmark work that introduced systematically the principle of the commonalities across chronic conditions in child health was the book commissioned for the Vanderbilt University study of children with chronic conditions and the services they require (Hobbs et al 1985). But even today, as we expand our clinical horizons to include non-categorical thinking and consider the implications for service delivery, we struggle to translate this approach into practice. This expanded view is especially important in an era in which insurance coverage and public policy should impact a wide range of chronic neurological and developmental conditions regardless of the specific diagnosis. For example, among the top research priorities for the health of children with disabilities is the need to identify facilitators and barriers to accessing health services, together with finding the best possible strategies to integrate their needs into primary healthcare systems. These findings show that addressing disease-specific impairments is judged to be secondary to ensuring adequate healthcare systems for all people with disabilities (Tomlinson et al 2009).

The non-categorical approach makes it possible to examine the impact of various neurological conditions throughout the developing years by studying the lives of young people and their families' adaptation as well as the impact of these conditions on education and social development and their influence on later adult life. This way of thinking also allows us to construct outcomes models that assess outcomes between, as well as within, groups of people with chronic conditions. Tools that evaluate outcomes in a non-categorical way can focus on multidimensional views of health that acknowledge the priorities of children and young adults with neurological and developmental conditions and their families.

Health of the individual

In 1948, the World Health Organization (WHO) defined health as 'a state of complete physical, mental and social well-being and not merely the absence of disease or infirmity'. Widening the idea of health to a multidimensional construct that encompassed the psychological and social dimensions of people's lives in addition to the biomedical was novel. Equally significant was a shift towards focusing positively on well-being. Some might view this definition as an unattainable utopian state to which we aspire only conceptually. Today scholars even view this definition as counterproductive because the phrase 'complete … well-being' declares people with chronic conditions to be ill and unhealthy.

In reality, clinicians vary in their opinion regarding what health is, based on their own values and beliefs as well as their day-to-day practice experience. However, scholars suggest that shifting from a definition to a conceptual framework broadens the perspective and allows us to view health in a realistic manner as a universal continuum that includes individual expectations and opportunities (Huber et al 2011). It becomes obvious that health cannot be measured simply in terms of anatomical, physiological, or mental attributes. The real measure of health is the ability of individuals to function in a manner acceptable to themselves and their close social network even if this means the presence of disease (Dubos 1959, 1979). While respecting health as a broad concept it is unrealistic and impractical to regard it as an epiphenomenon that includes all the domains of well-being in life, such as financial status, level of education, poverty, or political freedom, although the impact on health of these important elements of people's lives is undeniable.

Unfortunately, the lack of specificity of the 1948 WHO definition has not enhanced our understanding of the skills required to improve health for certain populations. Furthermore, the concept of a child or young adult's health is multifaceted and complex. Many processes additional to biomedical factors contribute to the variability in health, including the ways in which the dynamic aspects of continual development and change, and psychosocial adaptation, interact with the biological, psychological and social–environmental components. It is definitely worthwhile to consider that '… to be healthy does not mean that you are free of all diseases; it means that you can function, do what you want to do and become what you want to become' (Dubos 1981, cited by Levine et al 1983: 400).

Outcomes

Outcomes have been referred to as the extent and impact that programmes or interventions have on their participants in real-life situations, as well as the accomplishment of objectives as demonstrated by a wide range of indicators.

> *Health outcomes* can therefore be thought of as changes in the global health or any of its core dimensions of an individual, group or population, attributable to a planned intervention or series of interventions regardless of whether such an intervention

was intended to cause any change. Interventions may include government policies and consequent programs, laws and regulations, or health services and programs, including health promotion programs. It may also include the intended or unintended health outcomes of government policies in sectors other than health.

(Adapted from: www.definitionofwellness.com/dictionary/health-outcomes.html)

Because the terms *outcomes* and *prognosis* are often used interchangeably we recommend reserving the medical term 'prognosis' to refer to the medical end point of a health condition and its treatment. Hippocrates used the word prognosis to indicate foretelling of the course of a disease. Its origin comes from the Greek *progignoskein*, meaning 'come to know before-hand' or foreknowledge. Nowadays prognosis is often expressed in terms of life expectancy, chance of recovery, survival, or some other specifically defined end point. Each is considered an 'outcome' when it is affected by an intervention.

In studying health outcomes we want to advance our understanding of medical conditions and their management by attempting to answer the following questions: 'How can we tell whether our patients are in fact "better" after interventions?' 'What do we mean by "better" and who is judging?' 'By what yardsticks can we evaluate outcomes, or changes in health over time?' Equally significant is the need to know whose perspectives are important. Building upon Cassell's (1982) concept, reducing persons to the details of their medical conditions does not help us better understand the person, including their potential aspirations and suffering, or comprehend their most important life issues. We propose that in thinking about *outcomes* we need to identify and incorporate not only the realization or attainment of the actual and the perceived health state on a continuum between 'good health' and 'poor health' but also the person's life goals as influenced by a multitude of factors at any point in that person's lifespan. This broad viewpoint goes beyond the notion of health as expressed by the ICF framework (discussed below).

There is an increasing body of empirical evidence across various chronic conditions that suggests that it is difficult to attribute better or poorer health outcomes solely to the biologi-cal aspects of a disease and its medical treatment. From patients' perspectives, the relation between life quality outcomes and the biomedical impairment is not necessarily linear. Clinicians working with people with complex clinical realities now recognize that it is neces-sary but not sufficient to manage the biomedical components of disease 'severity' (e.g. reduc-ing seizures with minimal adverse effects of medication or reducing spasticity with botulinum toxin injections). Many additional factors influence overall outcomes in young people with chronic disorders – factors such as a child's psychosocial adaptation, problem-solving abili-ties, coping skills in adverse situations, social communication, educational issues, and delivery of services, as well as a host of environmental factors, of which family is the most important.

Clinicians collect and evaluate 'evidence' to assess 'health outcomes' regarding whether and under what circumstances treatments, e.g. medication to control seizures or the symptoms of attention-deficit–hyperactivity disorder (ADHD), do more good than harm. However, it is not clear whether patients share clinicians' views about what constitutes good versus harm, or if they have additional or different concerns about their well-being and life quality. This leads concerned professionals to ask: 'What frames of reference should guide our understanding and evidence gathering regarding patients' life quality outcomes, and what instruments should we use to assess these outcomes?'. Outcomes research refers to the study of experiences, determinants (e.g. facilitators and barriers), and processes that influence the life-course patterns of people with chronic conditions (including the impacts of health care); such research takes account of patients' experiences, preferences, and values. Patient-reported outcomes are reports of the patient's condition that come direct from the patient without any outsiders' interpretations. In this context the distinction between moderating and mediating factors is critical for planning useful interventions (Baron and Kenny 1986).

Systems theory models play a major role in outcomes research. An *outcomes system* is conceptualized as any system in which an attempt is made to intervene in a causal process in a real-life situation in order to change higher-level outcomes. Outcome system models contain cascading sets of anticipated factors and effects. These factors can either influence something to happen or can be 'negative' in the sense of preventing higher-level outcomes occurring. An *outcome* is something that is caused (or prevented) by a lower level step within an outcomes model (Duignan 2009) (for more on system theory see Chapter 20, p. 287). In the following chapters it will become apparent that evidence-based outcomes need to follow sound theoretical frameworks.

The International Classification of Functioning, Disability and Health

Following the United Nations Standard Rules on Equalization of Opportunities for Persons with Disability (1994), the development and dissemination of the ICF (World Health Organization 2001) provided a very useful framework for thinking about important dimensions of health outcomes, especially in people with chronic conditions.

The ICF describes health through the lens of functioning. It assesses interactions among body functions and structures, activities (tasks and demands of life), and participation (engagement in life situations) (Leonardi and Ustun 2002) (see also Chapter 4, in which these ideas are discussed in detail). These components of functioning are seen to be in a dynamic relationship with the contextual factors of environment (social, physical, and geographic) and personal factors (the unique characteristics of traits that make each human a unique individual). The ICF moves beyond the traditional view of disability arising as a direct consequence of medical conditions and residing in the individual. Rather, it views (good or desired) health as a harmonious interactive dynamic process among the interconnected components of functioning and contextual factors. In this model, disability results from an erosion in the interaction between a person's body functions and structures, their activities, and their participation in society as influenced by environmental and personal factors. Thus, disability is an umbrella term for impairments, activity limitations, or participation restrictions that impede a person's desired functioning within his or her environment and personal context, and it is in this way essentially personal.

The ICF has been heralded as an important step towards a shared understanding of functioning and disability, providing multidisciplinary concepts and terminology for a transcultural universal description of health. The creation of the children and youth version (ICF-CY) (World Health Organization 2007) complements the ICF framework by addressing the contribution of child development to the concept of disability. However, the ICF can be critiqued on a number of conceptual and practical issues, including the argument that, as an objective analytical assessment system, it overlooks the perceived experience of the individual (Ueda and Okawa 2003, Hemmingsson and Jonsson 2005). (Chapter 4 describes in detail the usefulness of adopting the ICF in a variety of clinical situations.)

Impairment and disability

There is general agreement that 'impairment' indicates reduced body function, whereas the term 'disability' has been undergoing a major transformation from its use in the WHO's International Classification of Impairments, Disabilities and Handicaps linear model of disease (→ impairment → disability → handicap) (World Health Organization 1980) to its current meaning influenced by the theoretical concepts of the ICF framework (World Health Organization 2001). A 2006 *Lancet* commentary suggested that 'to be able to stand up to scrutiny, a definition of disability should be: (1) applicable to all people, (2) without segregation into groups such as the "visually impaired" or those with a chronic illness, (3) be able to describe the experience of disability across many areas of functioning, (4) allow comparison of severity across different types of disability, (5) be flexible enough for different applications, (6) be able to describe all types of disability, (7) recognize the effect of the environment on a person's disability, and (8) not include stipulations about the causes of any disability' (Leonardi et al 2006). Those authors proposed to define disability as 'difficulty in functioning at the body, person, or society level, in one or more life domains, as experienced by an individual with a health condition in interaction with contextual factors'. Their definition is both congruent with that of the ICF and consistent with the thinking behind the non-categorical approach to health.

In the context of this book we propose to think about disability as a conceptual framework on which we will be able to expand and build. Accordingly, we can put forward our idea of classifying disability as 'present but not limiting' (mild) when the ICF transdimensional construct shows only increased tensions among the main components, 'impaired interaction' (moderate) when the interaction is severed but still present at some level, and 'interaction breakdown' (severe) when total system disintegration occurs. The introduction of the concept of capability provides an additional approach to disability that adds a dimension regarding whether the individual actually wants to participate in a specific life situation (Morris 2009).

There is currently no agreement as to how to label and describe situations or individuals with multiple disabilities. When patients present with multiple and often progressive disabilities, rather than using terms with negative connotations such as 'burden of disease' or 'catastrophic conditions', we prefer the use of the neutral-sounding phrases 'complexity' or 'complicated life'. The term *complexity* refers to the level of organization of a system and can be useful for understanding outcomes. An organizational level sets the problems and provides the potential for the system to maintain a dynamic steady state through interaction with sub- and supra-systems. Following this line of thinking, the greater the complexity of disability the greater the potential conflict within a person's state, or between persons, or between a person and their environment. On the other hand, the greater the complexity, the greater is the possibility of choice, of flexibility, of adaptive behaviour or system reorganization

(Antonovsky 1993). In other words, with greater complexity there is potentially greater instability in the systems around the disabilities, opening the system to potentially useful interventions.

Another perspective on *complexity* – currently being explored by Brehaut, Kohen, Rosenbaum, and Miller (Brehaut 2012, personal communication) – concerns the potential impact on parents and families of raising a child whose life situation is beset by 'complexity'. Such a child might, for example, have multiple impairments in body structure and function, associated with restrictions in activities and participation, with the cumulative effect on parents potentially creating enormous stresses and demands. Note that this idea differs importantly from 'severity' (a clinical designation that describes the extent of a specific disease or disorder), and attempts instead to capture a gestalt sense of how these realities impact on the daily lives of the person with the 'complex' situation and on their caregivers. This notion of complexity needs further exploration and elaboration, as well as a clear separation from the term 'burden of disease'.

The 'disability paradox'

When professionals think about outcomes in their patients they often compare these with outcomes of typical people (usually including themselves!). Able-bodied observers tend to focus on the discrepancy between what they perceive the 'disabled' person would like to do and what they believe that person can do. They may also imagine themselves in these states of 'disability', and make their (almost always negative) valuations with this perspective in mind. In measuring these outcomes health professionals are likely to interpret the findings by contrasting the scores with those reported by able-bodied people.

We argue, as others have, that this comparison can be misleading and is often unjustified for a number of reasons. Individuals with chronic neurological and developmental conditions are not likely to be cured of their medical impairment. Does this mean that their health outcomes are automatically and permanently poorer than those of a typically developing population? Are persons whom others score as less than perfect on a health attribute scale (measuring levels of severity of impairments developed by typical people) necessarily in peril of poor health (Feeny et al 1996)? Do patients who score less than zero on a health attribute scale truly believe that death is preferable to life (Patrick et al 1994). There are empirical data that show that many individuals with biomedical impairments consider their life trajectories to be as satisfactory and fulfilling as those of people without impairment, in apparent discordance with their externally perceived health (Albrecht and Devlieger 1999).

In contrast to a purely biomedical approach, life issues are highly individual. They differ from person to person, highlighting the fact that an apparently similar medical condition or even similar levels of functioning such as visual impairment can be valued or perceived by individuals in many different ways. Patients may report suffering when one does not expect it, or may not report suffering when one does expect it (Cassell 1982). Individuals with lasting impairments can be highly satisfied with at least some aspects of their lives, consider themselves healthy and independent, demonstrate success, and regard themselves as having satisfactory life quality outcomes. Albrecht and Devlieger (1999) explored this paradigm and introduced the term 'disability paradox'. Relying on earlier work they raised the question:

'Why do many people with serious and persistent disabilities (impairments in this book's terminology) report that they experience a good or excellent quality of life when to most external observers these people seem to live an undesirable daily existence?'. From patients' perspectives ratings of perceived health and of biomedical impairments have been found to be distinct concepts, demonstrating that perceptions of outcomes cannot be explained by biomedical variables alone, as illustrated in young people with cerebral palsy (Rosenbaum et al 2007) and with spinal muscular atrophy (de Oliveira and Araújo 2011).

Albrecht and Devlieger (1999) used semi-structured interviews with people with moderate and serious impairments. Among those people that reported excellent or good quality of life: (1) the impairment and capability present a personal, individual, and sometimes new standard against which success is measured (analogous to the processes that many immigrants go through in their new country); (2) satisfaction is derived from performing a good job with one's life (having a 'can do' approach to life) and experiencing a sense of achievement and fulfilment within the limits of impairment and the environment; (3) finding a purpose, meaning, and harmony in life is important; and (4) there is fulfilment in recognizing the value of still being in control over their body, mind, and life. These observations are all highly personal, and they provide evidence that the relationship between modern thinking about patient-reported outcomes and impairment or functions is not necessarily linear, and that 'outcomes' do not seem to be explained by denial of the consequences of impairment or disability.

Factors identified as contributing to poor or fair outcomes include suffering from pain, feeling fatigued and depressed, losing control over body and mind, and lacking any purpose in life. In addition, people with invisible impairments also had poorer outcomes than those with visible impairments. We consider any suffering to be associated with poor outcomes. According to Cassell (1982), *suffering* can be defined as the perception of a state of severe distress associated with events that threaten the intactness of the person or the perception of impending personal destruction. In order for a situation to be a source of suffering, it must influence the perception of future events (Cassell 1982). Albrecht and Devlieger (1999) interpreted their results by suggesting that among people with an impairment one dimension of the self may compensate for the poorer function in another dimension so that the relative balance of self is maintained whereby good outcomes may result. We believe that constructs that promote a positive adaptive attitude, such as self-efficacy, optimism, benefit finding, acceptance, mindfulness, and hope, are important moderator–mediator factors that may be helpful in explaining the disability paradox. It is conceivable, if not probable, that some of these variables are amenable to change and therefore could be enhanced by interventions that address strength-based functioning. (See Chapter 10 for more on strength-based approaches to health.)

Quality of life of the individual (see also Chapter 3)

The World Health Organization (WHOQOL 1993) defined quality of life as the 'individual's perceptions of their position in life in the context of the culture and value systems in which they live, and in relation to their goals, expectations and concerns'. In a theoretical model of outcomes systems, health would probably be ranked as a major component of the overall quality of life, whereas health-related quality of life (HRQL) would be both a component of the higher-ranked quality of life as well as the subordinate-ranked level of health. This is only one of the reasons why it is so difficult to reconcile the countless definitions of quality of life and HRQL that have been proposed over the years.

In the context of this book we will adhere, at both the conceptual and the operational levels, to the definition outlined above or any other description that is congruent with the WHO framework. This is true, for example, for the Centre for Health Promotion definition of quality of life as 'the degree to which a person enjoys the important possibilities of his or her life', with its major components of 'Being' (who one is), 'Belonging' (one's place in one's environment), and 'Becoming' (achieving one's goals) (Renwick et al 2003). The terms quality of life and HRQL represent a number of interacting dimensions (we therefore prefer to use the term transdimensional over multidimensional), which entail at least the three dimensions of the individual's perceptions: (1) of satisfaction; (2) of affect balance on the pleasant–unpleasant scale; and (3) of freedom from stress (Campbell 1976). The greatest desire and happiness of a human being is not necessarily a state in which he or she experiences physical vigour and a sense of well-being, nor even one giving him or her a long life. It is, instead, the condition best suited to reach goals or complete a worthwhile task that each individual formulates for herself or himself (Dubos 1959). Here the words desire and happiness, vague as they are, seem to denote better than any other words the values of quality of life. In our Western society health has been ranked the most important domain of life, and the perception of health has been found to be closely related to perceived quality of life (Ferrans and Powers 1992). Thus, when focusing on the quality of life of patients, and in the context of this book on patient outcomes, the concerns of both sociology and medicine converge (Levine 1987).

Health-related quality of life and its measurement

As indicated above, significant misconceptions remain about what constitutes quality of life and HRQL. In the late 1970s and in the 1980s the construct of 'quality of life' emerged as an important dimension for evaluating health interventions in general and medical interventions in particular (Levine 1987). During the subsequent years the healthcare community has acknowledged that chronic conditions cannot be cured and recognized that patients with chronic impairments can improve in their social functioning. In addition civil movements have advocated for social and health planners to take more responsibility for the weakest links in society and have campaigned for more humanized health care and help to integrate these individuals as fully accepted members within their social circle in order to help them to attain their social roles. Levine et al (1987) emphasized that the 'major historical function of medicine and other health professions has been to care, to heal, and to enhance the quality of life'.

The concept of quality of life has evolved beyond the idea of activities of daily living, important as they may be, and has directed attention to the more complete social and psychological being, the individual's performance of social roles, mental acuity, emotional state, and sense of well-being (Levine 1987). In the healthcare context, the construct of quality of life aims to explore the perceived experience of the patient, where expectations, values, and satisfaction about health are emphasized over the presence, absence, frequency, or severity of actual health problems or challenges for a young person living with a chronic condition. Researchers started 'distinguishing between quality-of-life aspects which are health related

(HRQL) from the quality of life which resides in the basic social conditions of our larger world' (Levine 1987). HRQL focuses specifically on the aspects of quality of life impacted by a health condition (Guyatt et al 1993). Significantly, HRQL is relatively independent from the construct of health status that incorporates the dynamic interactions among the major ICF components and may also include the patients' symptoms.

An emerging aim within the healthcare system is to be able to measure important non-biomedical and non-physiological aspects of health that focus on the indirect effects of disease or treatment and include the perceived experiences of the individual (Guyatt et al 1989). The initial measures developed and applied to evaluate these attributes were called 'HRQL instruments' although their content was similar, if not identical, to health status measures that focus on elements of functioning in today's ICF (Bergner 1985). Many of these instruments have useful properties, but their content is not congruent with current understanding of HRQL. Cella and Tulsky (1993) have recognized that conceptualizing quality of life as health status is limited from both a theoretical and a rehabilitation perspective, and cautioned not to confuse performance (and health status) scales with measures of quality of life. They have also specified that a single-item score of quality of life, though appealing by its simplicity of administration, is not acceptable as a quality of life measure because such an approach is dimensionless. A single-item measure makes it impossible to determine specific information about the nature of a score change (Cella and Tulsky 1993).

We argue that HRQL should be considered conceptually as either a sub-domain of the more global construct of quality of life (Spilker and Revicki 1996), and measured by generic HRQL scales, or a closely related but independent construct of quality of life concerning a person's particular health condition, whereby the HRQL dimensions of concern are identi-fied by the patients themselves regarding their life with the condition (and are measured by condition-specific HRQL scales) (Ronen et al 1999, 2003). We believe that the term HRQL should be used at the operational level specifically and exclusively to describe individuals' perceptions and valuations of the health-related domains of their life with a chronic condition and not to be used interchangeably with functional or health status, which focuses on objec-tive elements of functioning.

Today the overwhelming majority of HRQL and quality of life measures found in the health services literature are based on questions that arise from clinical practice (Varni et al 2005). Recent measures have combined qualitative and quantitative methodologies and include the patients' own perspectives of their values, expectations, and dilemmas of their life (known as patient-reported outcomes or PROs). Routine collection of HRQL data in our practice has enhanced our understanding of the daily lives of young people and their families from their perspective while providing guidance on which interventions to target in individual cases and which aspects of therapy to expand upon at a programmatic level (Ronen et al 2010). HRQL measures not only can lead to useful, concrete, documented evaluation of interventions but also can assist in strengthening and highlighting the 'real stuff' focus, providing legitimization and fulfilment to health professionals to delve deeper into these issues (Annells and Koch 2001). Among young people with neurological and developmental impairments of a chronic nature, life adjustment following intervention is quite possible. Quality of life and HRQL instruments that target satisfaction, expectations, standards, and concerns about health domains are likely to tell clinicians more about the life of our chronically impaired patients than health status instruments alone (Fayed et al 2011).

Summary

In this chapter we have highlighted the notion that for young people with long-lasting or permanent neurological and developmental conditions their medical impairments must be considered in the context of their aspirations and concerns for what they want to do or to become, irrespective of their underlying biomedical condition (non-categorical approach). Disability may be considered deprivation from the freedom to act as they want. For these individuals *health* is the possibility of the freedom to live a full life, even in the presence of biomedical impairments (disability paradox) (Dubos 1979, Albrecht and Devlieger 1999). For these people successful life quality outcomes represent the degree of realization of their goals at any point in their life. In addition to their important medical guidance, health professionals can and should embrace this opportunity and take ownership of the responsibility to make it possible for their patients to realize their own goals or at least to achieve an optimal balance in their lives.

Further reading

Ronen GM, Fayed N, Rosenbaum PL (2011) Outcomes in pediatric neurology: a review of conceptual issues and recommendations. The 2010 Ronnie Mac Keith Lecture. *Dev Med Child Neurol* 53: 305–312.

REFERENCES

Key references

*Albrecht GL, Devlieger PJ (1999) The disability paradox: high quality of life against all odds. *Soc Sci Med* 48: 977–988. http://dx.doi.org/10.1016/S0277–9536(98)00411–0

Annells M, Koch T (2001) 'The real stuff': implications for nursing of assessing and measuring terminally ill person's quality of life. *J Clin Nurs* 10: 806–812. http://dx.doi.org/10.1046/j.1365–2702.2001.00546.x

*Antonovsky A (1993) Complexity, conflict, chaos, coherence, coercion and civility. *Soc Sci Med* 37: 969–981. http://dx.doi.org/10.1016/0277–9536(93)90427–6

*Baron RN, Kenny DA (1986) The moderator-mediator variable distinction in social psychological research: conceptual, strategic and statistical considerations. *J Pers Soc Psychol* 51: 1173–1182. http://dx.doi.org/10.1037/0022–3514.51.6.1173

Bergner M (1985) Measurement of health status. *Med Care* 23: 696–704. http://dx.doi.org/10.1097/00005650–198505000–00028

Campbell A (1976) Subjective measures of well-being. *Am Psychol* 31: 117–124. http://dx.doi.org/10.1037/0003-066X.31.2.117

*Cassell EJ (1982) The nature of suffering and the goals of medicine. *N Engl J Med* 306: 639–645. http://dx.doi.org/10.1056/NEJM198203183061104

Cella DF, Tulski DS (1993) Quality of life in cancer: definition, purpose, and method of measurement. *Cancer Invest* 11: 327–336. http://dx.doi.org/10.3109/07357909309024860

Dubos R (1959) *Mirage of Health: Utopias, Progress and Biological Change*. Garden City New York: Anchor Books Doubleday & Company, Inc.

Dubos R (1979) Adapting man adapting: curing, helping, consoling. *Yale J Biol Med* 52: 211–218.

Dubos R (1983) Interview reported in 'Modern Maturity', August–September 1981, p. 35. Cited by Levine S, Feldman JJ, Elinson J. Does medical care do any good? In: Mechanic D, editor. *Handbook of Health, Healthcare and the Health Professions*. New York: The Free Press, p. 400.

Duignan P (2009) Definitions used in outcome theory. Outcomes Theory Knowledge Base Article No. 231. Available at: http://knol.google.com/k/paul-duignan-phd/definitions-used-in-outcomes-theory/2m7zd68aaz774/59.

Fayed N, Schiariti V, Bostan C, Cieza A, Klassen A (2011) Health status and QOL instruments used in child-hood cancer research: deciphering conceptual content using World Health Organization definitions. *Qual Life Res* 306: 639–645.

Feeny DH, Torrance GW, Furlong WJ (1996) Health Utilities Index. In: Spilker B, editor. *Quality of Life and Pharmacoeconomics in Clinical Trials*, 2nd edn. Philadelphia, PA: Lippincott-Raven, pp. 239–252.

Ferrans SE, Powers MJ (1992) Psychometric assessment of the Quality of Life Index. *Res Nurs Health* 15: 29–38. http://dx.doi.org/10.1002/nur.4770150106

Guyatt GH, Veldhuyzen Van Zanten SJO, Feeny DH, Patrick DL (1989) Measuring quality of life in clinical trials: a taxonomy and review. *Can Med Assoc J* 140: 1441–1448.

Guyatt GH, Feeny DH, Patrick DL (1993) Measuring health-related quality of life. *Ann Intern Med* 118: 622–629.

Hemmingsson H, Jonsson H (2005) An occupational perspective on the concept of participation in the International Classification of Functioning, Disability and Health – some critical remarks. *Am J Occup Ther* 59: 569–576. http://dx.doi.org/10.5014/ajot.59.5.569

Hobbs N, Perrin JM. (1985) *Issues in the Care of Children with Chronic Illness. A Sourcebook on Problems, Services and Policies*. San Francisco, CA: Jossey-Bass Publishers.

Huber M, Knottnerus JA, Green L, et al (2011) How should we define health? *BMJ* 343: d4163. http://dx.doi.org/10.1136/bmj.d4163

Leonardi M, Ustun TB (2002) The global burden of epilepsy. *Epilepsia* 43(Suppl. 6): 21–25. http://dx.doi.org/10.1046/j.1528-1157.43.s.6.11.x

*Leonardi M, Bickenbach J, Ustun TB, Kontanjsek N, Chatterji S (2006) The definition of disability: what is in a name? *Lancet* 368: 1219–1221. http://dx.doi.org/10.1016/S0140-6736(06)69498-1

*Levine S (1987) The changing terrains in medical sociology: emergent concern with quality of life. *J Health Soc Behav* 28: 1–6. http://dx.doi.org/10.2307/2137136

Levine S, Feldman JJ, Elinson J (1983) Does medical care do any good? In: Mechanic D, editor. *Handbook of Health, Healthcare and the Health Professions*. New York: The Free Press, pp. 394–404.

Morris C (2009) Measuring participation in childhood disability: does the capability approach improve our understanding? *Dev Med Child Neurol* 51: 92–94. http://dx.doi.org/10.1111/j.1469–8749.2008.03248.x

de Oliveira CM, Araújo AP (2011) Self-reported quality of life has no correlation with functional status in children and adolescents with spinal muscular atrophy. *Eur J Paediatr Neurol* 15: 36–39. http://dx.doi.org/10.1016/j.ejpn.2010.07.003

Patrick DL, Starks HE, Cain KC, Uhlmann RF, Pearlman RA (1994) Measuring preferences for health states worse than death. *Med Decis Making* 14: 9–18. http://dx.doi.org/10.1177/0272989X9401400102

Pless IB, Pinkerton P (1975) *Chronic Childhood Disorders: Promoting Patterns of Adjustment*. Chicago, IL: Year Book Medical Publishers.

Renwick R, Nourhaghighi N, Manns PJ, Rudman DL (2006) Quality of life for people with physical disabilities: a new instrument. *Int J Rehabil Res* 26: 279–287. http://dx.doi.org/10.1097/00004356-200312000-00005

Ronen G, Rosenbaum P, Law M, Streiner D (1999) Health-related quality of life in childhood epilepsy: the results of children's participation in identifying the components. *Dev Med Child Neurol* 41: 554–559.

Ronen GM, Streiner DL, Rosenbaum P, Canadian Pediatric Epilepsy Network (2003) Health-related quality of life in children with epilepsy: development and validation of self-report and parent proxy measures. *Epilepsia* 44: 598–612. http://dx.doi.org/10.1046/j.1528-1157.2003.46302.x

Ronen GM, Lach L, Streiner DL, et al (2010) Disease characteristics and psychosocial factors: explaining the expression of quality of life in childhood epilepsy. *Epilepsy Behav* 18: 88–93. http://dx.doi.org/10.1016/j.yebeh.2010.02.023

Rosenbaum PL, Livingston MH, Palisano RJ, Galuppi B, Russel DJ (2007) Quality of life and health-related quality of life of adolescents with cerebral palsy. *Dev Med Child Neurol* 49: 516–521. http://dx.doi.org/10.1111/j.1469-8749.2007.00516.x

Spilker B, Revicki DA (1996) Taxonomy of quality of life. In: Spilker B, editor. *Quality of Life and Pharmacoeconomics in Clinical Trials*, 2nd edn. Philadelphia, PA: Lippincott-Raven, p. 25.

Tomlinson M, Swartz L, Officer A, Chan KY, Rudan I, Saxena S (2009) Research priorities for health of people with disabilities: an expert opinion exercise. *Lancet* 374: 1857–1862. http://dx.doi.org/10.1016/S0140-6736(09)61910-3

Ueda S, Okawa Y (2003) The subjective dimension of functioning and disability: what is it and what is it for? *Disabil Rehabil* 25: 596–601. http://dx.doi.org/10.1080/0963828031000137108

Varni JW, Burwinkle TM, Lane MM (2005) Health-related quality of life measurement in pediatric clinical practice: an appraisal and precept for future research and application. *Health Qual Life Outcomes* 3: 34. http://dx.doi.org/10.1186/1477-7525-3-34

WHOQOL Group (1993) Study protocol for the World Health Organization project to develop a Quality of Life assessment instrument (the WHOQOL). *Qual Life Res* 2: 153–159. http://dx.doi.org/10.1007/BF00435734

World Health Organization (1980) *International Classification of Impairments, Disabilities and Handicaps*. Geneva: WHO Press.

World Health Organization (2001) *International Classification of Functioning, Disability and Health*. Geneva: WHO Press.

World Health Organization (2007) *International Classification of Functioning, Disability and Health – Children and Youth version*. Geneva: WHO Press.

3
QUALITY OF LIFE FOR YOUNG PEOPLE WITH NEUROLOGICAL AND DEVELOPMENTAL CONDITIONS: ISSUES AND CHALLENGES

Rebecca Renwick

Overview

Quality of life is a powerful construct that enjoys wide appeal because it resonates with many people. It is a familiar term used in daily life, for example in the media and advertisements as well as in government press releases and policies. Thus, it is often assumed that everyone knows what quality of life means. However, it is evident from the vast and diverse literature on quality of life that it is a complex, multidimensional, and somewhat elusive construct with many possible meanings. In fact, it can mean different things to different individuals, in diverse contexts (e.g. within fields of health, economics, demography, sociology) and during different periods of time. Given its many possible meanings, is quality of life an important and useful construct? What are its various meanings? How is it different from, or similar to, other constructs, such as health, functional status, participation, and well-being, that are often used in connection with quality of life? How has it been measured or assessed? Whose perspective of quality of life for individual children and young people with neurological and developmental conditions should be considered and emphasized? What are some of the ways that quality of life concepts and measures of quality of life can be used in research and practice with this group of young people?

This chapter addresses these questions and highlights the issues and challenges of understanding, conceptualizing, measuring, and applying quality of life in research and practice with young people living with neurological and developmental conditions.

Why is quality of life important?

Enhancing quality of life is frequently cited as the optimal, broad outcome of health interventions for children and young people with neurological and developmental conditions (Koot and Wallander, 2001, Renwick et al 2003). Medical treatments for individuals with acute and temporary conditions typically focus on reducing symptoms or on cure, while rehabilitation interventions aim to restore the person's usual levels of function and facilitate return to engagement in the usual activities of everyday life. However, for individuals with lasting conditions, impairments, and disabilities, the desired medical and rehabilitation outcomes usually include managing symptoms, improving function, and engagement in the person's meaningful life activities, often through the use of technical devices, adapted activities, appropriate resources, and support from others (Payot and Barrington 2011). Most importantly in the context of this chapter, the overall goal of medical, rehabilitation, and habilitation interventions for individuals with lasting conditions, impairments, and disabilities is to improve, or at least maintain, quality of life so that the individual can have a good life and, ideally, the best possible life. Therefore, it is critical to be able to measure and evaluate quality of life outcomes of such interventions (Renwick 2004, Tsoi et al 2011) and determine what other interventions might help address that goal (Payot and Barrington 2011). However, what constitutes quality of life and how it is measured depend on how quality of life is conceptualized. These issues are addressed in the sections that follow.

Having a life of high quality or the best life possible is a widely shared goal among people of all ages, with or without medical conditions, impairments, and disabilities. For young people with neurological conditions, fostering and supporting good quality of life over the lifespan requires some special considerations, especially because, as they progress through life's various transitions, they will also encounter challenges associated with their neurological conditions, impairments, and disabilities. As several perspectives on disability (e.g. the social model) maintain, environmental forces play a major role in the challenges they encounter (Whalley Hammell 2006). For example, typical urban and rural environments that are not completely accessible to people with neurological and developmental conditions may constrain their opportunities for full and meaningful engagement in community activities and participation in society. Further, societal, cultural, and community understandings of, and assumptions about, impairment and disability can be stigmatizing. Attitudinal barriers (e.g. about what young people with neurological and developmental conditions can and cannot do or should and should not do) may also play a role in their experienced quality of life (Whalley Hammell 2006). However, living with conditions and impairments is not necessarily associated with poorer quality of life for all individuals (Albrecht and Devlieger 1999, Colver 2008, Payot and Barrington, 2011). For the reasons noted in this section, it is essential to know and understand how quality of life is perceived by individual young people in the context of health outcomes.

What does quality of life mean?
Quality of life is an abstract concept that, in some cases, is fleshed out in terms of an explicit, detailed conceptual framework or model that can serve as the foundation for the creation of one or more measurement instruments. However, many quality of life instruments have only implicit conceptual underpinnings that must be inferred from their items and rating scales (Zeckovic and Renwick 2003, Davis et al 2006). This issue is discussed in the next section. For now, the emphasis will be on some constructs that are often associated with quality of life, and major approaches to understanding and conceptualizing quality of life.

CONSTRUCTS RELATED TO QUALITY OF LIFE

Quality of life is often discussed in conjunction, or even interchangeably, with other terms such as *well-being*, *participation*, *health*, and *functional status*. While a number of definitions for each of these terms appear in the literature, only selected ones will be noted here in order to highlight how they differ from quality of life. However, developers of conceptual approaches and measurement instruments, researchers, and professionals do not all agree on particular definitions for quality of life or for any of the constructs noted here. Nor is there consistent agreement on the nature of the relationships among these constructs. This multiplicity of perspectives contributes considerably to the complexity of the literature about quality of life.

In the literature on childhood impairment and disability, *participation* is often discussed in association with quality of life. The International Classification of Functioning, Disability and Health (ICF) framework (World Health Organization 2001) defines participation in terms of involvement in real-life situations (e.g. going to school, doing activities in the community, etc.). A conceptual analysis of participation for children with disabilities by Hoogsteen and Woodgate (2010) amplifies the ICF definition. Their analysis adds that participation requires the child to: take part in an activity or engage with another person; feel included; choose to take part; and move towards a meaningful goal (e.g. strengthening a skill or becoming more independent) by taking part. (For more details on participation see Chapter 5.)

Well-being is a term often used interchangeably with quality of life. However, Bowling (1991) conceptualizes it as being a broader construct than either quality of life or satisfaction with life but related to both. She notes that well-being refers to a harmonious state of life as a whole, or in one or more areas of life (e.g. material well-being, physical well-being, emotional well-being).

Health is defined in various ways but probably the best-known definition is offered by the World Health Organization (1948), which states that health is not simply 'the absence of disease' (p. 11). This definition also emphasizes that health includes not only physical aspects but also mental and social aspects. More recently, the Ottawa Charter for Health Promotion contextualized the construct of health by emphasizing the empowerment of people to exert more control over and improve their own health (World Health Organization 1986). *Functional status*, which is related to health but is a narrower construct, refers to the ability to carry out roles required to fulfil an individual's fundamental needs as well as to support health and well-being (Bowling 1991, Davis et al 2006). (For more details refer to Chapter 2.)

DEFINING AND CONCEPTUALIZING QUALITY OF LIFE

The notion of a *good life* or quality of life can be traced back as far as the writings of Aristotle (Megone 1990). The term seems to embody an essential idea that has had wide and enduring appeal, at least in Western countries. Since the 1960s, more than 100 definitions of quality of life and a number of conceptual approaches have appeared in the literature. Researchers have attempted to delineate points of agreement on a definition in order to reduce the potential confusion and difficulty associated with this complex literature (Hughes and Hwang 1996). However, there is still no general consensus on either a definition or a particular conceptualization (Bowling 1991, 1995, Pizzi and Renwick 2010).

There are many definitions and a number of conceptual frameworks or models of quality of life applicable to this group of young people (Davis et al 2006). These can be thought of as being on a continuum, anchored at one end by *health-related quality of life approaches* and at the other end by *life-focused or holistic approaches.* Some definitions and conceptualizations of quality of life include aspects of both but usually have characteristics that more closely align with one approach than the other.

Definitions of health-related quality of life vary considerably (e.g. see Davis et al 2006). However, two clear examples are presented here. The definition adopted by Graham et al (1997) describes it as the individual's evaluation of his own functioning and satisfaction or distress with his own functioning. Fekkes et al (2000), in accordance with earlier definitions by Guyatt et al (1993) and Spilker and Revicki (1996: 25), characterize it as the part of overall quality of life that is mainly impacted by an individual's health and may be affected by clinical interventions. In contrast, a definition of quality of life associated with a broader, holistic conceptual approach is that it consists of 'the discrepancy between a person's achieved and unmet needs and desires' (Brown et al 1994: 41). Another is: 'the degree to which a person enjoys the important possibilities of his/her life' (Renwick et al 2000: 10).

Quality of life can be conceptualized as arising from the ongoing, complex interplay of environmental or contextual factors (e.g. environmental conditions, resources, supports) and personal factors (e.g. experiences, beliefs, values) (Renwick et al 2000, Payot and Barrington 2011). Most conceptualizations include domains that can be subjectively determined (e.g. satisfaction with school and leisure activities) while a few also include domains that can be objectively measured (e.g. quality of education, type of housing, family structure) (Lindstrom and Eriksson 1993, Brown et al 1994, Hughes and Hwang 1996, Berntsson and Kohler 2001).

Health-related quality of life conceptualizations focus on aspects of life associated with function or health, or both (e.g. perceived impact on quality of life of pain, anxiety, and other symptoms; mobility; physical, psychological, and social functioning). This is the most typical approach reported in the literature relevant to young people with neurological and developmental conditions (e.g. see Ronen et al 1999, Cowan and Baker 2004, Narayanan et al 2005, White-Koning et al 2005, Davis et al 2006). *Life-focused or holistic quality of life* is less commonly used in relation to young people, including those with neurological and developmental conditions. Such approaches address life's broader aspects that extend beyond more traditional understandings of health (e.g. perceptions about quality of life related to social and family life, spiritual aspects of life, links with one's community, opportunities for personal development and fulfilment, opportunities for making choices and decisions) (e.g. see Brown et al 1994, Schalock 1996, Renwick et al 2003, Renwick 2004).

In the literature on young people with neurological and developmental conditions, the preponderance of attention to health-related quality of life is reflected in the focus of the measurement instruments that have been developed for this group. Further, while some of these health-related conceptual approaches are stated explicitly (e.g. Ronen et al 1999, 2003a, Narayanan et al 2005), most used with this population must be inferred from the instruments developed to measure quality of life. The relatively few holistic approaches that have been developed for or applied to help understand quality of life for young people with neurological or developmental conditions typically present a definition as well as an elaborated quality of life conceptual framework or model (see Renwick et al 2003, Davis et al 2006, Waters et al 2009).

It is clearly important for professionals, researchers, and parents to understand the impact of health and function on quality of life as experienced by this group of young people. However, it is also essential to understand how they experience their lives in a more holistic sense because, first and foremost, they are young people who are much more than their neurological or developmental conditions, impairments, and disabilities (Renwick et al 2003) (see also Chapter 6). Specifically, as these young people develop from childhood through adolescence to young adulthood, the aspects of life encompassed by a broader conception of quality of life may become more and more important in contributing to subjective experiences of a good life than those aspects of life more closely associated with health and function (see Albrecht and Devlieger 1999, Payot and Barrington 2011).

Historically, very few quality of life conceptualizations applicable to young people with neurological or developmental conditions have been developed in consultation with them or their families (Renwick et al 2003, Davis et al 2006). However, based on the growing recognition of the lived experience expertise of these young people and their families as a key source of information, doing so is becoming more common (e.g. see Ronen et al 1999, Renwick et al 2003, Narayanan et al 2005). This is a positive development because, as expert sources, they can contribute essential, nuanced information about what it means to live with a lasting neurological or developmental condition. This information can be used to guide the creation of conceptual approaches that can serve as a foundation for developing quality of life measures with greater relevance to this group of young people.

QUALITY OF LIFE AS A DYNAMIC CONSTRUCT

Quality of life is a dynamic or fluid construct. It evolves over time as life circumstances change, for instance through the process of development, especially during adolescence and life transitions (e.g. from home to elementary school and then to high school) (Hanson 2001). In addition, there are differences among children, young people, and adults in terms of their perceptions about what makes life good or not so good (i.e. their perceived quality of life). An individual's evolving understanding of what constitutes a good quality of life may be influenced by cognitive and emotional development as well as life experiences and adaptation in the context of a changing environment (e.g. family, school, community, society) (Hanson 2001). Different meanings are attached to quality of life at different stages of life, with physical factors becoming less important and psychological ones becoming more important during the trajectory from childhood to young adulthood (Payot and Barrington 2011). Different needs related to different aspects of quality of life may be more salient during a particular time in the lifespan than at other times. Accordingly, the types, intensity, and combination of resources and supports that contribute to maintaining or enhancing quality of life may also change across the lifespan (Stark and Faulkner 1996). However, much remains to be explored concerning this evolutionary aspect of quality of life and its implications. This temporal evolution of quality of life is also not adequately represented in most existing conceptual frameworks.

How has quality of life been measured?

Quality of life measurement instruments are grounded in their developers' understandings and assumptions about the construct, whether these are explicitly stated or implicit. Consequently, these instruments will reflect their conceptual underpinnings by focusing on certain aspects of life, and not on others. Relatively few generic and condition-specific measures of quality of life used with young people with neurological or developmental conditions are underpinned by explicit conceptual frameworks (Renwick et al 2003, Davis et al 2006). *Generic instruments* can be used with a variety of populations and allow for comparisons among them (e.g. comparisons of quality of life among young people with cardiac conditions, skin conditions, and neurological conditions). *Condition-specific* instruments focus on young people with a particular condition or diagnosis, such as epilepsy or cerebral palsy. They are particularly sensitive to aspects of that particular condition and its impacts on quality of life (and/or functioning) (Cowan and Baker 2004). Examples of specific instruments are the Quality of Life in Childhood Epilepsy Questionnaire (QOLCE; Sabaz et al 2000) and the CP QOL-Child (Waters et al 2007). Generic instruments are exemplified by the Child Health Questionnaire (Landgraf et al 1999, Vargas-Adams 2006) and the KIDSCREEN measure (Ravens-Sieberer et al 2001).

Most of these instruments can be grouped based on their implicitly or explicitly stated underpinnings, as previously described. Measures of *health-related quality of life* tap functional or health-related aspects of quality of life, or both. Examples of such measures are the CPCHILD (Narayanan et al 2005) and the Health-related Quality of Life in Children with Epilepsy measure (CHEQOL-25) (Ronen et al 2003b). *Life-focused or holistic quality of life measures* assess broader aspects of life that extend beyond the impacts on health and function. The Quality of Life Questionnaire (Schalock and Keith 1993), the KIDSCREEN (Ravens-Sieberer et al 2001), and the Quality of Life Measure for Children with Intellectual/ Developmental Disabilities – Parental Version (Renwick et al 2005) are examples of instruments tapping holistic quality of life. There is a greater number of health-related instruments available and appropriate for use with this group of young people. The conceptual foundations of many of these health-related instruments are not described in the literature (Zekovic and Renwick 2003, Cowan and Baker 2004, Davis et al 2006); however, there are some notable exceptions (e.g. Ronen et al 1999, 2003a,b, Narayanan et al 2005).

Psychometric evaluation for reliability and validity has been done, to varying degrees, for most of the health-related and holistic instruments used with young people with neurological and developmental conditions. However, the quality of their various psychometric properties ranges from highly acceptable to poor (see Chapters 14 and 15 for more detailed discussions on psychometric evaluation and measurement). Construct validity is frequently not reported, and this is a critical missing piece of information concerning the soundness of an instrument (Cremeens et al 2006, Davis et al 2006). Further, responsiveness to changes in quality of life over time has not been adequately tested, or has not been reported, for many of these instruments (Cowan and Baker 2004, Cremeens at al 2006, Carlon et al 2010). Therefore, considerable care must be exercised when selecting an instrument that is reliable, valid, and sensitive with respect to detecting change, an essential characteristic for outcome measures employed in clinical assessment or research. Although a detailed discussion of the properties of particular instruments is beyond the scope of this chapter, there are comparative appraisals available of generic and specific instruments used to measure quality of life for young people with neurological conditions (e.g. Speith and Harris 1996, Cowan and Baker 2004, Cremeens et al 2006, Waters et al 2009, Carlon et al 2010, Fayed et al 2012).

Whose perspective should be considered?
Recently, international organizations that promote health and well-being have published documents clearly highlighting the rights of young people, both with and without health conditions, impairments, and disabilities, to express their own views and choices as well as to be heard (World Health Organization 2009, 2011, United Nations Children's Fund 2010). The collective message of these documents points to the ethical aspects of including and heeding the perspectives of young people about matters affecting their health and quality of life.

Eliciting their perspectives about their own quality of life also has practical value in that it contributes to professionals' understanding of young people's most important issues and concerns. It can also help to determine whether they experience current or recent health interventions as effective and whether the issues they perceive as important might be addressed by other kinds of health interventions (Colver 2008). Professionals may observe, or assume, that quality of life for individual young persons is compromised; however, those young persons may evaluate their own lives quite differently (Payot and Barrington 2011). In addition, because they are at a different stage of cognitive development and life experience than professionals and their parents, they are likely to focus on and prioritize the various aspects of their lives (e.g. social relationships, engagement in school and leisure activities, opportunities for making their own decisions) differently than adults do. Young persons also know first hand the content of their own thoughts, feelings, concerns, and life experiences, and, therefore, are essential and direct sources of information about their own quality of life (Renwick and Fudge Schormans 2011).

Obtaining young people's self-reports about their perceived quality of life is paramount whenever that is possible, but doing so with some young people with neurological or developmental conditions poses challenges. Therefore, proxy or indirect reports (typically by parents, less often by professionals) about quality of life have routinely been used to assess quality of life for younger children, depending upon their level of cognitive maturity, and for young people who have cognitive impairments or developmental conditions and are non-speaking, or both (Eiser and Morse 2001, Renwick and Fudge Schormans 2011). However, proxy reports have also been used when it is or may have been possible for a young person to provide their own self-report if an appropriate instrument or method had been identified or available. In recent years, more emphasis has been given to developing standardized quality of life instruments with more 'user-friendly' items and rating scales for completion by young people from a wider age range, including young children (e.g. Ronen 2003a,b, Peterson et al 2005, Varni et al 2006). For example, alternative rating scales and instrument formats have been used (Cremeens et al 2006) and alternative methods to respond to standardized instruments have been developed that are more comprehensible to, and effective in eliciting responses from, young people with cognitive impairments and who are non-speaking (e.g. Renwick and Fudge Schormans 2011).

A review by Gates et al (2010) concluded that parents' proxy reports have been found to be more reliable than those of teachers and health professionals, based on higher levels of concordance between the ratings of young people and their parents. However, concordance between parents' proxy reports and their children's self-reports tends to be higher for more readily observable areas of life, such as those associated with cognitive and physical function and pain. On the other hand, proxy reports also reflect parents' standards and beliefs with respect to the young person's quality of life (Ronen et al 2003a) as well as their concerns and anxiety about their children's condition (White-Koning et al 2005). For example, there are differences between proxy and self-reports with respect to the young person's social, psychological, and emotional function and well-being (Varni et al 2005, Gates et al 2010). Overall, parents also tend to provide lower ratings of their children's quality of life than young people themselves (Gates et al 2010). White-Koning et al (2005) point out that lack of agreement between ratings by parents and young persons does not necessarily signify inaccuracy. Rather, such discrepancies may be indicative of different perceptions or interpretations on the part of young people and their parents (White-Koning et al 2005, Waters et al 2009).

Despite the challenges posed by the use of proxy reports, their use in conjunction with young people's self-reports has been commonly recommended (Davis et al 2006, Gates et al 2010, Tsoi et al 2011). Note, however, that it has not been suggested that they replace self-reports. Young people should be asked to express their own perspectives when at all possible (White-Koning et al 2005). Doing so respects their rights to be heard about issues concerning their own health and quality of life (Renwick and Fudge Schormans 2011) and also can highlight motivational issues that may influence intervention outcomes (Gates et al 2010). It is argued that proxy reports from parents can potentially provide additional information to inform decisions about appropriate interventions (Gates et al 2010). In combination with one or more proxy reports a young person's self-report could provide several different types of information. The value of eliciting multiple perspectives is that it may provide additional insights about, and a more complete and detailed picture of, a young person's quality of life, how it should be considered in planning interventions, and how it may be affected by interventions (Gates et al 2010). (For a more detailed discussion on self- and proxy raters see Chapter 17.)

What can qualitative approaches contribute?
Much of the contemporary scientific and professional literature on quality of life assessments and outcomes for young people with neurological and developmental conditions concentrates on standardized measures and statistical results. However, qualitative approaches can contribute valuable information and new insights about both experienced quality of life and the effects of interventions (e.g. to inform development and refinement of outcome measures) (see also Chapter 16). Of course, there are challenges posed by using qualitative approaches. Most notably, these approaches are more labour intensive and time consuming for researchers and professionals (e.g. to gather and analyse information) than using standardized measures. However, they typically yield different and more in-depth, nuanced information than numerical scores from standardized instruments alone. They also have the potential to capture the voices of a wider range of young people with neurological conditions (e.g. younger children,

young people with cognitive impairments and developmental conditions) as well as detailed contextual information from their families. Several illustrative examples of such contributions of qualitative approaches are presented here.

In both practice and research settings, it is often difficult to interpret a lack of agreement between the ratings of young people and those of their parents on standardized outcome measures of quality of life that they both have completed (White-Koning et al 2005, Waters et al 2007). Waters et al (2007) suggest the use of qualitative methods to help explain low concordance rates between these self- and proxy reports. For example, separate 'cognitive interviews' with young people and their parents, using open-ended questions and probes, can explore how they each understood the questionnaire items and illuminate the reasons for their ratings in ways that could not be inferred from their numerical ratings. Such interviews can reveal differences and similarities that young people and their parents may have with respect to expectations, perceptions, and priorities associated with particular aspects of life (e.g. independence, social relationships, school and leisure activities) (White-Koning et al 2005). This qualitative information can provide a more meaningful context for interpreting seemingly incongruent numerical ratings made by young people and their parents.

Creation of conceptual frameworks of health-related and holistic quality of life, established through use of rigorous qualitative methods, can offer a coherent set of rich, essential themes concerning the experiences, concerns, expectations, and priorities of young people with neurological conditions and those of their families. These conceptual frameworks also offer valuable foundations on which to ground development of standardized measures and can contribute to both the face and construct validity of those measures. Methods such as semi-structured interviews or video-based methods for accessing the perspectives of young people and their families and systematic qualitative analysis of the findings have been effectively employed to construct frameworks or measures, or both. Several research groups have provided details of such qualitative work (e.g. Ronen et al 1999, 2003a,b, Renwick et al 2003, 2005, Narayanan et al 2005, Morris et al 2007, Waters et al 2007, Renwick and Fudge Schormans 2011).

Conceptual frameworks of quality of life developed through such qualitative methods can be used as guides for research and practice. For example, a particular conceptual framework may serve as the theoretical underpinning for a programme of research. It can also provide the basis for generating and formulating the research questions that investigators address in a particular study. Further, it can help to determine the specific standardized measures or qualitative methods, or both, that are selected for use in a study. In practice settings, a conceptual approach that is congruent with the goals of service provided by an organization or clinical unit can be employed to guide the various stages of health service provision, including assessment, goal setting with individuals, programme planning for individuals and groups, intervention, and evaluation of programme effectiveness (Renwick et al 2000, Renwick 2004). At each of these stages of service provision qualitative or quantitative strategies, or both, can be employed (e.g. initial and post-intervention quality of life assessments using both a standardized instrument and a qualitative interview with the young person and his or her parents).

Summing up: issues and challenges

Because of the considerable size, scope, and complexity of the literature on quality of life relevant to young people with neurological and developmental conditions, it is rather daunting to select and do justice to delineation of all the associated major issues and challenges affecting research and practice. Given this context, several selected key issues and challenges alluded to in this chapter are highlighted here.

In addition to important research already undertaken, attention is needed to more fully conceptualize quality of life, especially health-related quality of life. Further, most existing holistic and health-related conceptual frameworks of quality of life do not adequately address the issue of its evolution and change over time, from early childhood to young adulthood. In particular, more research is needed to capture the perspectives of young people with neurological and developmental conditions and their families about changes in their quality of life over time. Longitudinal and cross-sectional studies that employ both qualitative and quantitative measures could contribute both new knowledge and new or refined conceptualization concerning these temporal aspects of quality of life. Such studies could also illuminate patterns of support and resources needed to enhance quality of life as it evolves. This kind of research is typically costly as well as time and labour intensive but would yield much rich information about quality of life for this group of young people and their families.

There is considerable diversity in the quality of life literature on conceptualizations relevant to this group of young people, particularly in terms of its definition and the elements purported to constitute quality of life. Greater agreement based on shared commonalities in existing definitions and frameworks could help to clarify the essence of what is meant by health-related and holistic quality of life for these young people. Having such a consensus could facilitate interpretation of multiple reports of research findings and offer some agreed-upon definitions and common essential elements of quality of life that could be adopted for use in future studies

Taking a multimodal approach that employs various combinations of methods and information-gathering strategies in the contexts of both research and practice can contribute to a fuller understanding of quality of life. One example of this approach is to include both self- and proxy reports for both standardized measures and qualitative open-ended questions related to quality of life. Other examples include using a generic instrument in combination with a condition-specific one or combining a holistic measure with a health-related measure. While it is not feasible to employ all of these combinations in all assessments conducted in practice settings or during any given research study, using even two well-chosen methods or strategies can reveal additional information.

As elaborated in Section B on Methods and Measurement, it can be challenging for both healthcare providers and researchers to select psychometrically sound quality of life measures that are suitable for a specific intended purpose (e.g. assessment, outcomes of research interventions, comparisons across groups with different types of conditions) and individuals to be assessed (e.g. children, adolescents, parent proxies), and that can also be administered within a reasonable amount of time. Many quality of life measures relevant to this group of young people require further psychometric testing. Two areas in particular that need further attention are psychometric evaluation of construct validity and the ability to detect changes in quality of life. For practitioners and investigators who wish to include qualitative information about quality of life in their assessments, finding an appropriate, existing, semi-structured interview protocol may be difficult. Some protocols that have been tested and refined are reported in the literature, but not all describe their full range of questions and probes. Therefore, sometimes the most fruitful solution is to modify an existing protocol or develop, pilot-test, and refine one tailored to the intended purpose and requirements.

Qualitative methods can help to enrich our understanding of quality of life from the personal perspectives of a broader range of children in the group. As noted earlier, it has been challenging to elicit perceptions and experiences of young children as well as young people who have cognitive impairments or developmental conditions or are non-speaking. There is considerable scope and potential to apply existing approaches, or to create alternative innovative methods and strategies for doing so, such as those that are image based (e.g. photographic, video based, computer based). However, many of these have yet to be explored and further developed in the context of quality of life research.

Based on the issues and challenges identified here, much work remains to be accomplished. However, it is clear that researchers and professionals working to advance knowledge and practice relevant to quality of life for young people with neurological and developmental conditions can look forward to an exciting future as they address these issues and challenges.

REFERENCES

Key references

*Albrecht G, Devlieger PJ (1999) The disability paradox: high quality life against all odds. *Soc Sci Med* 48: 977–988. http://dx.doi.org/10.1016/S0277-9536(98)00411-0

Berntsson LT, Kohler L (2001) Quality of life among children aged 2–17 years in the five Nordic countries. *Eur J Pub Health* 11: 437–445. http://dx.doi.org/10.1093/eurpub/11.4.437

Bowling A (1991) *Measuring Health: A Review of Quality of Life Measurement Scales*. Buckingham, UK: Open University Press.

Bowling A (1995) *Measuring Disease: A Review of Disease-Specific Quality of Life Measurement Scales*. Buckingham, UK: Open University Press.

Brown RI, Brown PM, Bayer MB (1994) A quality of life model: new challenges arising from a six-year study. In: Goode D, editor. *Quality of Life For Persons with Disabilities: International Perspectives and Issues*. Cambridge, MA: Brookline, pp. 39–56.

*Carlon S, Shields N, Yong K, Gilmore R, Sakzewski L, Boyd R (2010) A systematic review of the psychometric properties of quality of life measures for school aged children with cerebral palsy. *BMC Pediatr* 10: 81. http://dx.doi.org/10.1186/1471-2431-10-81

Colver A (2008) Measuring quality of life in studies of disabled children. *Pediatr Child Health* 18: 423–426. http://dx.doi.org/10.1016/j.paed.2008.05.011

*Cowan J, Baker GA (2004) A review of subjective impact measures for use with children and adolescents with epilepsy. *Qual Life Res* 13: 1435–1443. http://dx.doi.org/10.1023/B:QURE.0000040796.54498.69

Cremeens J, Eiser C, Blades M (2006) Characteristics of self-report measures for children three to eight years: a review of the literature. *Qual Life Res* 15: 739–754. http://dx.doi.org/10.1007/s11136-005-4184-x

*Davis E, Waters E, Mackinnon A, et al (2006) Pediatric quality of life instruments: a review of the conceptual framework on outcomes. *Dev Med Child Neurol* 48: 311–318. http://dx.doi.org/10.1017/S0012162206000673

Eiser C, Morse R (2001) The measurement of quality of life in children: past and future. *J Dev Behav Pediatr* 22: 248–256. http://dx.doi.org/10.1097/00004703-200108000-00007

Fayed N, de Camargo OK, Kerr E, et al (2012) Generic patient-reported outcomes in child health research: a review of conceptual content using World Health Organization definitions. *Dev Med Child Neurol* 54: 1085–1095. http://dx.doi.org/10.1111/j.1469-8749.2012.04393.x

Fekkes M, Theunissen NC, Brugman E, et al (2000) Development and psychometric evaluation of the TAPQOL: a health-related instrument for 1–5 year old children. *Qual Life Res* 9: 961–972. http://dx.doi.org/10.1023/A:1008981603178

*Gates P, Otsuka N, Sanders J, McGee-Brown J (2010) Functioning and health-related quality of life of adolescents with cerebral palsy: self versus parent perspectives. *Dev Med Child Neurol* 52: 843–849. http://dx.doi.org/10.1111/j.1469-8749.2010.03666.x

Graham P, Stevenson J, Flynn D (1997) A new measure of quality of life for children: preliminary findings. *Psychol Health* 12: 655–665. http://dx.doi.org/10.1080/08870449708407412

Guyatt GH, Feeny DH, Patrick DL (1993) Measuring health-related quality of life. *Ann Intern Med* 118: 622–629.

Hanson CL (2001) Quality of life in families of youths with chronic conditions. In: Koot J, Wallander JL, editors. *Quality of Life in Child and Adolescent Illness: Concepts, Methods, and Findings*. New York, NY: Taylor and Francis, pp. 181–209.

Hoogsteen L, Woodgate RL (2010) Can I play? A concept analysis of participation in children with disabilities. *Phys Occ Ther Pediatr* 30: 325–339. http://dx.doi.org/10.3109/01942638.2010.481661

Hughes C, Hwang H (1996) Attempts to conceptualize and measure quality of life. In Schalock RI, editor. *Quality of Life: Volume 1. Conceptualization and Measurement*. Washington, DC: American Association on Mental Retardation, pp. 51–61.

Koot J, Wallander JL, editors (2001) *Quality of Life in Child and Adolescent Illness: Concepts, Methods, and Findings*. New York: Taylor and Francis.

Landgraf JM, Abetz L, Ware JE (1999) *The CHQ User's Manual* (second printing). Boston, MA: Health Act.

Lindstrom B, Eriksson B (1993) Quality of life among children in the Nordic countries. *Qual Life Res* 2: 23–32. http://dx.doi.org/10.1007/BF00642886

Megone, CB (1990) The quality of life starting from Aristotle. In: Baldwin S, Godfrey C, Popper C, editors. *Quality of Life: Perspectives and Policies*. London: Routledge, pp. 28–41.

Morris C, Liabo K, Wright P, Fitzpatrick R (2007) Development of the Oxford ankle foot questionnaire: finding out how children are affected by foot and ankle problems. *Child Care Health Dev* 33: 559–568. http://dx.doi.org/10.1111/j.1365-2214.2007.00770.x

Narayanan UG, Fehling DL, Campbell K, Weire S, Knights S, Kivan S (2005) *Caregiver Priorities and Child Health Index of Life with Disabilities (CPCHILD): Development and Validation of an Outcome Measure of Health Status and Well-being in Children with Cerebral Palsy*. Toronto, ON: The Canadian Orthopaedic Research Society and The Canadian Orthopaedic Association.

*Payot A, Barrington KJ (2011) The quality of life of young children and infants with chronic medical problems: review of the literature. *Curr Probl Pediatr Adolesc Health Care* 41: 91–101. http://dx.doi.org/10.1016/j.cppeds.2010.10.008

Peterson C, Schmidt S, Power M, Bullinger M, the DISABKIDS Group (2005) Development and pilot testing of a health-related quality of life chronic generic module for children and adolescents with chronic health conditions: a European perspective. *Qual Life Res* 14: 1065–1077. http://dx.doi.org/10.1007/s11136-004-2575-z

Pizzi MA, Renwick R (2010) Quality of life and health promotion. In: Scaffa ME, Reitz SM, Pizzi MA, editors. *Occupational Therapy in the Promotion of Health and Wellness*. Philadelphia, PA: F.A. Davis, pp. 122–134.

Ravens-Sieberer U, Gosch A, Abel T, et al (2001) Quality of life in children and adolescents: a European public health perspective. *Soc Prevent Med* 46: 294–302. http://dx.doi.org/10.1007/BF01321080

Renwick R (2004) Quality of life as a guiding framework for occupational intervention. In: Bachner S, Ross M, editors. *Adults with Developmental Disabilities: Current Approaches in Occupational Therapy*, 2nd edn. Bethesda, MD: American Occupational Therapy Association, pp. 20–38.

Renwick R, Fudge Schormans A (2011) *Using Video Methods to Access Voices of Children with Intellectual/ Developmental Disabilities*. Toronto, ON: Quality of Life Research Unit, University of Toronto.

Renwick R, Brown I, Raphael D (2000) Person-centred quality of life: Canadian contributions to an international understanding. In: Keith KD, Schalock RL, editors. *Cross-cultural Perspectives on Quality of Life*. Washington, DC: American Association on Mental Retardation, pp. 5–21.

Renwick R, Fudge Schormans A, Zekovic B (2003) Quality of life: a new conceptual framework for children with disabilities. *J Dev Dis* 10: 107–121.

Renwick R, Fudge Schormans A, Zekovic B (2005) *Quality of Life Measure for Children with Intellectual and Developmental Disabilities – Parental Version*. Toronto, ON: Quality of Life Research Unit, University of Toronto.

Ronen GM, Rosenbaum P, Streiner P, Law M, Streiner DL (1999) Health-related quality of life in childhood epilepsy: the results of children's participation in identifying the components. *Dev Med Child Neurol* 41: 554–559. http://dx.doi.org/10.1017/S0012162299001176

Ronen GM, Streiner DL, Rosenbaum P (2003a) Health-related quality of life and epilepsy: moving beyond 'seizure control with minimal adverse effects'. *Health Qual Life Outcomes* 28: 1–36. http://dx.doi.org/10.1186/1477-7525-1-36

Ronen GM, Streiner DL, Rosenbaum P, Canadian Pediatric Epilepsy Network (2003b) Health-related quality of life in children with epilepsy: development and validation of self-report and parent proxy measures. *Epilepsia* 44: 598–612. http://dx.doi.org/10.1046/j.1528-1157.2003.46302.x

Sabaz M, Cairns DR, Lawson JA, Nheu N, Bleasel AF, Bye AM (2000) Validation of a new quality of life measure for children with epilepsy. *Epilepsia* 41: 765–774. http://dx.doi.org/10.1111/j.1528-1157.2000.tb00240.x

Schalock RL, editor (1996) *Quality of Life: Volume 1. Conceptualization and Measurement*. Washington, DC: American Association on Mental Retardation.

Schalock RL, Keith KD (1993) *The Quality of Life Questionnaire*. Washington, OH: IDS Publishing Co.

Speith LE, Harris CV (1996) Assessment of health-related quality of life in children and adolescents: an integrative review. *J Pediatr Psychol* 21: 175–193. http://dx.doi.org/10.1093/jpepsy/21.2.175

Spilker B, Revicki DA (1996) Taxonomy of quality of life. In: Spilker B, editor. *Quality of Life and Pharmacoeconomics in Clinical Trials*, 2nd edn. Philadelphia, PA: Lippincott-Raven, p. 25.

*Stark JA, Faulkner E (1996) Quality of life across the life span. In: Schalock RI, editor. *Quality of Life: Volume 1. Conceptualization and Measurement*. Washington, DC: American Association on Mental Retardation, pp. 23–32.

Tsoi WS, Zhang LE, Wang YW, Tsang KL, Lo SK (2011) Improving quality of life with cerebral palsy: a systematic review of clinical trials. *Child Care Health Dev* 38: 21–31. http://dx.doi.org/10.1111/j.1365-2214.2011.01255.x

United Nations Children's Fund (2010) *Facts for Life*. New York: UNCF.

Vargas-Adams J (2006) Longitudinal use of the Child Health Questionnaire in childhood cerebral palsy. *Dev Med Child Neurol* 48: 343–347. http://dx.doi.org/10.1017/S0012162206000752

Varni JW, Burwinkle TM, Lane MM (2005) Health-related quality of life measurement in pediatric clinical practice: an appraisal and precept for future research and application. *Health Qual Life Outcomes* 3: 1–34. http://dx.doi.org/10.1186/1477-7525-3-34

Varni JW, Burwinkle TM, Berrin S, et al (2006) The PedsQL in pediatric cerebral palsy: reliability, validity, and sensitivity of the generic core scales and the cerebral palsy module. *Dev Med Child Neurol* 48: 442–449. http://dx.doi.org/10.1017/S001216220600096X

Waters E, Davis E, MacKinnon A, et al (2007) Psychometric properties of the quality of life questionnaire for children with CP. *Dev Med Child Neurol* 49: 49–55. http://dx.doi.org/10.1017/S0012162207000126.x

*Waters E, Davis E, Ronen GM, Rosenbaum P, Livingstone M, Saigal S (2009) Quality of life instruments for children and adolescents with neurodisabilities: how to choose the appropriate instrument. *Dev Med Child Neurol* 51: 660–669. http://dx.doi.org/10.1111/j.1469-8749.2009.03324.x

Whalley Hammell K (2006) *Perspectives on Disability and Rehabilitation: Contesting Assumptions, Challenging Practice*. Philadelphia, PA: Elsevier.

*White-Koning M, Arnaud C, Bourdet-Loubère S, Bazex H, Colver A, Grandjean H (2005) Subjective quality of life in children with intellectual impairment – how can it be assessed? *Dev Med Child Neurol* 47: 281–285. http://dx.doi.org/10.1017/S0012162205000526

World Health Organization (1948) *Charter*. Geneva: WHO Press.

World Health Organization (1986) *Ottawa Charter for Health Promotion*. Geneva: WHO Press.

World Health Organization (2001) *International Classification of Functioning, Disability and Health*. Geneva: WHO Press.

World Health Organization (2009) *Child and Adolescent Health and Disability: Progress Report: Highlights*. Geneva: WHO Press.

World Health Organization (2011) *World Report on Disability*. Geneva: WHO Press.

Zekovic B, Renwick R (2003) Quality of life as a framework for evaluating public policy for children with disabilities. *Dis Soc* 18: 19–34. http://dx.doi.org/10.1080/713662199

4
'HEALTH STATUS' AND THE USEFULNESS OF THE ICF FRAMEWORK: CLINICAL AND PROGRAMME PERSPECTIVES

Olaf Kraus de Camargo and Nora Fayed

Overview

The International Classification of Functioning, Disability and Health (ICF) is a conceptual framework and a universal language that can be used to structure and organize clinical findings, research observations, and the life situations of people with medical conditions. The framework is based on a broad definition of health, which includes body functions and structures, activities, participation, and contextual factors, derived from the biopsychosocial model. At the level of healthcare provision, the ICF helps people to understand how to improve patients' participation in their roles in life, describing the functioning of individual patients within their unique context to generate meaningful goals for intervention. When used as a tool for communication the ICF can assist in facilitating an interdisciplinary understanding of the priority areas of functioning in order to identify needs.

Case scenario 1

Aaron is an 8-year-old male who was diagnosed with neurofibromatosis type 1 (NF-1) after a number of café-au-lait spots were noted on his skin. The clinical examination also revealed coarse facial features, down-slanting palpebral fissures, and the absence of left lateral gaze. He was also found to have an optic glioma with a retinal mass requiring chemotherapy, a common presentation in NF-1. Aaron attends regular classes, feels successful at school, and is well integrated with his classmates. The main difficulties reported by his parents include access to hospital services due to lack of finances, transport constraints, and a disability suffered by Aaron's father, who has his own needs. His mother is a waitress who frequently works night shifts. Signs of NF-1 are absent in Aaron's younger brother and the rest of the family.

Case scenario 2

Bruno is a 9-year-old male who was also diagnosed with NF-1, based on café-au-lait spots and a small optic glioma. Bruno presents with developmental problems that are frequently found in children with NF-1, such as speech and reading delay, learning difficulties at school, and behavioural and interpersonal issues. He tends to have frequent emotional outbursts and tantrums and is poorly integrated with his peers.

Part I: Applying the ICF to the assessment and management of children with chronic health conditions

This chapter discusses how to apply the ICF framework and its accompanying classification to typical scenarios in health services for children with neurological and developmental conditions such as those presented above, and the rationale for doing so. The ICF will be used to conceptualize clinical cases in order to illustrate how professionals can use this approach to collaborate on common ground, set goals, evaluate children, and expand the horizons of population health using this international framework of concepts.

The ICF concept of health provides perspectives on people's lives through the lens of functioning. This view of health, described in Chapter 2, promotes integration of a child's *body functions and structures*, *activities* performed in daily life, and the personal and social roles that constitute his or her *participation* in life situations. A child's functioning occurs within the context of the *environment* as well as *personal factors* such as age, culture, personal preferences, and educational status. According to this framework, when there is discordance among these components of functioning, disability ensues (see Fig. 4.1 and Chapter 2).

The ICF framework is simple, but applying it in clinical practice has multifaceted implications. The way we choose to define and conceptualize health affects the way in which both Aaron and Bruno are assessed and provided with health services. More importantly, Aaron and Bruno's clinicians, health services researchers, parents, and community-based supporters will evaluate the success of these services based on their own understanding of what it means for a child to be healthy. The concepts of the ICF explain and organize health with a common language that all stakeholders can use to understand and evaluate the health of children.

As was noted in Chapter 2, current challenges to health providers extend beyond the frontiers of acute illnesses. Many conditions are chronic and incurable, and this poses challenges to our traditional conceptualization of health as merely 'the absence of disease' (see also Chapter 2). However, we know that children with chronic or recurring neurological conditions can receive medical treatment that emphasizes their potential to be happy and healthy citizens with capabilities, competence, and the ability to adjust to the challenges of society, despite the complication of a health condition (Rosenbaum and Gorter 2011).

For many clinicians, children, parents, and the general public, it is becoming increasingly inappropriate to decide that children like Aaron and Bruno have poor health or even have no value (*invalide* in French) or less value (*menos valido* in Spanish) (see Fig. 4.2) simply

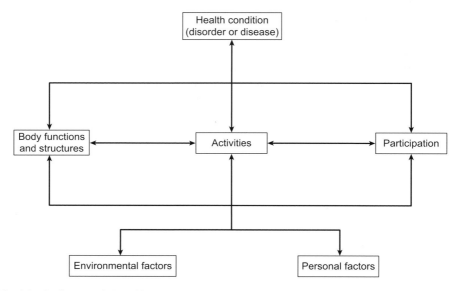

Fig. 4.1 ICF framework (World Health Organization 2001).

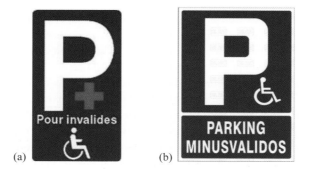

Fig. 4.2 French (a) and Spanish (b) parking signs for people with impairments.

because they have a medical condition associated with impairment. Many people involved in the lives of children with ongoing health conditions are concerned about their emotional well-being, their adaptations in daily life, and the quality of their relationships. These are elements that *they* see as relevant to a child's health. This realization that health involves many factors (only some of which are medical) promotes a shift in the way in which we think about health to include the biological, psychological, and social aspects of people's lives that are associated with a health condition.

USING THE ICF FRAMEWORK TO CONCEPTUALIZE OR UNDERSTAND CARE FOR THE
INDIVIDUAL CHILD WITH A NEUROLOGICAL CONDITION

We applied the functioning perspective to the case scenarios of Aaron and Bruno using components of the ICF. The results are illustrated in Figs 4.3. and 4.4, respectively. Lesions and impairments are related to *body functions* and *body structures*; abilities and limitations regarding the execution of tasks or involvement in life roles are classified as *activities* and *participation*, respectively; and the contextual factors that facilitate or restrict participation are categorized in the chapter of the ICF on *environmental factors*.

The impairments described for Aaron (Fig. 4.3) consist of the skin manifestations of NF-1 and the optic nerve glioma. His eye movements are impaired, with a lack of left lateral gaze (body function). He has no activity limitations: he has good mobility, communicates well, and can learn and perform various tasks. Aaron's participation as a patient is restricted by his father's own disability, the financial strain on his family, endless phone calls to the insurance company, time constraints, and the inaccessibility of the hospital. At the present time Aaron and his family would benefit from transport subsidies and support from a healthcare or social worker to keep his appointments when his parents are unable to do so. These interventions are as important to his functioning and health as a traditional medical approach targeting his physical impairments.

Bruno (Fig. 4.4) displays similar body structure and function characteristics to Aaron. Although his oculomotor functions are intact, he displays impairments in the cognitive

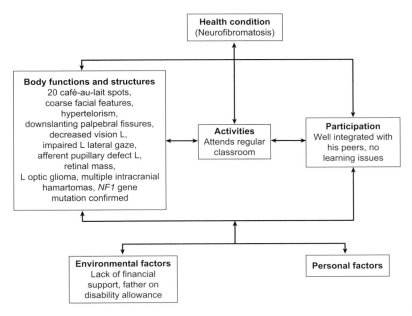

Fig. 4.3 The effects of Aaron's health condition (see Case scenario 1). L, left; *NF1*, neurofibromatosis type 1.

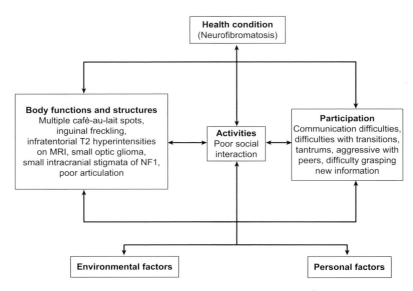

Fig. 4.4 The effects of Bruno's health condition (see Case scenario 2). MRI, magnetic resonance imaging; NF1, neurofibromatosis type 1.

functions necessary for focusing attention, memory, and regulating his emotions. His level of participation is restricted in the classroom by these cognitive challenges, and as a result of his difficulties with emotional regulation he has few friends. People in his environment, such as his parents and teachers, might be unaware of his limitations and expect a level of performance and behaviour that he is not able to perform. Further assessment of his cognitive and learning functions is indicated.

The components of functioning and health in the ICF are useful not only for assessment but also have the potential to direct interventions at the body function, activities, participation, as well as environment levels. Thus, interventions based on the ICF approach to assessment could involve an accommodated learning plan, a support facilitator at school, and potentially a pharmacological approach to improve Bruno's attention function (see Table 4.1 for a summary of both cases).

TABLE 4.1
Applying the ICF to facilitate interprofessional communication and documentation

Patient	Needs	Possible supports	Services involved
Aaron	Restricted accessibility to services	Transport subsidy	Social service
		Health support worker	Health service
Bruno	Limited cognitive functions	Psychometric assessment and counselling	Education service
	Reduced attention functions	Pharmacological intervention	Health service

The utility of the ICF in clinical practice was further assessed by comparing it with the framework of the recommendations in the Consensus Statement for Health Supervision in Neurofibromatosis, published by the American Academy of Pediatrics (AAP) in 2008. The guidelines from the AAP are recommended for Aaron and Bruno based on their age (Hersh and the American Academy of Pediatrics 2008). By applying the ICF to the consensus statement we identified aspects of participation and the impact of environmental factors beyond the regular screening recommendations for changes in body structures and functions (mostly skin and nervous system), as shown by the following excerpts:

AAP *Review the child's development and appropriateness of school placement.*

ICF The topic *school placement* is addressed within the ICF in environmental factors. *Development* is a broad concept, in this case referring to what is expected for a child's age and stage. A review of the child's cognitive and adaptive functions (body functions, activities, and participation) relative to his or her school placement (environment) is the ICF approach.

AAP *Refer the child to a clinical psychologist or child psychiatrist for further evaluation and therapy should problems with self-esteem related to his or her physical findings or developmental problems exist.*

ICF Here, additional medical or allied health services (environmental factors) should be considered, based on clinical findings such as difficulties with academic expectations, mood swings, or withdrawn behaviour (personal factors).

AAP *Review the effects of puberty on the disease.*

ICF The anticipatory quality of this topic is not part of the ICF, as the ICF describes only a person's current state of functioning and not the future or potential developmental trajectories (and prognosis). However, as Rosenbaum and Gorter (2011) point out, there always needs to be an awareness of the importance of the 'future' in our work with children and young people with chronic conditions.

AAP *Discuss the possibility of the growth of neurofibromas during adolescence and pregnancy.*

ICF This topic is also anticipatory. In the ICF, service providers and the information they provide are part of the environment, which can facilitate or promote a child's health.

AAP *Counsel the parents about how and when to discuss the diagnosis with their child.*

ICF This issue directly affects environmental factors influencing the attitudes of parents towards their child's diagnosis. If the diagnosis is to be discussed from an ICF perspective, the discussion should also include disability and how it can be influenced by the context (see Chapter 2). Parents can be counselled to appreciate that they can have a positive impact on their child's functioning not only by being well informed about NF-1 but also by understanding that the social and physical environment in which their child lives has a significant impact on his or her functioning.

AAP *Assess the quality of life of the patient ...*

ICF Although 'quality of life' is not formally part of the ICF (see McDougall et al 2010), a child's perception of his or her life should form part of the thinking of all service providers working with children and young people with impairments and chronic conditions.

The case scenarios of Aaron and Bruno are two common presentations of NF-1. Despite the same diagnosis, they experience their condition in very different ways. In traditional medical paradigms, a diagnosis was thought to convey enough information for the clinicians to be able to decide upon the most appropriate treatment and on the probable prognosis. A diagnosis (in acute care) is often sufficient for making immediate decisions about the use of resources needed for the care of a patient: the appropriate medications, interventions, and professional support. The publication of consensus statements such as that from the AAP shows that the diagnosis of a chronic condition such as NF-1, which has a variable presentation, needs a broader approach that includes aspects relevant to issues of participation and the influence of the environment. In this way, many aspects of the biopsychosocial model have already been introduced into modern clinical thinking.

The ICF provides a standardized and internationally agreed way of discussing, collecting, and documenting health-related information regarding our patients. Describing Aaron and Bruno with the ICF concepts draws attention to additional factors that need to be considered in order to address the functioning of the two boys. Comparing the ICF with the AAP guidelines shows that each approach demonstrates some elements the other does not. For Aaron, the possibility of providing social support is not mentioned in the AAP statement. Bruno requires a review of his school placement and psychological support, which is addressed by the AAP. We observe that, although broad in its approach, the AAP consensus statement still misses some primary concerns encountered by patients with NF-1, especially issues of cognition and behaviour that are addressed only in the school context. In this sense the ICF allows people to take a more individualized approach when assessing patients' needs than does the consensus statement. On the other hand, the ICF alone does not identify the *future* implications of the diagnosis or how to proceed to prevent further complications or disabilities. The developmental aspect of functioning is one area that can serve as a barrier to the ICF's uptake for describing the functioning of children.

When it comes to planning what support is needed for a patient and what services should be activated, the ICF can play an important role as a tool for clarifying how different types of support will impact a patient's functioning. In our two examples, the organization of the findings helps us to determine the interactions (as illustrated by the bidirectional arrows between the boxes in the ICF diagram, Fig. 4.1) and decide which types of support and interventions are appropriate, as well as what potential impacts these might have on the life and functioning of the person described. Although traditionally support services outside the health system have determined the eligibility of people to receive benefits if they fulfilled certain diagnostic criteria, we might expect that this practice would have to change with the adoption of a functioning approach using the ICF as the common language and approach to documentation across different service systems. Eligibility for services would then depend on the ability of those services to match a patient's needs and improve his or her functioning.

The ICF framework has been presented as a tool for conceptualizing and understanding individual children. The ICF classification gives users who have adopted the framework a common language that can be applied to clinical practice on the programmatic level for the purpose of interprofessional communication and documentation.

In this context the ICF is a taxonomy providing a uniform vocabulary organized in a standardized way according to the different components of the observed phenomena. In some respects it constitutes a universal language with its own words and rules. The goal of this taxonomy is to facilitate understanding between professionals and patients about aspects of functioning that might be relevant to the health of patients irrespective of diagnosis, language, culture, or service provision setting.

It is important to point out that the adoption of the ICF does not guarantee that practitioners will be more thorough or detailed or provide better assessments and interventions. However, a consequence of adopting the ICF is that we are stimulated to think about aspects of health in a broad sense. Many new adopters of the ICF comment that they have always been cognizant of health components such as participation or environmental factors but did not have a way of documenting and communicating them as they did with results of the findings of magnetic resonance imaging or electroencephalography (Kaffka-Backmann et al 2007).

The examples above discuss the application of the concepts of the ICF to individuals. The use of the ICF classification as a common language for a service will be further illustrated within the context of a feeding programme and case scenarios associated with it.

Part II: Applying the concepts of the ICF within a clinical programme

Case scenario 3

A feeding team in a children's rehabilitation facility has decided to apply the ICF to their programme in the hopes of facilitating improved communication with each other and with families. The team includes a developmental paediatrician, a radiologist, a nurse, a speech–language pathologist, an occupational therapist, a dietician, and a dentist. They receive consultancy from a social worker and a psychologist in their facility on request. The team members want to develop consistency across their practice processes, documentation, and reports.

Health professionals have varied disciplinary language, training, and culture that all emphasize certain domains of children's functioning over others. However, adoption of the ICF implies that all members of a clinical team are motivated to improve a child's functioning within a common conceptual approach. In the scenario above, the feeding team is dedicated to improving the functioning of children's feeding in the context of each child's life, and they are using the ICF as an interdisciplinary opportunity to describe their roles explicitly.

As a starting point for a discussion of roles, each provider on the feeding team spent a week of their practice keeping track of what functioning domains they commonly addressed in their assessments and interventions. The members came together with their list, reviewed the chapters of the ICF, and mapped out their assessments and interventions relative to the classification of functioning. All professionals acknowledged the expertise of the parents in knowing their child, how their child is performing in the home environment, previous intervention strategies that were either effective or ineffective, and issues that need to be addressed in order to improve the life situation of their child.

Once the team had linked their assessments and interventions to the ICF and identified their involvement relative to those domains of functioning, there was a basis for determining the areas of overlap and the unique contributions of everyone involved. The overlapping area of functioning did not automatically result in the reassignment of duties to one profession, because the team discovered that it was positive to have certain important domains addressed using more than one perspective. For example, in some manner all of the team members were concerned with swallowing safety. The radiologist performed and interpreted video swallow procedures; the nurse assessed medical history (e.g. aspiration pneumonia); the paediatrician provided and coordinated swallowing recommendations and performed clinical examinations (cervical auscultation of swallowing); the occupational therapist determined how the utensils and feeding of each child impacted upon the delivery to, and flow of foods and liquids in, the mouth prior to swallowing, as well as the consistency of solids and liquids; the speech pathologist performed clinical observations of swallowing functioning through listening and observing for pharyngeal coordination with various solids and liquids and textures; the dietician assessed whether all caloric and nutritional needs could be met with existing pharyngeal abilities; and the dentist conducted an assessment of oral hygiene and its potential impact on head and lung symptomatology. Although all of these role components were performed to improve swallowing function (category b510 in the ICF), each professional contributed to this goal in a manner valued by the team and the children's family. These ideas are outlined in Table 4.2.

Mapping each professional's areas of clinical assessment and intervention to the ICF was useful for highlighting the uniqueness of each contribution to the functioning of the children and families serviced by the programme. The occupational therapist's knowledge of assistive devices, equipment, and positioning was important to the safety and comfort of eating, while the speech pathologist's assessment of language capability was important to facilitate choice making, autonomy, and problem solving at mealtimes. This mapping exercise increased the team's awareness of each other's and their own roles in providing comprehensive care.

Finally, the list of roles identified relative to enabling functioning was useful for describing the comprehensiveness of the feeding team's service provision within a biopsychosocial

TABLE 4.2
Mapping the service domains covered by team members in the feeding clinic to ICF domains

Domain of assessment/intervention	Professional assessing or intervening	ICF Domain	ICF Code
		Body functions	*b*
Emotional aspects of feeding (e.g. frustration, pleasure, apprehension)	All	Emotional functions	b152
Sensory preferences and sensitivities (hyper-/hyposensitivity to flavours, textures, appearance and smell of food, and feeding environment)	OT	Sensory functions and pain	b2
Safety with eating and drinking/dysphagia	All	Ingestion functions	b510
Assessment of reflux and digestive functions	MD	Ingestion functions	b510
Weight, height, nutrition, and growth	Dietician, MD, nurse	Weight maintenance functions	b530
Monitor pain/discomfort associated with digestion	MD (primary) All (secondary)	Sensations associated with the digestive system	b535
Metabolic function	Dietician, MD	General metabolic functions	b540
Hydration	Dietician, MD, nurse	Water, mineral, and electrolyte balance functions	b545
Overall muscle tone and coordination	OT	Muscle tone functions, control of voluntary movement functions	b735, b760
		Activities and participation	*d*
Capacity for self-feeding	OT	Acquiring skills	d155
Capacity for making food choices	SLP, OT, dietician	Making decisions	d177
Behavioural strategies to promote feeding	SLP, OT	Managing one's own behaviour	d250
Positioning while eating	OT	Maintaining a body position	d415
Utensil use	OT	Fine hand use	d440
Hand and mouth coordination	OT	Hand and arm use	d445
Oral hygiene maintenance	Dentist, OT	Caring for body parts	d520
Oral motor development with solids and liquids	SLP (primary) All (secondary)	Eating, drinking, ingestion functions	d550, d560, b510
Cup use	OT	Drinking	d560
Nutrition	Dietician, MD, nurse	Looking after one's health	d570
Social situations and feeding (including family mealtimes, at school with peers)	All	Interpersonal interactions and relationships	d7
		Environment	*e*
Caregiver knowledge of feeding	All	Immediate family, personal care providers, and personal assistants	e310, e340

Domain of assessment/intervention	Professional assessing or intervening	ICF Domain	ICF Code
School supports for feeding (e.g. educational assistant)	SLP, OT	Personal care providers and personal assistants, education and training services, systems, and policies	e340, e585
Coordination with other professionals or support involved with feeding issues	All	Health professionals	e355
Family readiness to explore oral feeding alternatives if applicable	All	Individual attitudes of immediate family members	e410
Caregiver attitude about feeding	All	Individual attitudes of immediate family members, individual attitudes of personal care providers and personal assistants	e410, e440
		Body structure	*s*
Oral status and oral health	Dentist	Structure of mouth	s320

MD, doctor; OT, occupational therapist; SLP, speech–language pathologist.

approach. For example, the team could see that there was excellent coverage of body function and of activities issues traditionally addressed by their service provision. Participation-based domains such as feeding among peers, or environment domains such as eligibility for feeding support at school, were open opportunities for providing even more comprehensive care. Following this mapping, the team made plans to request funds to gather systematic qualitative feedback about the priority areas of functioning from the perspective of families and children. The team would then be able to contrast the functioning domains currently assessed and implemented by their programme with the priority areas identified by families and children. Once this comparison has been made (Fig. 4.5), using the common language of the ICF, the gaps between the services currently provided and the priorities for families can be a starting point to improving family-centred services. Such an approach will result in a continuous learning process for all involved, providing a good example of a transdisciplinary process in which all members, including families, can contribute more than simply their own specialized knowledge.

Example: Using the ICF to Structure Individual Patient Goal Setting and Documentation

---

Case scenario 4

Andrea is a 14-year-old female with cerebral palsy who walks independently but with difficulty (Gross Motor Function Classification System level II) (Palisano et al

---

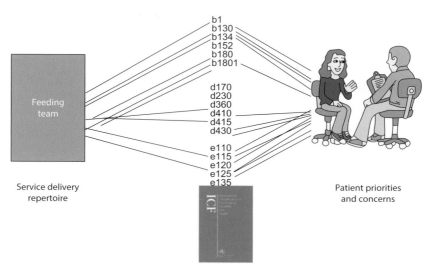

Fig. 4.5 Comparing and contrasting the feeding team's repertoire with child and family concerns.

2008) with a body mass index of 16, which puts her at the 10th centile for her age. She attends an integrated classroom. Andrea was referred to an interdisciplinary feeding team by her family physician, who wanted specialized information about her safety with feeding, weight gain, and oral motor abilities. At her first visit she was seen by the developmental paediatrician, occupational therapist, dietician, speech–language pathologist, and dentist. Her mother was also in attendance at the visit.

The domains outlined by the chapters of the ICF were used for goal setting as they pertained to feeding (Table 4.3). The ICF domains that were relevant to Andrea were recorded and reviewed with Andrea and her family after assessment. Once Andrea, the team, and the family had reviewed the goals, they could be prioritized so that Andrea could elucidate areas of importance from her perspective. This form was also useful for providing cues to Andrea and her family regarding the comprehensiveness of the team's service delivery in terms of body functions, activities, participation, and environment.

Identifying areas for evaluation
The areas that were identified as a priority for Andrea, Andrea's mother, and the team should also be the basis for evaluation. Both an individualized and a group approach to evaluating ICF domains will be useful. An individualized approach based on the goals set and prioritized in Table 4.3 will provide the team with awareness of Andrea's progress relative to herself, while a group approach with a comprehensive measure will provide information about children who are served by the programme in general.

TABLE 4.3
Action plan for Andrea

ICF Domain	Goal	Approach	Outcome	Professionals involved	Patient's rating[a]
Body structure and function	Maintain appropriate weight for height and growth	Provide a high-calorie, high-nutrient, and low-ingestion cost diet composed of smaller more frequent meals and snacks	Andrea will become skilled in identifying the nutrient value vs oral motor challenge of different foods and monitoring an adequate intake	Dietician (clinic doctor, family doctor, nurse, OT, SLP)	*
Activity	Safety with eating and drinking	Assess a range of food consistencies and intake methods with clinical observation and swallowing studies and create a plan for 'safe' foods with Andrea's input at all stages	Andrea and her parents will have firm knowledge of the types of foods and methods of food intake that are safe

Andrea will have a working list of her favourite foods in the safe range of swallowing ability | All | ** |
Participation and environment (school)	More frequent meals and snacks	Meeting with teachers and vice-principal: Andrea will have strategies to discuss or explain eating in class and the attitudes of peers	Andrea can have snacks during class	Clinic doctor, dietician, OT, school staff	***
Environment (family and family physician)	Family and family physician will learn about acceptable weight for height individualized to Andrea	Dietician and clinic doctor review Andrea's growth and weight history, hydration, and nutritional status with Andrea, family, and doctor to determine what is 'healthy' for her	A target range of healthy weight for height will be established for Andrea	Clinic doctor, family doctor, family	*
Environment (peers)	Peer understanding and acceptance of Andrea's nutritional needs and strategies	Identify two close peers as mediators and supporters	The peers will accept Andrea's nutrition breaks as necessary for her health	Teacher, dietician	***

[a]Patient's rating: *least important to ***most important. OT, occupational therapist; SLP, speech–language pathologist.

Part III: Applying the ICF in child and health services evaluation

In adopting the ICF, it is impractical to evaluate care using the entire classification system. We would also not recommend using the World Health Organization ICF checklist, which was created with a general population of adults as the target population. Rather, the ICF framework can be used as a means of identifying what domains are included in goal-setting tools and health status measures, and we can try to ensure that the content of the measures chosen matches the ICF concepts being assessed (Fayed 2012).

An individualized approach to health status evaluation can be useful when we want to assess the progress of a child relative to him- or herself. The advantage of such an approach is that improvements are easily noted, but the disadvantage is that the improvements are not comparable across children when programmatic assessments are required. We can always cross-reference the goals identified through popular goal-setting tools such as the Perceived Efficacy and Goal Setting system (PEGS: Missiuna et al 2006), the Canadian Occupational Performance Measure (COPM: Law et al 2005), and goal attainment scaling (GAS) with the ICF to demonstrate which goals are set by the children and families in a programme (Nijhuis et al 2008, Fayed and Kerr 2009, McDougall and Wright 2009). The above systems of goal identification (PEGS, COPM, and GAS) all have quantitative methods for comparing a child's progress to him- or herself before and after an intervention or service has been provided. It is important always to note how these goals relate to the overall conception of functioning in the ICF. For example, were only body function-type goals set, or were activity, participation, and/ or environment factors included as the basis for individualized evaluation of a particular child? When we choose to adopt an ICF approach to clinical practice, a comprehensive approach to goal setting and individualized evaluation should be included in the assessment of health.

Although goal-setting tools are highly sensitive to the needs, challenges, and functional changes of each particular child, standard instruments that evaluate the health status of children within a group and across groups are needed for programme or research evaluation (see Chapter 15). Generic health status measures for children are readily available and can be applied to children irrespective of diagnosis. The content of those measures can vary considerably, and applying the ICF conception of functioning to any health status instrument being considered is highly useful in order to achieve a good match between the domains of functioning that a programme or team needs or wants to measure and what is actually measured by the instrument (Fayed et al 2012). For example, the Child Health Questionnaire focuses on body functions such as emotions, and activities and participation such as socializing, as well as some features relating to personal factors and the environment, whereas the Health Utilities Index III emphasizes body function attributes such as vision, hearing, cognition, and emotion and activities and participation items such as walking, hand function, and communication without the direct assessment of environment domains. This variability in the content of currently used health status instruments shows that one cannot rely solely on the name of an instrument as a 'health status' tool as sufficient evidence that it is a comprehensive measure of ICF concepts of functioning. A specific example on matching ICF domains to the content of an instrument is available in Chapter 15 on choosing measurement scales.

Conclusion

The ICF can be used as a framework to facilitate professional understanding, patient assessment, communication, service provision, and documentation in patient care. The ICF can also provide a conceptual basis for individual and programme evaluation and help determine an agenda for population health in an era of increasing awareness of chronic health issues. A notable limitation in applying the ICF to children and young people is that developmental issues that require the anticipation of future problems are poorly identified in the framework. Nonetheless, international experience supports its use and utility and demonstrates the potential of the ICF for expanding horizons in health care (Cerniauskaite et al 2011).

REFERENCES

Key references

Cerniauskaite M, Quintas R, Boldt C, et al (2011) Systematic literature review on ICF from 2001 to 2009: its use, implementation and operationalisation. *Disabil Rehabil* 33: 281–309. http://dx.doi.org/10.3109/096 38288.2010.529235

Fayed N, Camargo DE, Kerr E, et al (2012) Generic patient-reported outcomes in child health research: a review of conceptual content using World Health Organization definitions. *Dev Med Child Neurol* 54: 1085–1095. http://dx.doi.org/10.1111/j.1469-8749.2012.04393.x

Fayed N, Kerr EN (2009) Identifying occupational issues among children with intractable epilepsy: individualized versus norm-referenced approaches. *Can J Occup Ther* 76: 90–97.

Hersh J, American Academy of Pediatrics (2008) Health supervision for children with neurofibromatosis. *Pediatrics* 121: 633. http://dx.doi.org/10.1542/peds.2007-3364

Kaffka-Backmann M, Simon L, Grunwaldt A (2007) Praktische Erfahrungen mit der Verwendung einer ICF-Checkliste für die Interdisziplinäre Frühförderung ("ICF-Checkliste IFF"). *Frühförderung interdisziplinär* 26: 167–172.

Law M, Baptiste S, Carswell A, McColl M, Polatajko H, Pollock N (2005) *The Canadian Occupational Performance Measure*, 4th edn. Ottawa: CAOT Publications.

*McDougall J, Wright V (2009) The ICF-CY and Goal Attainment Scaling: benefits of their combined use for pediatric practice. *Disabil Rehabil* 31: 1–11. http://dx.doi.org/10.1080/09638280802572973

*McDougall J, Wright V, Rosenbaum P (2010) The ICF model of functioning and disability: incorporating quality of life and human development. *Dev Neurorehabil* 13: 204–211. http://dx.doi.org/10.3109/17518421003620525

Missiuna C, Pollock N, Law M, Walter S, Cavey N (2006) Examination of the Perceived Efficacy and Goal Setting System (PEGS) with children with disabilities, their parents, and teachers. *Am J Occup Ther* 60: 204–214.

*Nijhuis BJ, Reinders-Messelink HA, de Blecourt AC, et al (2008) Goal setting in Dutch paediatric rehabilitation. Are the needs and principal problems of children with cerebral palsy integrated into their rehabilitation goals? *Clin Rehabil* 22: 348–363. http://dx.doi.org/10.1177/0269215507083055

Palisano RJ, Rosenbaum P, Livingston MH (2008) Content validity of the expanded and revised Gross Motor Function Classification System. *Dev Med Child Neurol* 50: 744–750. http://dx.doi.org/10.1111/j.1469-8749.2008.03089.x

*Rosenbaum P, Gorter JW (2011) The 'F-words' in childhood disability: I swear this is how we should think! *Child Care Health Dev* 37: 1–7. http://dx.doi.org/10.1111/j.1365-2214.2011.01338.x

World Health Organization (2001) *International Classification of Functioning, Disability and Health*. Geneva: WHO Press.

5

THE ROLE OF PARTICIPATION IN THE LIVES OF CHILDREN AND YOUNG PEOPLE WITH NEUROLOGICAL AND DEVELOPMENTAL CONDITIONS

Dana Anaby and Mary Law

Overview

Over the past 15 years, children's participation in daily activities has gained increasing attention in the research and clinical communities and is now considered one of the most important outcomes of habilitative interventions. In fact, the notion of participation and its benefits is pertinent to many stakeholders, including patients, parents, teachers, and policy makers. In this chapter we discuss the concept and definition of the construct of participation, with a special focus on leisure participation, and suggest relevant assessments of participation. In addition, we provide a summary of the research evidence on the nature of participation of children and young people with neurological and developmental conditions while accounting for the factors that affect these participation patterns. Finally, a case scenario is presented to illustrate participation-based assessment and intervention.

Introduction

Participation has become an important term in neurodevelopmental (re)habilitation over the past 15 years. Whereas in everyday language the word 'participation' means 'to take part', its inclusion in the International Classification of Functioning, Disability and Health (ICF) (World Health Organization 2001) has increasingly led people to focus on participation in rehabilitation medicine (see Chapter 4). The inclusion of participation in the ICF represents a shift towards a social model of disability in which the environment plays an important role. With increasing knowledge, it has become clear that participation is a complex concept.

The ICF does not distinguish between activities and participation within its model. Whereas activity is defined as 'the execution of a task or action by an individual', activities and participation share the same organizational structure and chapters within the ICF. There has been considerable discussion in the literature about ways in which to separate activities and participation (Whiteneck and Dijkers 2009), but no consensus has emerged. Most researchers tend to think about participation as clusters or sets of activities that involve the person within the societal context.

In the ICF, participation is defined as 'involvement in life situations' such as personal care, community life, education, work, or play. The list of the ICF participation chapters is summarized in Table 5.1. The ICF model also conceptualizes participation as being influenced by a person's health condition and personal and environmental factors. According to the World Health Organization (WHO), participation restriction, which reflects one component of disability, is the product of the interaction of a health condition, body function and structure, and personal and environmental factors (see also Chapters 2 and 4).

In an attempt to clarify the concept of participation, Coster and Khetani (2008) suggested defining participation as 'sets of organized sequences of activities directed toward a personally or socially meaningful goal'. Other definitions emphasize the subjective aspects

TABLE 5.1
ICF chapters concerning activity and participation

Chapter	Description	Example
Learning and applying knowledge	Learning, applying learned knowledge, thinking, problem solving and decision making	*d155*: acquiring skills; following rules and coordinating movement for playing games
General tasks and demands	Carrying out simple and complex tasks, as well as dealing with stress and organizing routines	*d230*: carrying out a daily routine; managing time, fulfilling daily roles such as waking up, dressing, eating, etc.
Communication	Communication by language, signs, conversation, and devices	*d360*: using communication devices/techniques (e.g. calling someone on the telephone, emailing)
Mobility	Movement of body by changing position, moving objects, walking, running, and using transport	*d470:* using transport as a passenger, e.g. a public bus
Self-care	Caring for oneself, including dressing, eating, washing, caring for one's health and body	*d5400:* putting on clothes (coordination of clothes with proper body parts, i.e. arms and head in neck and sleeves of shirt)
Domestic life	Carrying out domestic and everyday tasks	*d6300*: preparing light meals (selecting ingredients, heating, and serving)
		d6506: taking care of pets (exercising, feeding, playing with, grooming)
Interpersonal interactions and relationships	Fulfilling actions and tasks for basic/complex social interactions with others	*d7200*: forming and maintaining relationships with others (e.g. peers, family) for short/long periods of time
Major life areas	Carrying out tasks related to education, employment, and economic transactions	*d820*: school education; learning course material, attending class, working with other students
Community, social, and civic life	Actions and tasks required to engage in social life in the community and civic areas, outside the family	*d920*: recreation and leisure; sports, museums, cinemas, touring, crafts

of participation such as choice, control, and meaning. Thus, researchers have identified that participation for children and young people involves the experiences of choice, control, belonging, and active involvement or being a part of daily activities (Eriksson and Granlund 2004, Almqvist and Granlund 2005, Heah et al 2007, Harding et al 2009). Examples of how participation has been defined in the literature are listed in Table 5.2.

Participation of children and young people with neurodevelopmental conditions focuses on more than just performance, as participation is defined not solely by what the child can

TABLE 5.2
Definitions of 'participation'

Online Etymology Dictionary	Particeps = part taking Pars + capere = to take or to share in
Fougeyrollas et al 1998: 133	Life habits are 'activities of daily living and social roles recognized by the socio-cultural context of a person according to age, sex, and social and personal identity'
World Health Organization 2001: 10	'involvement in life situations'
Perenboom and Chorus 2003: 578	'involvement in life situation which includes being autonomous to some extent or being able to control your own life, even if one is not actually doing things themselves. This means that not only the actual performance should be the key indicator, but also the fulfilment of personal goals and societal roles'
Eriksson and Granlund 2004: 240	'Participation is a means to define well-being'
Hemmingsson and Jonsson 2005: 574	'The experience of meaning, autonomy and self-determination are components of participation along with the actual performance'
Almqvist and Granlund 2005: 306	'The experience of participation has three interactive dimensions: to experience (to have positive experiences of control and belonging through active interaction with the environment); to act (both physically and mentally in a life situation); context (availability of activities and opportunities for interaction with the environment) ... to successfully participate, there must be a feeling of being a part of something, an ability to act, and availability of activities in a particular context'
Rochette et al 2006: 1233	'"optimal" participation relies on a perfect fit between the reality (how activities and roles are actually realised) and expectations (how activities and roles should be realised)'
Heah et al 2007: 41	'"Successful participation" is associated with four themes: having fun, feeling successful, doing and being with others, and doing things myself'
Coster and Khetani 2008: 643	'sets of organized sequences of activities directed toward a personally or socially meaningful goal'
Hammel et al 2008: 1445	'A cluster of values that includes active and meaningful engagement/being apart of, choice and control, access and opportunities, personal and societal responsibilities, having an impact and supporting others, and social connection, inclusion and membership'
Whiteneck and Dijikers 2009: S24	'Participation is more complex than activity; it involves role performance at the societal level and is more likely to be influenced by the environment. Activity, on the other hand, occurs at the personal level and is more result-oriented and a means to an end'

or cannot do. Children or young people with persistent chronic conditions can still experience participation even if they are receiving assistance and not completing an activity by themselves. For example, an adolescent with quadriplegic cerebral palsy can experience participation when engaged in a recreational dance class. He or she may not perform the dance movements independently, and at first glance may seem quite 'passive'; however, an exploration of the subjective experience may reveal that he or she enjoys the activity very much and finds meaning in the music and the social context. Such an activity is an excellent opportunity to make friends and develop a sense of belonging to one's peer group.

In other words, children can feel fully involved and completely immersed in an activity even though they do not perform it independently. Moreover, there is more than one way of engaging in a dance class, and one should not be limited to executing the movements: for example, choosing the music or choreographing the steps are other ways in which people can participate. Hence, participation is a complex process that involves the orchestration of multiple activities, is likely to involve other people and is often environmentally dependent. When considering participation, we must take into account the types of activities, where and with whom they occur, and other aspects of participation such as frequency, involvement, meaning, and desire for change.

The benefits of participation
Participation plays a key role in children's development, particularly in leisure activities outside of school. Through participation in activities of a recreational nature, outside of school, children and young people acquire skills and competency, achieve physical and mental health benefits, and develop a sense of meaning and purpose in life (Larson and Verma 1999). There is empirical evidence to suggest that participation in activities that are enjoyable and that promote skill development can protect at-risk children and young people from developing mental health, academic, and social problems (Rutter 1987, Mahoney and Cairns 1997, Mahoney et al 2002, Eccles at al 2003). Participation – notably in out-of-school activities – is a positive force for health, quality of life, and well-being, as it provides the context in which children and young people develop and prepare for life transitions. As Eriksson and Granlund (2004) indicate, participation 'is a means to define well-being'.

Other areas of participation, such as school participation, are also important and known to be restricted. While our focus is primarily on leisure participation, readers interested in further information regarding the school setting are invited to read the work of Almqvist and Granlund (2005), as well as that of Simeonsson et al (2001).

How to measure participation? (see Table 5.3)
Participation is a challenging concept to operationalize and measure because of all the many definitions of the construct and the lack of conceptual clarity. It is agreed, however, that participation is a complex concept of a multidimensional, highly individualized, and subjective construct guided by one's preference and interests (Whiteneck and Dijikers 2009).

A handful of measures are available to assess the participation of children across different settings, i.e. home, school, and community, and across developmental ages and stages. Some of the measures examine specific areas or domains such as leisure (Children Assessment

TABLE 5.3
Measures of participation

Measure		Purpose/ Domain	Targeted population (age range, years)	Items	Scales	Psychometric properties
CAPE	Children's Assessment of Participation and Enjoyment	Out-of-school activities: recreational, physical, social, skill-based, and self-improvement activities	6–21	55 activities	Diversity Intensity Enjoyment With whom Where	King et al 2007
APCP	Assessment of Preschool Children's Participation	Out-of-school activities: play, skill development, active physical recreation, and social activities	2–6	45 drawing on everyday activities	Diversity Intensity	Law et al 2012a
CASP	Child and Adolescent Scale of Participation	Home, community, school	>5	20	Age-expected participation	Bedell 2004
LIHE-H	Assessment of Life Habits for Children – Frequency of Participation Questionnaire	Daily activities, social roles	5–13	64 life-habits	Accomplishment satisfaction	Fougeyrollas et al 1998
LAQ-CP	Lifestyle Assessment Questionnaire	Physical independence, mobility, schooling, clinical burden, economic burden, social integration	>5	46	The impact of disability on the life of children and families	Mackie et al 1998
PACS	Preschool Activity Card Sort	Self-care, community mobility, leisure, social interaction, domestic chores, and education	3–6	85 activity photographs	Five activities are chosen by parents to guide intervention	Berg and La Vasser 2006
PEM-CY	Participation and Environment Measure of Children and Youth	Home, school, community	5–17	25	Count, frequency, involvement, desire for change; environmental supports and barriers	Coster et al 2011

TABLE 5.3
(Continued)

Measure		Purpose/ Domain	Targeted population (age range, years)	Items	Scales	Psychometric properties
CHORES	Children Helping Out: Responsibilities, Expectations and Supports	Home setting: self-care, family care	School-aged children	34 tasks	Performance, assistance	Dunn 2004
SFA	School Function Assessment	School activities/ settings	Elementary school-aged children	Six different school settings	Participation, task support, performance	Coster et al 1998
COPM	Canadian Occupational Performance Measure	Self-care, play, and productivity	All ages	Depending on number of selected activities/ goals	Performance, satisfaction	Law et al 2005
GAS	Goal Attainment Scaling	All domains	All ages	Depending on number of selected goals	Goal achievement	Kiresuk and Sherman 1968

of Participation and Enjoyment – the CAPE), school (School Function Assessment – the SFA), and home (Children Helping Out: Responsibilities, Expectations and Supports – the CHORES), whereas others include a variety of settings (Participation and Environment Measure for Children and Youth – the PEM-CY; Child and Adolescent Scale of Participation – the CASP). Most of the available measures examine the quantitative dimensions of participation that can be observed using counts and frequency data. Other participation measures consider the qualitative aspects of participation or the subjective experience that is derived from participation, assessing the attributes such as enjoyment (CAPE), satisfaction with performance (Life Habits – LIFE-H), and level/degree of involvement (PEM-CY).

As with most highly individualized constructs, no norms exist against which to measure participation, and there is a considerable debate in the literature about what optimal participation is and whether norms for the concept of participation are appropriate. There is a lack of clarity about the concept of 'successful or adequate participation', because participation varies so much across individuals and is based on and reflects personal values and subjective perspectives. One can be perfectly satisfied and experience 'full participation' by taking part in what others may consider a limited number of activities (potentially with assistance), as long as the activities in which one is engaged are rewarding, are imbued with personal meaning, and allow for control and choice (see Chapter 2 for more on the concept of the 'disability paradox'). As Bedell and Coster (2008: 222) state, 'a great extent of participation is not necessarily better unless the situation is one that matters to the child or the family.'

Thus, it is worthwhile to use measures that address both aspects of participation: the actual quantity and the perception of quality. For example, measures can include the extent to which a child is participating (quantity aspect) as well as his or her satisfaction with the extent of participation (quality aspect). A newer measure, the PEM-CY (Coster et al 2011) also examines the gap between the actual and desired participation in addition to the quantity (e.g. frequency) and quality (e.g. level of involvement) facets. In this assessment, parents are asked if they would like to see a change in their child's participation and to indicate the type of change desired. Such information adds one more piece to the puzzle and can help parents and clinicians to identify participation issues and expectations, and consequently design more effective interventions.

Is participation of children with neurological or developmental conditions different from or similar to their typically developing peers, and, if so, in what ways?

Despite the known benefits of participation, the literature has demonstrated that children and young people with various types of physical impairments (Bult et al 2010, King et al 2010), cerebral palsy (Imms et al 2008, Engel-Yeger et al 2009), and acquired brain injury (Bedell and Dumas 2004, Law et al 2011a) experience greater restrictions to participation in leisure activities than their typically developing peers. More specifically, young people with impairments tend to participate more in informal activities at home and alone, for example by reading or completing a puzzle, and less in formal community-based activities such as organized sports or planned groups or lessons (Law et al 2006, Majnemer et al 2008, Klaas et al 2010). Similar patterns were identified among children following acquired brain injury: greater participation restriction was reported in structured events in the community and social and leisure activities with peers either at school or in the community (Bedell and Dumas 2004, Galvin et al 2010). Finally, striking differences were recognized in a study that included 576 children and young people with and without various types of impairments. For example, 37% of children and young people with impairments never took part in organized physical activities in the community compared with only 10% among their typically developing peers (Bedell et al 2013).

School participation

Over the last 15 years a number of studies have explored the participation of children and young people with a variety of impairments in various school-related activities. In the school setting, children with impairments have fewer friends and lower levels of participation in structured and unstructured activities (Simeonsson et al 2001, Eriksson et al 2007). It is important to note that school participation is not limited to academic activities in class but also encompasses other activities, more social in nature, such as field trips, clubs/teams, lunch/recess, and special roles in school (Coster et al 2012). School participation of disabled children and young people is restricted in comparison to typically developing children (W. Coster, personal communication, 2012): for example, twice as many children with impairments (62%) never took part in school-sponsored teams, clubs, and organizations compared with one-third (31%) among their typically developing peers.

Similar participation patterns, with less profound differences, are evident in the *home setting*, in which children with impairments tend to take part in less complex, quieter, and more sedentary activities than their counterparts (Law et al 2012b). Lower levels of participation in household tasks were also evident among children with attention-deficit–hyperactivity disorder (Dunn et al 2009).

What factors affect participation?

Several factors – in particular those that relate to the child, family, and their environment – affect children's participation. Among *child* characteristics, the child's age is one of the important factors. Participation changes as children move into adolescence, around the age of 12 years, when one observes a decline in participation in most types of activity except social activities. This pattern is similar for children both with and without impairments (Jarus et al 2010, King et al 2010) and may reflect a typical developmental change.

Another important factor for participation is sex. Girls tend to participate in more social activities and skill-based activities, whereas boys prefer physical activities (Engel-Yeger et al 2009). Participation is also influenced by child function and abilities such as gross motor function, measured by the Gross Motor Function Measure (Majnemer et al 2010), manual abilities (Imms et al 2009), behavioural, cognitive, and physical function (King et al 2006), and severity of injury (Anaby et al 2012). Overall, children with more severe functional limitations (gross motor, fine motor, intellectual, and communication) have lower participation scores (Fauconnier et al 2009).

The child's preferences are another important factor determining participation; children's participation is greater when they engage in activities of their own choosing and interests (King et al 2006). There is some evidence that a child's temperament or personality influences participation; children with cerebral palsy who are more persistent and have higher levels of mastery motivation participate more intensely (Majnemer et al 2008). However, in regression analyses when the child's function is included temperament does not seem to exert any effect on participation (Imms et al 2009).

The *family* also has an important role in determining children's participation (see also Chapter 11). Children and young people tend to participate more intensely when their families value recreational activities (King et al 2006) and provide physical and emotional support to their child and to one another (Lawlor et al 2006, Anaby et al 2012) and when household income is higher, with lower levels of parental stress (Majnemer et al 2008).

Finally, the *environment* is gaining growing recognition as a key factor in participation. One of the common barriers to participation is a negative attitude by others including peers and service providers (Law et al 1999, Lawlor et al 2006), whereas greater social support from family, peers, and friends increases participation (Harding et al 2009). Children's participation is often extremely limited due to lack of accessibility to buildings and transport, limited services, and non-inclusive policies. To illustrate, a study conducted in Canada and the USA (*n*=576) established that 36% of caregivers of children and young people with impairments reported no access to, or a lack of availability of, programmes and services in comparison to only 3% of caregivers of children without impairments (Law et al 2012b).

The impact of the environment on children's participation was very clearly demonstrated by a research team in Europe (Colver et al 2011), which reported substantial variation in participation across the nine European regions among 818 children with cerebral palsy. The authors highlight social and legislative differences within these regions and illustrate the considerable impact that policy can have on children's participation.

How does participation change over time?

Two studies have examined how participation in leisure changes over time among children and young people with physical impairments (King et al 2009) and following acquired brain injury (Anaby et al 2012). These studies show that specific activities, such as recreational, physical, and social activities, are more likely to change than skill-based and self-improvement activities.

Future directions: the need for intervention studies and knowledge translation activities

Although there is growing evidence about the factors that affect participation, little is known about how to promote children's participation. To date, interventional studies among children and young people with neurological conditions have tended to focus on promoting body function, e.g. upper extremity skills (Imms 2008), or functional performance of an activity, e.g. ability to get dressed independently (Lammi and Law 2003), rather than examining the more complex but key construct of participation engagement (e.g. frequency of taking part/ participating in Scouts events). There is little evidence that improving body function or activity performance directly affects participation (Wright et al 2008). Moreover, studies tend to address participation domains related to self-care and mobility, whereas the area of leisure – an area that is believed to have a positive effect on children's development and well-being – is less evident (Larson and Verma 1999).

With the growing evidence regarding the impact of the environment on children's participation, attention is directed towards an environment-focused approach as a strategy to promote participation. In this approach, also known as the context approach (Darrah et al 2011), rather than focusing exclusively on changing the child's abilities, interventions can also be directed towards modifying environmental conditions (physical, social, attitudinal, familial) to foster the child's participation. A randomized controlled trial involving 128 young children with cerebral palsy examined the context approach, in which change was targeted towards the environment rather than the child. The study found that the context approach was as useful as a conventional therapy in promoting performance (Law et al 2011b). Further examination of this strategy to increase participation among other interventional plans is warranted across ages and neurological conditions.

Knowledge translation of current evidence surrounding participation is another important line of enquiry that requires attention. Increasing awareness regarding the importance of participation is of interest to many stakeholders and is not limited to the research and clinical communities; patients, parents, teachers, and policy makers can all benefit from such knowledge in order to foster change towards participation-based communities and policies (readers can learn more about knowledge translation in Chapter 19).

Take home messages

- Participation is a complex, highly individualized construct that is hard to define and consequently difficult to measure.
- Participation is influenced by a variety of factors that are not limited to children's characteristics (health condition, abilities, motivation) but also include factors related to their family and the broader aspects of the environment.
- Interventional studies and knowledge translation activities are areas that require future research.

Case scenario: promoting Rachel's participation in community participation

Rachel is a 13-year-old female with cerebral palsy who walks at home with support but uses a wheelchair outdoors (Gross Motor Function Classification System level III) and has challenges with mobility in the community; completing the PEM-CY (see Table 5.3) indicated that she is engaged in an array of activities at home yet participates much less frequently in activities in her community and at school. Rachel and her parents wish to see changes in community-based activities. For example, she wishes to participate more frequently in organization, group, and club activities and organized physical activities and be more involved in getting together with other children in the community. Environmental barriers that were identified included: physical layout of the setting and the demands of the activity in terms of physical, social, and cognitive demands. Support included: access to transport, family support, adequate equipment, availability of programmes, and money. Attitudes and access to information were reported as sometimes helping and sometimes hindering.

Rachel and her family were seen by an occupational therapist who administered the Canadian Occupational Performance Measure (COPM: Law et al 2005) to enable her to identify specific participation goals. The following goals were identified:

- join an after-school club
- go to the local YMCA for swimming
- hang out with her friends at the mall.

Intervention

Guided by the context therapy approach (Darrah et al 2011), which focuses on changing task and/or the environment while drawing on family-centred principles and educational strategies, the following action plan was developed:

- The occupational therapist will assess the environment barriers and supports of the specific setting in which participation goals are to be carried out (i.e. YMCA, club, mall) while analysing the physical, social, and cognitive demands of the activity (i.e. task analysis).

- Solutions for overcoming these barriers will be suggested to enable engagement in that activity by modifying environmental conditions. For example, if Rachel's participation in a youth club is restricted due to negative attitudes towards her impairment from her peers, an intervention can be targeted to increase her peers' knowledge of impairments (e.g. preparing a presentation about cerebral palsy, initiating an awareness day for inclusion at the community centre). The intervention can also address the physical layout of the community centre to improve its accessibility; this may involve contacting municipal services and negotiating for accommodations.
- Finally, intervention can occur at the level of the organization, which involves contacting programme managers, describing Rachel's needs, and suggesting alternative activities and equipment to include her in the programme.
- Providing education about useful strategies to overcome environmental barriers and utilizing support, information, and advocacy for her inclusion will empower Rachel and her parents. For example, a handout promoting self-advocacy and outlining accessibility requirements for Rachel's participation can be prepared, as well as a reference guide to accessibility when searching for activities.

Intervention outcomes

Participation goals can be monitored over time using the COPM to see if a satisfactory change in performance has been achieved. Overall participation patterns can be reassessed using the PEM-CY to further evaluate the effect of the intervention.

REFERENCES

Key references

Almqvist L, Granlund M (2005) Participation in school environment of children and youth with disabilities: a person-oriented approach. *Scand J Psychol* 46: 305–314. http://dx.doi.org/10.1111/j.1467-9450.2005.00460.x

*Anaby D, Law M, Hanna S, Dematteo C (2012) Predictors of change in participation rates following acquired brain injury: results of a longitudinal study. *Dev Med Child Neurol* 54: 339–346. http://dx.doi.org/10.1111/j.1469-8749.2011.04204.x

Bedell GM (2004) Developing a follow-up survey focused on participation of children and youth with acquired brain injuries after discharge from inpatient rehabilitation. *NeuroRehabilitation* 19: 191–205.

Bedell G, Coster W (2008) Measuring participation of school-aged children with traumatic brain injuries: considerations and approaches. *J Head Trauma Rehabil* 23: 220–229. http://dx.doi.org/10.1097/01.HTR.0000327254.61751.e7

Bedell GM, Dumas HM (2004) Social participation of children and youth with acquired brain injuries discharged from inpatient rehabilitation: a follow-up study. *Brain Inj* 18: 65–82. http://dx.doi.org/10.1080/0269905031000110517

Bedell G, Litjenquist K, Coster W, et al (2013) Community participation, supports and barriers of school age children with and without disabilities. *Arch Phys Med Rehabil* 94: 315–323. http://dx.doi.org/10.1016/j.apmr.2012.09.024

Berg C, La Vasser P (2006) The Preschool Activity Card Slot. *OTJR Occup Particip Health* 26: 143–151.

Bult M, Verschuren O, Gorter J, Jongmans M, Piskur B, Ketelaar M (2010) Cross-cultural validation and psychometric evaluation of the Dutch language version of the Children's Assessment of Participation and Enjoyment (CAPE) in children with and without physical disabilities. *Clin Rehabil* 24: 843–853. http://dx.doi.org/10.1177/0269215510367545

*Colver AF, Dickinson HO, Parkinson K, et al (2011) Access of children with cerebral palsy to the physical, social and attitudinal environment they need: a cross-sectional European study. *Disabil Rehabil* 33: 28–35. http://dx.doi.org/10.3109/09638288.2010.485669

*Coster W, Khetani MA (2008) Measuring participation of children with disabilities: issues and challenges. *Disabil Rehabil* 30: 639–648. http://dx.doi.org/10.1080/09638280701400375

Coster W, Deeny T, Haltiwanger J, Haley S (1998) *School Function Assessment User's Manual*. San Antonio, TX: The Psychological Corporation/Therapy Skill Builders.

*Coster W, Bedell G, Law M, et al (2011) Psychometric evaluation of the Participation and Environment Measure for Children and Youth. *Dev Med Child Neurol* 53: 1030–1037. http://dx.doi.org/10.1111/j.1469-8749.2011.04094.x

*Coster W, Law M, Bedell G, Khetani M, Cousins M, Teplicky R (2012) Development of the Participation and Environment Measure for Children and Youth: conceptual basis. *Disabil Rehabil* 34: 238–246. http://dx.doi.org/10.3109/09638288.2011.603017

*Darrah J, Law MC, Pollock N, et al (2011) Context therapy: a new intervention approach for children with cerebral palsy. *Dev Med Child Neurol* 53: 615–620. http://dx.doi.org/10.1111/j.1469-8749.2011.03959.x

Dunn L (2004) Validation of the CHORES: a measure of school-aged children's participation in household tasks. *Scand J Occup Ther* 11: 179–190. http://dx.doi.org/10.1080/11038120410003673

Dunn L, Coster WJ, Cohn ES, Orsmond GI (2009) Factors associated with participation of children with and without ADHD in household tasks. *Phys Occup Ther Pediatr* 29: 274. http://dx.doi.org/10.1080/01942630903008327

Eccles JS, Barber BL, Stone M, Hunt J (2003) Extracurricular activities and adolescent development. *J Soc Issues* 59: 865–889. http://dx.doi.org/10.1046/j.0022-4537.2003.00095.x

Engel-Yeger B, Jarus T, Anaby D, Law M (2009) Differences in patterns of participation between youths with cerebral palsy and typically developing peers. *Am J Occup Ther* 63: 96–104. http://dx.doi.org/10.5014/ajot.63.1.96

Eriksson L, Granlund M (2004) Conceptions of participation in students with disabilities and persons in their close environment. *J Dev Phys Disabil* 16: 229–245. http://dx.doi.org/10.1023/B:JODD.0000032299.31588.fd

Eriksson L, Welander J, Granlund M (2007) Participation in everyday school activities for children with and without disabilities. *J Dev Phys Disabil* 19: 485–502. http://dx.doi.org/10.1007/s10882-007-9065-5

*Fauconnier J, Dickinson HO, Beckung E, et al (2009) Participation in life situations of 8–12 year old children with cerebral palsy: cross sectional European study. *BMJ* 338: b1458. http://dx.doi.org/10.1136/bmj.b1458

Fougeyrollas P, Noreau L, Bergeron H, Cloutier R, Dion SA, St-Michel G (1998) Social consequences of long term impairments and disabilities: conceptual approach and assessment of handicap. *Int J Rehabil Res* 21: 127–141. http://dx.doi.org/10.1097/00004356-199806000-00002

Galvin J, Froude EH, Mcaleer J (2010) Children's participation in home, school and community life after acquired brain injury. *Aust Occup Ther J* 57: 118–126. http://dx.doi.org/10.1111/j.1440-1630.2009.00822.x

Hammel J, Magasi S, Heinemann A, Whiteneck G, Bogner J, Rodriguez E (2008) What does participation mean? An insider perspective from people with disabilities. *Disabil Rehabil* 30: 1445–1460. http://dx.doi.org/10.1080/09638280701625534

Harding J, Harding K, Jamieson P, et al (2009) Children with disabilities' perceptions of activity participation and environments: a pilot study. *Can J Occup Ther* 76: 133–144.

Harter S, Pike R (1984) The Pictorial Scale of Perceived Competence and Social Acceptance for Young Children. *Child Dev* 55: 1969–1982. http://dx.doi.org/10.2307/1129772

Heah T, Case T, Mcguire B, Law M (2007) Successful participation: the lived experience among children with disabilities. *Can J Occup Ther* 74: 38–47. http://dx.doi.org/10.2182/cjot.06.10

Hemmingsson H, Jonsson H (2005) An occupational perspective on the concept of participation in the International Classification of Functioning, Disability and Health – some critical remarks. *Am J Occup Ther* 59: 569–576. http://dx.doi.org/10.5014/ajot.59.5.569

Imms C (2008) The evidence-base for upper extremity intervention for children with cerebral palsy. In: Eliasson AC, Burtner PA, editors. *Improving Hand Function in Cerebral Palsy: Theory, Evidence and Intervention.* London: Mac Keith Press.

Imms C, Reilly S, Carlin J, Dodd K (2008) Diversity of participation in children with cerebral palsy. *Dev Med Child Neurol* 50: 363–369. http://dx.doi.org/10.1111/j.1469-8749.2008.02051.x

Imms C, Reilly S, Carlin J, Dodd KJ (2009) Characteristics influencing participation of Australian children with cerebral palsy. *Disabil Rehabil* 31: 2204–2215. http://dx.doi.org/10.3109/09638280902971406

*Jarus T, Anaby D, Bart O, Engel-Yeger B, Law M (2010) Childhood participation in after-school activities: what is to be expected? *Br J Occup Ther* 73: 344–350. http://dx.doi.org/10.4276/030802210X12813483277062

*King G, Law M, Hanna S, et al (2006) Predictors of the leisure and recreation participation of children with physical disabilities: A structural equation modeling analysis. *Child Health Care* 35: 209–234. http://dx.doi.org/10.1207/s15326888chc3503_2

King GA, Law M, King S, et al (2007) Measuring children's participation in recreation and leisure activities: construct validation of the CAPE and PAC. *Child Care Health Dev* 33: 28–39. http://dx.doi.org/10.1111/j.1365-2214.2006.00613.x

King G, Mcdougall J, Dewit D, Petrenchik T, Hurley P, Law M (2009) Predictors of change over time in the activity participation of children and youth with physical disabilities. *Child Health Care* 38: 321–351. http://dx.doi.org/10.1080/02739610903237352

King G, Law M, Hurley P, Petrenchik T, Schwellnus H (2010) A developmental comparison of the out-of-school recreation and leisure activity participation of boys and girls with and without physical disabilities. *Int J Disabil Dev Educ* 57: 77–107. http://dx.doi.org/10.1080/10349120903537988

Kiresuk TJ, Sherman RE (1968) Goal attainment scaling: a general method for evaluating comprehensive community mental health programs. *Community Ment Health J* 4: 443–453. http://dx.doi.org/10.1007/BF01530764

Klaas SJ, Kelly EH, Gorzkowski J, Homko E, Vogel LC (2010) Assessing patterns of participation and enjoyment in children with spinal cord injury. *Dev Med Child Neurol* 52: 468–474. http://dx.doi.org/10.1111/j.1469-8749.2009.03552.x

Lammi BM, Law M (2003) The effects of family-centred functional therapy on the occupational performance of children with cerebral palsy. *Can J Occup Ther* 70: 285–297.

Larson RW, Verma S (1999) How children and adolescents spend time across the world: work, play, and developmental opportunities. *Psychol Bull* 125: 701–736. http://dx.doi.org/10.1037/0033-2909.125.6.701

Law M, Haight M, Milroy B, Willms D, Stewart D, Rosenbaum P (1999) Environmental factors affecting the occupations of children with physical disabilities. *J Occup Sci Aust* 6: 102–110. http://dx.doi.org/10.1080/14427591.1999.9686455

Law M, Baptiste S, Carswell A, Mccoll MA, Polatajko H, Pollock N (2005) *Canadian Occupational Performance Measure.* Ottawa, ON: CAOT Publications ACE.

Law M, King G, King S, et al (2006) Patterns of participation in recreational and leisure activities among children with complex physical disabilities. *Dev Med Child Neurol* 48: 337–342. http://dx.doi.org/10.1017/S0012162206000740

Law M, Anaby D, Dematteo C, Hanna S (2011a) Participation patterns of children with acquired brain injury. *Brain Inj* 25: 587–595. http://dx.doi.org/10.3109/02699052.2011.572945

*Law M, Darrah J, Pollock N, et al (2011b) Focus on function: a cluster, randomized controlled trial comparing child- versus context-focused intervention for young children with cerebral palsy. *Dev Med Child Neurol* 53: 621–629. http://dx.doi.org/10.1111/j.1469-8749.2011.03962.x

*Law M, King G, Petrenchik T, Kertoy M, Anaby D (2012a) The assessment of preschool children's participation: internal consistency and construct validity. *Phys Occup Ther Geriatr* 32: 272–287. http://dx.doi.org/10.3109/01942638.2012.662584

Law M, Coster W, Bedell G, Arnaby D, Teplicky R, Khetani MA (2012b) Participation in occupations: profiles for children with and without disabilities. Paper presented at the Canadian Association of Occupational Therapists conference, June 2012, Montreal, QB.

Lawlor K, Mihaylov S, Welsh B, Jarvis S, Colver A (2006) A qualitative study of the physical, social and attitudinal environments influencing the participation of children with cerebral palsy in northeast England. *Pediatr Rehabil* 9: 219–228.

Mackie P, Jessen E, Jarvis S (1998) The lifestyle assessment questionnaire: an instrument to measure the impact of disability on the lives of children with cerebral palsy and their families. *Child Care Health Dev* 24: 473–486. http://dx.doi.org/10.1046/j.1365-2214.1998.00083.x

Mahoney JL, Cairns RB (1997) Do extracurricular activities protect against early school dropout? *Dev Psychol* 33: 241–253. http://dx.doi.org/10.1037/0012-1649.33.2.241

Mahoney JL, Schweder AE, Stattin H (2002) Structured after-school activities as a moderator of depressed mood for adolescents with detached relations to their parents. *J Community Psychol* 30: 69–86. http://dx.doi.org/10.1002/jcop.1051

Majnemer A, Shevell M, Law M, et al (2008) Participation and enjoyment of leisure activities in school-aged children with cerebral palsy. *Dev Med Child Neurol* 50: 751–758. http://dx.doi.org/10.1111/j.1469-8749.2008.03068.x

Majnemer A, Shikako-Thomas K, Chokron N, et al (2010) Leisure activity preferences for 6-to 12-year-old children with cerebral palsy. *Dev Med Child Neurol* 52: 167–173. http://dx.doi.org/10.1111/j.1469-8749.2009.03393.x

Perenboom RJM, Chorus AMJ (2003) Measuring participation according to the International Classification of Functioning, Disability and Health (ICF). *Disabil Rehabil* 25: 577–587. http://dx.doi.org/10.1080/0963828031000137081

Rochette A, Korner-Bitensky N, Levasseur M (2006) 'Optimal' participation: a reflective look. *Disabil Rehabil* 28: 1231–1235. http://dx.doi.org/10.1080/09638280600554827

Rutter M (1987) Psychosocial resilience and protective mechanisms. *Am J Orthopsychiatry* 57: 316–331. http://dx.doi.org/10.1111/j.1939-0025.1987.tb03541.x

Simeonsson RJ, Carlson D, Huntington GS, Mcmillen JS, Brent JL (2001) Students with disabilities: a national survey of participation in school activities. *Disabil Rehabil* 23: 49–63. http://dx.doi.org/10.1080/096382801750058134

Whiteneck G, Dijkers MP (2009) Difficult to measure constructs: conceptual and methodological issues concerning participation and environmental factors. *Arch Phys Med Rehabil* 90: S22–S35. http://dx.doi.org/10.1016/j.apmr.2009.06.009

World Health Organization (2001) *International Classification of Functioning, Disability and Health*. Geneva: WHO Press.

Wright FV, Rosenbaum PL, Goldsmith CH, Law M, Fehlings DL (2008) How do changes in body functions and structures, activity, and participation relate in children with cerebral palsy? *Dev Med Child Neurol* 50: 283–289. http://dx.doi.org/10.1111/j.1469-8749.2008.02037.x.

6
A DEVELOPMENTAL PERSPECTIVE ON CHILDHOOD NEUROLOGICAL CONDITIONS

Peter L. Rosenbaum and Gabriel M. Ronen

Overview

Traditional clinical perspectives on childhood neurodisabilities have focused almost exclusively on the biomedical aspects of these many conditions. The emphasis has been on diagnosis and 'treatment' of the underlying impairments, with the implicit assumption that improvements in body structure and function would result in enhanced functioning, as currently understood in the context of the World Health Organization's (WHO's) International Classification of Functioning, Disability and Health (ICF) framework.

These assumptions are not only of questionable validity but also fail to recognize the developmental implications and impacts of these many conditions. In this chapter perspectives on child development are presented, and it is argued that, in addition to whatever evidence-based biomedical interventions are available to children with these 'neurodevelopmental disabilities', it is essential that professionals and parents keep a constant focus on child and family development as a guiding principle in all their work with children with neurological conditions and their families.

Introduction

Paediatrics is the branch of clinical medicine devoted to the growth, development, health, and well-being of infants, children, and young people. The modern era of child health is only about 150 years old and reflects, among other factors, the relatively recent recognition that children are not small adults, but rather require, and deserve, consideration in their own right. The thesis of this chapter is that all professionals who work with children need to be aware of this concept and to tailor their thinking and actions appropriately.

Childhood is a vitally important foundational stage of one's lifetime development. We hope and expect to continue to develop throughout our lives, but the most dramatic manifestations of human development occur in the first two decades. This is the period of life that is most sensitive to the biological and social forces that shape who we become as adults. During this time, humans evolve from totally dependent beings, in the first few years, into full physical maturity in the second decade and towards an emerging capacity for complete independence.

It is a witticism that 'paediatrics is a branch of child development' – and yet, upon reflection, one can recognize the truth of that statement. Children's physical, psychological, and social health and well-being are clearly important elements in the processes of 'becoming' that are the essential components of children's journey towards adulthood in their first 20 to 30 years of life (as discussed in in Chapters 1, 9, and 22).

People who work in the field of childhood disability – what some people refer to as 'applied child development' – have too often neglected the 'developmental' aspects of these conditions (Rosenbaum 2009). This is particularly the case in thinking about children with 'neurodevelopmental' conditions – long-lasting health challenges that affect the development of the central nervous system. The traditional clinical emphasis has been on the biomedical aspects of these conditions – making the specific diagnosis, identifying the underlying aetiology and pathophysiological mechanisms, planning appropriate treatments, and so on. We have usually assumed that, by directing attention at remediation of the underlying impairments of body structure and function, our therapeutic efforts would lead to improvements in human functioning – changes in what the WHO's ICF (World Health Organization 2001) refers to as 'activity' (what people can do) and 'participation' (engagement in meaningful aspects of one's life) (see also Chapter 5). Unfortunately, evidence suggests that this linear connection does not happen as we would hope (Wright et al 2007).

No one would dispute the importance of the best of these biomedical interventions; we would, however, argue that they are necessary but certainly not sufficient perspectives. In the rest of this chapter our ideas are outlined concerning the ways that developmental considerations about childhood disability can complement the biomedical components of our work and help us to expand our thinking. This will include what we see to be huge opportunities to be helpful to children with neurodevelopmental conditions and their families.

Concepts to inform thinking and action in developmental impairments and disabilities

DEVELOPMENT IS A LIFE FORCE IN ALL CHILDREN

It is the nature of children to grow, develop, and change over the initial decades of their lives. If one reflects for a moment on the huge variability in the development of 'typical' children one quickly realizes that the range of 'typical' (we try to avoid the word 'normal') people's capabilities varies enormously – presumably based at least partly on variations in intrinsic neurodevelopmental capacity. Perhaps because we too easily divide the world into categories of 'normal' and 'abnormal' (a distinction we believe is unhelpful and potentially stigmatizing), we rarely stop to consider how these variations in all aspects of human development are part of the fabric of the human experience (Rosenbaum 2006).

As children's capacities develop, they typically take the initiative to explore these emerging abilities – and rarely ask permission to do so. Think of the relentlessly busy 2-year-old, exploring his or her physical environment with speed and passion (referred to by adults as 'terrible' because they are so 'motor-minded'), or of the 3-year-old ceaselessly asking 'Why?' because he or she has learned that there are cause-and-effect connections and needs to make sense of the world. One of the major roles of parents is to provide a safe and nurturing environment in which these amazing processes unfold.

It is important to remember that the forces of growth and development are also operating in children with neurodevelopmental conditions – though the trajectories of both their growth and development may be more or less significantly influenced by their neurological impairment. Thus, in addition to the biomedical implications of neurodevelopmental conditions, as assessed and formulated by health professionals, we must identify the emerging 'natural' development of which children with these conditions may be capable, and take advantage of every opportunity to capitalize on these abilities, even when they may be expressed in ways that are not 'typical'. Later in the chapter there are a few illustrations of this important principle.

RECOGNIZING THE 'TRANSACTIONAL' NATURE OF CHILD DEVELOPMENT
Child development was traditionally viewed as a 'top-down' process in which parents (usually mothers) exerted a powerful influence on the ways in which their children developed. The child was considered a blank slate ('tabula rasa') on which the hand of adult experience wrote the script. (The analogy of the sculptor shaping a lump of clay is quite apt here.) A palpable example of the power of this thinking was the belief, popular in the 1960s, that autism was caused by cold, distant, unengaged mothers, whose failure to relate warmly to their child led to the child's withdrawal from the world. We now recognize that idea to have been both incredibly naive – autism is caused by any of a number of biological impairments and is not a condition acquired from an unfeeling family environment – and very destructive to parent and family well-being by blaming caring parents who were completely bemused by their children's impairments in social communication which precluded interpersonal engagement.

In the past 40 years our changing understanding of child development has led to a seismic shift in how we perceive parenting and the role of child factors in how parents and children interact. The 'transactional' model of child development posits that even infants and young children are not empty vessels (Sameroff and Chandler 1975). Rather they are recognized as highly complex beings who bring individual features – personality and temperamental characteristics, abilities and limitations, even factors as obvious as sex and eye colour – to their relationships with the animate world around them. The idea is that the infant or child continually influences the human environment in powerful ways, and that this changed human environment (parents and others) constantly reacts back on the child in a 'transactional' manner over the dimensions of time and space. More colloquially, we like to say that 'parenting is a dance led by the children'! The implications of these perspectives for the development of children with neurodevelopmental conditions are discussed below.

DEVELOPMENT IS POWERFULLY INFLUENCED BY NEURODEVELOPMENTAL CONDITIONS
We see two important considerations in addressing this question. *First*, early onset neurological conditions virtually always have an impact on children's development. This impact can operate directly, by virtue of how the brain might be impaired and thus influence how, and how easily, functions emerge. As we have suggested elsewhere, this is of course true for typically developing people! Some of us are skilled at mathematics, or art, or music, while others are

less able. Some people are physically gifted as athletes or dancers, while others, despite all the lessons to which our parents expose us, lack the extra dimensions of aptitude and passion that are needed for 'success' in these fields. This does not mean that people without 'talent' are brain damaged – simply that the infinite variation in the human experience expresses itself very broadly in the range of human achievement.

Children with neurodevelopmental conditions are of course equally variable – despite their nervous system-induced impairments. It is therefore highly inappropriate to judge the book by the cover and assume that someone with a neurodevelopmental condition will be limited simply because he or she has some functional limitations in some aspect(s) of life. It is equally prejudicial (in both the literal and colloquial senses of that word) to assume that any problems a person with a neurodevelopmental condition may experience are 'caused' by his or her neurodevelopmental disorder, and thus to attribute any difficulties solely to the condition.

There is a *second* important way in which development may be affected by a neurodevelopmental condition. This requires us to recognize the potential 'secondary' impacts of these conditions – the many ways that functional limitations may create 'deprivation' of experience. One has simply to watch typically developing infants and young children at 'play' to realize how hard they actually work at things! They practise endlessly, exploring variations of an activity, be it fine motor play or gross motor exploration or experimentation with language. These skills are constantly being refined through repetition and trial and error, building on previous experience.

Children with neurodevelopmental conditions may have similar interests and inclinations to experiment and practise, but can often be 'deprived' of opportunities to engage with the world around them because of functional limitations imposed by their condition. Imagine a 2-year-old with severe visual limitation, or one with a significant mobility restriction, seeking to learn about his or her world. We too easily take it for granted that the 'usual' ways that children do this are the only ways and fail to appreciate the challenges that the child with impairment will face – or identify how the world around the child can be adapted in an effort to compensate for these natural impediments.

Insofar as these two young children may not be very good 'dancers', their parents may have difficulty knowing what to do to enhance their child's development. Professionals have an important role to play by recognizing the 'developmental' implications of the functional limitations associated with a neurodevelopmental condition and advising parents about how they can structure their child's environment to enhance learning opportunities. Thus, for example, a visually impaired child can learn about the environment using sound (e.g. sound-making toys and other cueing), smells (to orient the child to different rooms in the home), and touch (using temperature, texture, and shapes to learn to distinguish objects). The motor-challenged 2-year old can be provided with a mobility device such as an adapted motorized wheelchair that literally and figuratively may empower the child to explore the world, exert some physical control over the environment, and gain life experiences that he or she would have been having had it not been for the mobility restriction. There is sound support from research for these ideas, illustrating that with enhanced mobility capacity come important developments in play, social, and language skills, and even increased efforts at self-directed movement (Butler et al 1984, Butler 1986).

How Can We Link Social and Biological Impacts on Child Development?

In the last decade, epidemiological, psychological, basic neuroscience, and molecular genetic studies have all helped us to understand how experiences in early life affect subsequent child development and behaviour. Psychosocial influences, in concert with biological and nutritional influences, have been shown to affect the timing and pattern of genetic expression, which can alter brain structure and function. Poverty, poor maternal care, excessive stress, and maternal depression are all risk factors that affect brain development negatively (Walker et al 2011). Children with neurodevelopmental conditions are even more prone to many of these risk factors that compromise early child development in every society. These environmental factors operate as signals, particularly during early development, and affect gene transcription.

Advances in neurosciences demonstrate that the period of 'brain growth spurt', which extends from the sixth month of gestation to several years of age, is characterized by elaborate dynamic functional remodelling involved in synaptogenesis (the formation of synapses between neurons). This process permits the immature brain to develop in a manner directed by the environmental interaction of the child and facilitates the 'plastic' characteristics of the immature brain. Exposure to biological and psychosocial risk factors, prenatally and during early childhood, affects brain structure and function and compromises children's development and subsequent developmental trajectories. However, by eliminating or reducing the threats of biological and psychosocial risks, and within a caregiving environment that supports cognitive and social–emotional development, children experience healthier brain development that enables them to reach towards their developmental potential (Shen and Cowan 2009, Morrison et al 2012).

Epigenetic mechanisms may play a major role here. Epigenetics refers to a set of biochemical signals that directly or indirectly control genomic structure and function (i.e. transcription) without an alteration of the nucleotide sequence (Caldji et al 2011). The fact that these epigenetic mechanisms are important mediators of environmental influences on brain development opens many windows for interventions. Illustrative examples are randomized controlled trials that reveal a more positive attitude following interactive group therapy in the parents of children with intellectual impairments in India (Russell et al 1999) and in the adaptation of mothers of children with cerebral palsy in Bangladesh (McConachie et al 2000), which increase developmentally facilitative activities and probably benefit children's cognitive and psychosocial development.

The Time-course of Development Extends Beyond Childhood

One of the many tyrannies in the field of child development – be it in our teaching or in what is 'out there' for parents in books and on the Internet – is the expectation of a specific timing of development events as expressed by milestones. Milestones are the quantitative markers of children's achievements – a child's first tooth, first steps, first words, being toilet trained, and the onset of menarche are but a few examples. Parents of typically developing children, and many professionals, often fail to recognize the considerable variation that is associated with all these milestones and become concerned when a child appears to lag behind. The 5- to 6-year variation in the onset of menarche is our favourite example of how incredibly wide is the window for the onset of a physiologically 'normal' and significant development in the lives of females at some point during their first two decades of life.

Thus, we believe that it is very important to counsel parents about this kind of variability in quantitative markers of the developmental march, and to focus at least as much on qualitative indicators of emerging skills. The development of communication serves as a good example of how this can be done. Imagine a 3-year-old with a neurodevelopmental condition who has no words, a 'failure' that might cause great parental (and often professional) distress. However, that child might well manifest other evidence of communicative capacity – attentiveness, verbal comprehension, eye gaze to indicate interests, and so on – all of which would be important markers of communicative development despite the absence of conventional verbal 'output'. Parents of such a child would be well advised to provide the child with 'alternative and augmentative communication' tools such as sign language, picture boards, or other systems that enable the child both to express 'what's on his or her mind' and to receive the social, linguistic, and cognitive feedback that such encounters demand. (This is of course simply another illustration of the transactional model of child development at work!)

Another implication of the issue of the time-course of development in children with neurological conditions – relevant for both parents and professionals – is the potential for considerable variation in the emergence of skills in different dimensions of children's development. For example, a child with a mobility restriction may have typical language and cognitive skills that appear discrepant with his or her impaired movement development; a child with cognitive limitations might have good fine and gross motor abilities. Thus, it is important to look at each aspect of a child's development separately, manage each on its own merits, and not make assumptions about either capacity or impairment based on any specific dimension of development.

These examples of the variability of timing in child development hopefully serve to remind us of the need to help parents recognize that the development of the child with a neurodevelopmental condition might follow a different trajectory from that they experienced with their other children. It must be emphasized to them that 'different' is not necessarily 'abnormal', but that they may need patience as their child's skills and abilities develop and are refined with time and experience. The patterns of language development in visually impaired children have been shown to differ from those of typically developing children, but these children's abilities may eventually be highly functional, presumably based on the alternative ways by which these children learn about the world around them (Reynell and Zinkin 1975). Parents also need to realize that children with apparently similar conditions may show different developmental trajectories and should not be discouraged by what they observe of other children's development or behaviour in clinic or in a rehabilitation facility.

WHAT ARE PARENTS' NEEDS?
Adults develop and change. This happens simply because development is part of the human condition, even after adolescence. In the case of parents experiencing a child's development, the transactional realities of the 'parenting dance' mean that parents are constantly being

challenged to adapt to the rapidly changing capacities of their developing children. This is what makes parenting an infinitely fascinating and kaleidoscopic experience.

These factors are of course more complex for parents raising a child with a neurodevelopmental condition. To the extent that the counselling offered to parents about their child's predicament emphasizes that 'the glass is half empty', parents can easily be left with a sense of hopelessness about both their child's situation and their own possibilities as parents. Insofar as we cannot 'cure' neurodevelopmental conditions, it is easy for professionals to be pessimistic about possibilities for change and development. On the other hand, when we present parents with an understanding of the processes associated with child development we believe that we can empower them to take an active role in shaping their children's lives and experiences while accommodating the differences that are imposed by the presence of a neurodevelopmental condition (Rosenbaum and Gorter 2012).

One implication, for professionals, is that the interventions we recommend need to be considered in a 'developmental' as well as a biomedical context. For example, what might be appropriate goals for a preschool child might be quite inappropriate later on, when developmental considerations in the child's life force us to consider the 'impairment' and 'developmental' issues differently. The nature of 'treatment' should always be tempered by appropriate identification and implementation of activities relevant to that child's stage of development. This also includes engaging the child as an active participant in his or her 'therapy' – giving the child the opportunity to make *choices* about *how* things are done within the context of the *decisions* that have been made by parents and professionals about *what* is needed at that stage of life (Darrah et al 2011).

We indicated earlier that children rarely ask permission to practise and exploit their emerging capacities. In typically developing children much of the work of parents is reactive – keeping up with our children's initiatives. Children with neurodevelopmental conditions may have many fewer opportunities to initiate these explorations, and parents may not recognize the need to promote their children's independence. We have often talked about the need to 'prescribe mischief' – helping parents to recognize opportunities for the child with a neurodevelopmental condition to take chances, make mistakes, and learn from experience, as happens with most children. This clearly does not give parents a licence to allow recklessness or danger; it does, however, remind them of the need for children to have opportunities for engaged learning and choice making and the possibility of having an active role in their own development. Anecdotally we know that parents can understand and support this approach to parenting and that they are excited by their children's 'mischief' with its attendant social consequences and its apparent 'normality'.

There are of course many additional ways that parents can be reminded of how their children with neurodevelopmental conditions can be given opportunities for self-discovery – all with the aim of promoting the development of self-esteem and a sense of personal competence. For example, parents can have expectations that their child will take on graded responsibilities for his or her own day-to-day life – dressing, toileting, eating, cleaning his or her room, undertaking appropriate household chores – all of which give the child a chance to become competent and acquire a 'can do' approach to life. Needless to say, the more that parents perceive their children as competent beings the less likely they are to focus on the 'impairment'. (One might add here that this is equally true for typically developing children: when we hear from the parents of our children's friends, or from teachers, about how polite/friendly/helpful/responsible our children are in other settings we gain an insight into how our children are incorporating lessons from home life into their own experience – and we are often pleasantly surprised!)

THE ROLE OF ENVIRONMENT

Children's most important environmental context is their family, including the extended family, in which grandparents may often play a special role. Thus, professionals should seek parental permission to involve the grandparents of the child with a neurodevelopmental condition. This is important because, among other realities, the child's parents are often living in a 'generational sandwich', being simultaneously parents to their child with a neurodevelopmental condition and 'children' of their own parents. Grandparents often have resources of time, money, life experience, and love for their (adult) child and can represent an important source of help and support to the young nuclear family as they embark on the career of parenting a child with a neurodevelopmental condition.

Of course children also experience other important environments – the preschool or school they attend, community-based recreational programmes, and the homes of their family and hopefully friends. It is important to advise people in these environments about the developmental dimensions of neurodevelopmental conditions, as discussed here, so that they too provide developmentally appropriate opportunities for children to thrive and do not simply treat them as impaired and dependent beings. Consistency from place to place and person to person generally serves children well; for children with neurodevelopmental conditions, with less flexibility in their capacities, it is essential.

Conclusion

In our work with children with neurodevelopmental conditions and their families we of course value and endorse the application of appropriate evidence-informed biomedical interventions that are known to enhance functioning and quality of life. Ultimately, however, we believe that our most important goal should be the long-term developmental, functional, and life quality outcomes of children with neurodevelopmental conditions and the well-being of their families. We see the processes involved in supporting parents and their children with these conditions along their journey to be vital, and to provide opportunities to support child and family development along the way.

REFERENCES

Key references

*Butler C (1986) Effects of powered mobility on self-initiated behaviors of very young children with locomotor disability. *Dev Med Child Neurol* 28: 325–332. http://dx.doi.org/10.1111/j.1469-8749.1986.tb03881.x

Butler C, Okamoto GA, McKay TM (1984) Motorized wheelchair driving by disabled children. *Arch Phys Med Rehabil* 65: 95–97.

Caldji C, Hellstrom IC, Zhang TY, Diorio J, Meaney MJ (2011) Environmental regulation of the neural epigenome. *FEBS Lett* 585: 2049–2058. http://dx.doi.org/10.1016/j.febslet.2011.03.032

*Darrah J, Law MC, Pollock N, et al (2011) Context therapy – a new intervention approach for children with cerebral palsy. *Dev Med Child Neurol* 53: 615–620. http://dx.doi.org/10.1111/j.1469-8749.2011.03959.x

McConachie H, Huq S, Munir S, Ferdous S, Zaman S, Khan NZ (2000) A randomized controlled trial of alternative modes of service provision in young children with cerebral palsy in Bangladesh. *J Pediatr* 137: 769–776. http://dx.doi.org/10.1067/mpd.2000.110135

Morrison G, Fraser DD, Cepinskas G (2012) Mechanisms and consequences of acquired brain injury during development. *Pathophysiology* 731:

Reynell J, Zinkin P (1975) New procedures for the developmental assessment of young children with severe visual handicaps. *Child Care Health Dev* 1: 61–69. http://dx.doi.org/10.1111/j.1365-2214.1975.tb00203.x

*Rosenbaum P (2006) Variation and 'abnormality': recognizing the differences. Invited editorial. *J Pediatr* 149: 593–594. http://dx.doi.org/10.1016/j.jpeds.2006.08.030

Rosenbaum P (2009) Putting child development back into developmental disabilities. *Dev Med Child Neurol* 51: 251. http://dx.doi.org/10.1111/j.1469-8749.2009.03275.x

*Rosenbaum P, Gorter JW (2012) The 'F-words' in childhood disability: I swear this is how we should think! *Child Care Health Dev* 38: 457–463. http://dx.doi.org/10.1111/j.1365-2214.2011.01338.x

Russell PS, al John JK, Lakshmanan JL (1999) Family intervention for intellectually disabled children: randomized controlled trial. *Br J Psychiatry* 174: 254–258. http://dx.doi.org/10.1192/bjp.174.3.254

*Sameroff AJ, Chandler MJ (1975) Reproductive risk, and the continuum of caretaking casualty. In: Horowitz FD, Harrington M, Scarr-Salapatek S, Siegel G, editors. *Review of Child Development Research*, Volume 4. Chicago: University of Chicago Press, pp. 184–244.

Shen K, Cowan CW (2009) Guidance molecules in synapse formation and plasticity. *Cold Spring Harb Perspect Biol* 2: a001842.

Walker SP, Wachs TD, Grantham-McGregor S, et al (2011) Inequality in early childhood: risk and protective factors for early child development. *Lancet* 378: 1325–1338. http://dx.doi.org/10.1016/S0140-6736(11)60555-2

*World Health Organization (2001) *International Classification of Functioning, Disability and Health.* Geneva: World Health Organization.

*Wright FV, Rosenbaum PL, Goldsmith CH, Law M, Fehlings DL (2008) How do changes in body functions and structures, activity, and participation relate in children with cerebral palsy? *Dev Med Child Neurol* 50: 283–289. http://dx.doi.org/10.1111/j.1469-8749.2008.02037.x

7
PSYCHOLOGICAL IMPACT OF LIVING WITH A NEURODEVELOPMENTAL CONDITION

Michele C. Thorne and David Dunn

Overview

Individuals with neurodevelopmental conditions face many struggles owing to the chronicity and the often progressive nature of these conditions. Chief among these difficulties are psychological concerns such as depression and anxiety, problems adjusting to increasing medical needs, cognitive impairments, behaviour problems, attention and concentration difficulties, academic concerns, and social challenges with both adults and peers. This chapter examines some of the more significant psychological outcomes and ways in which having a lifelong neurodevelopmental condition impacts all areas of an individual's life. We discuss the importance of creating multidisciplinary teams, which include a range of members from the health services community, the individual with the neurodevelopmental condition, and his or her loved ones, in order to increase the likelihood of successful life quality outcomes and help these individuals to reach their potential. Although this chapter draws particularly on our extensive experience of children and young people with epilepsy, it also presents and discusses evidence from other neurodevelopmental conditions to make the point that the psychological impacts of these conditions are broad and wide ranging.

Introduction

Parents and caregivers of children with neurodevelopmental conditions know all too well the struggles their children face. The lifelong nature of many of these conditions necessitates a close partnership with a team of individuals focused on ensuring that the child can reach his or her potential and navigate the obstacles that may arise. In order that these individuals can develop this crucial working relationship with children and their families, they must understand the myriad of difficulties the children face. These challenges may affect the children's physical, psychological, and emotional well-being. This chapter focuses on the psychological outcomes of living with a neurodevelopmental condition and the ways in which those involved in their care can assist children to have successful outcomes. First, it will address the cognitive impact that many neurodevelopmental conditions have on intellectual and academic functioning; then there will be a discussion of the emotional challenges that many of these individuals face and the effects that these conditions have on behaviour and social functioning.

Cognitive impact

As Ronen and Rosenbaum outlined in the introductory chapter of this book (Chapter 1), the central nervous systems (CNSs) of individuals with neurodevelopmental conditions often mature relatively late in life. This has a significant impact not only on these individuals' cognitive and educational abilities but also on how they understand and process the world around them. Much research has focused on the effects of neurodevelopmental impairments on academic achievements and health outcomes. For example, children with epilepsy have been found to be at significant risk for academic underachievement and problems with attention (Rodenburg et al 2011). Individuals with epilepsy are known to have decreased processing speed and an impairment of short-term memory. Risk factors for problems such as these include early onset, and continued progression, of the disorder. To complicate this issue even further, many individuals with neurodevelopmental conditions must take medications to address their medical concerns: these medications may also cause disruption in short-term memory and affect concentration and attention (Salpekar and Dunn 2007, Rodenburg et al 2011).

IQ AND MEMORY

Conditions such as cerebral palsy and neurofibromatosis have been shown to have considerable impact on overall brain functioning, and the resulting brain pathology that conditions such as these may cause can have significant impact on individuals' ability to learn and adapt to their environment (Sigurdardottir et al 2010, de Vries and Bolton 2010). Indeed, individuals with intellectual impairment often have comorbid neurodevelopmental conditions. One-third of individuals who fall into the severely intellectually impaired range have a seizure disorder and 30% to 60% of severely intellectually impaired individuals have cerebral palsy (Harris 2006).

Studies examining cognitive abilities in children with conditions such as epilepsy have found that these children often have significantly lower IQ scores than children without epilepsy (Williams et al 1998, Moore and Baker 2002, Smith et al 2002, Salpekar and Dunn 2007). Research has indicated that IQ scores tend to be fairly stable over time, but problems with memory and consolidation of learned material can lead to longer-term cognitive impairments (Borden et al 2006, Salpekar and Dunn 2007). While memory deficits have been highlighted in children with neurodevelopmental conditions, studies often have not controlled for IQ, making it difficult to ascertain whether memory deficits are actually a result of lower cognitive functioning rather than being indicative of global memory impairment. Future research should evaluate the benefits of cognitive rehabilitation programmes, which have shown promise in treating children with memory impairments associated with chemotherapy and CNS radiation treatments for childhood cancer.

ACADEMIC PERFORMANCE: SPECIFIC LEARNING IMPAIRMENT

In addition to the cognitive difficulties caused by intellectual impairment, children with neurodevelopmental disorders are at increased risk for specific learning impairments. The learning difficulties may be due to structural CNS changes, a manifestation of syndromes or chromosomal and gene disorders, the effects of seizure disorders, or the secondary effects of impaired early life experience (see Chapter 6 on developmental perspectives).

The impairment in learning abilities is part of the phenotype of many syndromes and chromosomal disorders. Children with neurodevelopmental conditions may show learning abilities that are substantially below what might be expected based on their global cognitive ability and are seen as part of the cognitive behavioural phenotypes of genetic syndromes (Moldavsky et al 2001). As an example, children with Down syndrome have marked deficits in verbal short-term memory but better developed visuospatial short-term memory. In contrast, children with Williams syndrome have impairment in spatial cognition but a relative strength in language (Gathercole and Alloway 2006). Children with fetal alcohol syndrome may have severe difficulties with complex executive functioning, and males with fragile X syndrome have severe deficits in social cognition and expressive language (Moldavsky et al 2001, Hoyme et al 2005).

Specific learning impairments are common in children with epilepsy and affect even children with normal intelligence. Approximately half of children with epilepsy have evidence of a specific learning impairment. The higher prevalence of learning disorders is found regardless of the criteria used to define a specific learning disorder. Fastenau et al (2008) found that 48% of children with epilepsy and normal intelligence had at least one learning impairment as defined by achievement test scores one standard deviation or more below IQ scores. Low reading, mathematics, or writing achievement scores, defined as one standard deviation below normal with or without a discrepancy with IQ scores, were seen in 41% to 62%.

The aetiology of specific learning impairments in the child with epilepsy is probably multifactorial. Impairment may be present at onset of seizures, suggesting that underlying CNS dysfunction results in both seizures and neuropsychological impairment. Fastenau et al (2009) found that 27% of children with normal intelligence and new-onset seizures had a neuropsychological deficit compared with 18% of siblings. Neuropsychological deficits were noted in 40% of children with a second seizure, a symptomatic or cryptogenic aetiology, epileptiform activity on electroencephalogram, and use of antiepileptic drugs. At baseline, although there were lower scores in neuropsychological functioning, there was no difference in academic achievement in children with new-onset seizures compared with siblings.

Over time, risk for specific learning impairment may increase with repeated persistent seizures and, apparently paradoxically, with treatment of epilepsy. Hermann et al (2006) found academic underachievement and mild diffuse cognitive impairment on neuropsychological testing 1 year after the onset of idiopathic epilepsy. Dunn et al (2010) reassessed the children initially described by Fastenau et al (2009) 36 months after seizure onset and found a relative drop in academic performance in reading and mathematics. There was no difference in scores in children with seizures compared with siblings at baseline, but significant differences were present by 36 months after onset of seizures.

Emotional impact

Individuals with neurodevelopmental conditions have been found to have a significant increase in risk for the development of mood problems and anxiety. Indeed, the Isle of Wight Childhood Epidemiology Study, conducted in the late 1960s and early 1970s, found that the prevalence of mental health problems in children with conditions such as epilepsy was double the rate of mental health concerns in children with other chronic medical conditions (i.e. those that do not directly affect the brain) (Rutter et al 1970). A survey of children enrolled in schools for the intellectually impaired found a prevalence of DSM-IV (*Diagnostic and Statistical Manual of Mental Disorders*, 4th edition) symptoms as follows: anxiety disorders 21.9%, mood disorders 4.4%, and disruptive behaviour disorders 25.1% (Dekker and Koot 2003). There appear to be two distinct phenomena contributing to the development of internalizing symptoms: the first involves actual neurobiological changes that occur as a result of the condition, while the second involves the individual's psychological responses to having a neurodevelopmental condition (Salpekar and Dunn 2007).

A primary problem is the difficulty of identifying internalizing problems in a child with a neurodevelopmental condition. The symptom most likely to lead to psychological assessment is aggression. The presence of aggression towards others or self-injurious behaviours does not necessarily mean that the child has a disruptive behaviour disorder. Children with depression may have irritable mood instead of obvious sadness. Anxiety may be easily misinterpreted as oppositionality. A history should be taken from both child and parent with an expectation that there may be differences in reporting. Children may be more aware of depression and anxiety than their parents. However, the child with a cognitive limitation may not be able to identify emotions. Occasionally, a child with cognitive limitations may be overly agreeable and may respond 'yes' to any question from the examiner. Parents and others who know the child (e.g. teachers) can provide information on behaviour, changes in functioning, precipitating causes for aberrant behaviours, and characteristic coping mechanisms. Factors that may be important in assessing changes in behaviour include health difficulties such as painful processes, sensory impairments that may lead to frustrations, new medications that may cause adverse effects, and changes in environment.

In part, the prevalence of internalizing disorders may be due to the stresses of a chronic condition. Rodenburg et al (2005) reviewed studies of psychopathology in children with epilepsy and found that when the comparison group was children with other chronic illness there were only small to medium differences in the occurrence of psychopathology. Other studies have shown that children with CNS involvement are more likely to experience difficulties. Davies et al (2003) found emotional problems in 16% of children with complicated epilepsy, 16% of those with uncomplicated epilepsy, 6% of children with diabetes, and 4% of controls. Breslau (1985) found that children with chronic conditions due to brain dysfunction had more problems than children with cystic fibrosis. In that study, the rate was related to degree of cognitive impairment, but even controlling for IQ the children with CNS problems experienced more social isolation.

In children with neurodevelopmental impairment, the prevalence of anxiety and depression varies by condition and age. Children with Down syndrome have a relatively low rate of psychopathology, but by adolescence and emerging adulthood the rate of internalizing symptoms and the prevalence of depression increase substantially (Dykens 2007). Anxiety is prominent in both males and females with fragile X syndrome and is present in Prader–Willi, Williams, velocardiofacial, and Turner syndrome. Children with Prader–Willi, velocardiofacial, and Turner syndrome and older adolescents with Williams syndrome have an increased risk for depression (Moldavsky et al 2001). Anxiety and depression are also problems for children and adolescents with epilepsy. Caplan et al (2005a) found that 33% of children with complex partial seizures or absence epilepsy had symptoms of anxiety. Dunn et al (2009) reported symptoms of phobias, obsessions, post-traumatic stress, and panic disorders in more than 30% of children with epilepsy. A review of depressive disorders in children with epilepsy noted a prevalence range of 12% to 26% (Barry 2008). Often both anxiety and depression go unrecognized and untreated.

Other behaviours of importance include suicidal ideation and suicide attempts. Children with neurodevelopmental conditions such as epilepsy have been shown to be at significantly higher risk for suicide compared with age-matched peers without epilepsy and compared with adults with older-onset epilepsy. Risk factors include early age of epilepsy onset and prevalence of mood problems (Nilsson et al 2002, Rodenburg et al 2011).

Treatment should begin with a careful search for the aetiology of the anxiety or depression. Symptoms of anxiety and depression may be reduced by modifications in the environment, changes in medication, or psychoeducation. Psychotherapy, behavioural interventions, and psychopharmacology are possible treatment options (Harris 2006). For pharmacological treatment of anxiety and depression, the effectiveness of selective serotonin reuptake inhibitors (SSRIs) has been demonstrated in double-blind, placebo-controlled trials. The most common side effects are nausea and sedation. A meta-analysis found only a minimal increase in suicidal ideation and attempts in children on SSRIs compared with placebo (Bridge et al 2007). Furthermore, there is no lowering of the seizure threshold with SSRIs (Alper et al 2007). In children with epilepsy, antiepileptic drug levels should be monitored when SSRIs are added. Bupropion and tricyclic antidepressants may lower the seizure threshold and should be used cautiously if at all.

Behavioural impact

An increased prevalence of mood and anxiety problems is found in children with chronic illness regardless of aetiology, but problems with attention seem specific to conditions involving the CNS. Symptoms of attention-deficit–hyperactivity disorder (ADHD) are significantly more common in children and adolescents with fetal alcohol syndrome, fragile X syndrome, Williams syndrome, velocardiofacial syndrome, tuberous sclerosis, neurofibromatosis, traumatic brain injury, and other disorders affecting the CNS. Children with epilepsy have a higher prevalence of ADHD than children in the general population. One population-based study found symptoms of ADHD in 44% of the children with epilepsy, and clinic-based studies have reported prevalence in the range of 11% to 40% (Turky et al 2008, Dunn et al 2011). Symptoms of ADHD in children with epilepsy are found more often in those with additional neurological dysfunction and in those with severe intractable seizures (Davies et al 2003, Sherman et al 2007). Symptoms of ADHD are more common in children with epileptic encephalopathies, but are not otherwise associated with any specific seizure type or syndrome. Impaired attention may be associated with antiepileptic drugs such as barbiturates, benzodiazepines, and topiramate (Loring and Meador 2004). Children with absence epilepsy have been found to have more attention problems when receiving valproate than are seen with lamotrigine or ethosuximide (Glauser et al 2010).

Treatment of inattention is essential because of its significant association with academic problems. Studies in children with epilepsy have shown that academic problems are more strongly associated with inattention than with memory, that difficulties in reading and mathematics are associated with symptoms of ADHD, and that children with epilepsy and ADHD have lower cognitive scores at baseline and at follow-up 2 years later than children with epilepsy and no symptoms of ADHD (Williams et al 2001, Fastenau et al 2008, Hermann et al 2008).

The treatment of ADHD in children with epilepsy is similar to that recommended for ADHD in children without seizures. Stimulants are the first choice for psychopharmacological treatment. Open-label trials have been reported for stimulant use in children with fetal alcohol syndrome, fragile X syndrome, velocardiofacial syndrome, neurofibromatosis, and traumatic brain injury (Kledzik and Dunn 2010). One placebo-controlled trial of stimulants in children with autistic spectrum disorders found that 49% responded to methylphenidate (Research Units on Pediatric Pharmacology Autism Network 2005). Although the package inserts warn against using stimulants in children with epilepsy, there are open-label studies showing that methylphenidate in children with ADHD and well-controlled seizures does not cause an increase in seizure number (Gross-Tsur et al 1997, Gucuyener et al 2003). Nevertheless, children with intractable seizures and ADHD should be monitored closely. One placebo-controlled trial reported a trend towards increased seizure frequency with the highest dose of OROS (osmotic-controlled release oral delivery system) methylphenidate (Gonzalez-Heydrich et al 2010).

However, treatment of attention problems may not be as effective in children with neurodevelopmental conditions as in children with ADHD alone. Studies in children with fetal alcohol syndrome and ADHD and children with traumatic brain injury and ADHD have shown response to stimulants, but the response was less robust than that seen in uncomplicated ADHD. In the treatment trial using methylphenidate for children with autistic spectrum disorder, the effect size was 0.20 to 0.54 and 18% withdrew because of adverse effects (Research Units on Pediatric Pharmacology Autism Network 2005). When methylphenidate was used to treat ADHD in children with complex partial seizures plus ADHD compared with children with ADHD alone, the scores of the children with ADHD alone normalized whereas in those with complex partial seizures plus ADHD the scores improved but remained 1.5 standard deviations below normal (Semrud-Clikeman and Wical 1999).

For most neurodevelopmental conditions, the data on alternative medications for the treatment of ADHD are limited. Atomoxetine is approved for treatment of ADHD and has not resulted in a significantly increased risk of seizures in patients with ADHD but no prior epilepsy (Wernicke et al 2007). Open-label studies have suggested that atomoxetine is safe and effective, although less effective than stimulants in children and adolescents with epilepsy (Hernández and Barragán 2005, Torres et al 2011). Bupropion and the tricyclic antidepressants are effective in the treatment of ADHD but can lower the seizure threshold and should be avoided.

Oppositional defiant disorder consists of defiance, anger, and irritability, while conduct disorder manifests as major violation of standards such as stealing, property destruction, and assault. Dekker and Koot (2003) found symptoms of oppositional defiant disorder or conduct disorder in 17% of a sample of children with borderline to moderate intellectual impairment. The prevalence of these disorders in children with epilepsy is less well established than in those with ADHD. A clinical series of children 9 to 14 years of age with epilepsy found oppositional defiant disorder in 21% and conduct disorder in 18% (Dunn et al 2009). One epidemiological study found conduct disorder in 24% of children with complicated epilepsy and 17% of children with uncomplicated epilepsy (Davies et al 2003). In comparison, the prevalence of oppositional defiant disorder and conduct disorder in the general population ranges from 2% to 16%.

Social impact

SOCIAL COGNITION

Social competence includes the ability to develop and participate in social interaction, to demonstrate social reciprocity, and to meet one's own needs while respecting the needs of others. Individuals with neurodevelopmental conditions may have difficulties with social competence related to cognitive impairments, language, and behaviour. Zadeh et al (2007) found that language was the mediating variable between externalizing disorders and impaired social cognition. In children with epilepsy, Caplan et al (2005b) showed that lower social competence scores were predicted by externalizing behaviours and lower IQ but not by seizure variables. In children with seizures, both inattention and anxiety are related to difficulties with peer relationships (Drewel et al 2008). Although the main predictor of social limitations is specific learning impairment, adults with epilepsy and no additional cognitive or behavioural problems are more likely to be unemployed or underemployed and are less likely to be married or to have children (Jalava and Sillanpää 1996, Chin et al 2011).

PEER RELATIONSHIPS

Extensive research has documented the importance of positive peer interactions in childhood and adolescence, in terms of both academic achievement and the development of meaningful adult relationships (i.e. Parker and Asher 1993, Birch and Ladd 1996, Newcomb and Bagwell 1998). Individuals who have neurodevelopmental conditions such as epilepsy, cerebral palsy, and spina bifida are at significantly increased risk for having social impairments and difficulties in social interactions (Lavigne and Faier-Routman 1993, Salpekar and Dunn 2007). Such difficulties may include poorer social skills, difficulties in initiating social interactions with peers, increased social isolation and social stigma associated with these conditions, and social restrictions owing to comorbid physical impairments (Warchausky et al 2003, Cunningham et al 2007, Parkes et al 2008). Elementary school-aged children with epilepsy are less likely to be named as a best friend by classmates, are more likely to be bullied, and are more likely to be reported to have poor social skills by teachers when compared with their peers (Hamiwka et al 2009, 2011) (these issues are discussed further in Chapters 8 and 12).

Social stigma exists not only at the peer level but also at the level of adults caring for children with neurodevelopmental conditions. For example, teachers of children with epilepsy often state that they do not feel adequately prepared to manage children with seizures and tend to view them as having lower academic skills than children without epilepsy (Salpekar and Dunn 2007). In addition, some studies have shown that teachers prefer more restrictions on recreation and physical activities than may actually be warranted by the chronic condition.

FAMILY RELATIONSHIPS

The association between behavioural problems in children with neurodevelopmental conditions and difficulty within the family is bidirectional. The child's condition and behaviour can be disruptive to parents and family. The psychological response of the child with a neurodevelopmental condition may be accentuated or ameliorated by parent and family factors.

Family life and the parents' hopes and expectations for the future may be disrupted by the birth of a child with CNS dysfunction or the initial diagnosis of a neurodevelopmental condition. Harris (2006) reports that behavioural and emotional problems in the child with a neurodevelopmental condition are better predictors of family functioning than age or level of cognitive ability. Other factors that may disrupt the family include a lack of predictability of the condition, the time demands of caring for and monitoring the child, and stigma associated with the condition.

Problems within the family in turn influence child behaviour and academic functioning. Rodenburg et al (2006) showed that the quality of the parent–child relationship was a stronger predictor of behavioural problems in the child than epilepsy-related factors. Austin et al (2004), in a study of children with new-onset seizures, found that parents' lack of a sense of mastery and parental uncertainty about child discipline were associated with child behaviour problems at baseline and 24 months later. Anxiety and depression in parents have been associated with poorer quality of life in children with epilepsy (Ferro et al 2011, Stevanovic et al 2011). Lower neuropsychological scores had less effect on the academic achievement of children from more competent families than on those from more disorganized or unsupportive families (Fastenau et al 2009). Also, parental anxiety contributed to lower academic achievement 36 months after onset of seizures (Dunn et al 2010). (Family issues are discussed more fully in Chapter 11.)

RELATIONSHIP WITH THE MEDICAL TEAM

One of the most critical elements of care for individuals with neurodevelopmental conditions is continuity of care. Many individuals with chronic illnesses with childhood onset face difficulty as they attempt to transition their care to the adult medical world (see also Chapters 22 and 23). Barriers to successful transition include a lack of transition clinics and adolescent clinics, doctors who specialize in adult disorders generally having less experience and familiarity with paediatric-onset conditions, and lack of communication between the multidisciplinary paediatric and adult teams (Rodenburg et al 2011). The standard of care for individuals with neurodevelopmental conditions should include an extensive proactive plan for adolescence and transition into the adult medical world. Development of a standard treatment protocol during the adolescent years would be beneficial (as discussed in greater detail in Chapter 22).

Conclusions

Despite the multiple challenges faced by individuals with neurodevelopmental conditions and their families, many are able to navigate successfully through childhood and adolescence and lead successful, healthy, and happy lives as adults. Factors associated with such outcomes include having a supportive family, having a positive perception about themselves and their capabilities, having access to up-to-date medical care and information, and learning and applying self-management techniques and strategies to cope with difficulties that arise as part of these conditions or other life situations. Although much work still needs to be done, interventions that strive to encourage these characteristics and help individuals learn to focus on the aspects that they can control have been successful in improving individuals' overall quality of life and confidence in their ability to manage their conditions (Dunn and Austin 2004, Wagner et al 2010). Interventions targeting the school system and decreasing the social stigma associated with these conditions are crucial, as is providing caregivers such as teachers and aides with information and tools to use to best assist the children in their care to reach their academic potential. Social skills groups and interventions targeting peer relations are also critical to the emotional and social well-being of individuals with neurodevelopmental conditions. Parent training and family interventions should also continue to be developed and evaluated for their ability to enhance family relationship quality, teach healthy coping strategies, and help foster independence and responsibility for medical care.

Mental health concerns have been identified as occurring at a much higher rate in individuals with neurodevelopmental conditions than in other children and young people. As a result, earlier screening and intervention should become a standard component of primary healthcare providers' involvement with these individuals. Tools such as questionnaires and checklists should routinely be employed to assess for common psychiatric concerns, including attention problems, specific learning impairments, depressive symptoms, and anxiety. Connections to mental health providers who specialize in working with children with comorbid psychiatric and medical problems are essential to ensure that children are referred to the appropriate healthcare provider to address symptoms and assist in creating appropriate treatments to address specific learning problems.

The transition to adulthood has been cited as an area of significant challenge for many individuals with neurodevelopmental conditions. Programmes should continue to be developed that aim to decrease the barriers associated with the transition to adult care, including better communication between paediatric and adult healthcare providers, transition programmes that focus on helping individuals understand and learn to manage their healthcare needs, and family education to help parents encourage and foster independence in their children. Finally, support groups for adults living with neurodevelopmental conditions can help foster a sense of community and provide social support and connections.

While much more research is needed to ascertain the exact pathways to enhance quality of life and provide comprehensive care for individuals with neurodevelopmental conditions, multidisciplinary care is gradually becoming the rule rather than the exception. Healthcare providers are realizing the need for multidisciplinary care teams to promote the best possible outcome in children with chronic conditions, including those with a neurodevelopmental basis. This chapter has served merely to highlight the myriad of difficulties faced by individuals with neurodevelopmental conditions, to suggest ways to improve overall quality of life and mental health, and to stress the importance of multidisciplinary approaches to the management of these conditions.

REFERENCES

Key references

*Alper K, Schwartz KA, Kolts RL, Khan A (2007) Seizure incidence in psychopharmacological clinical trials: an analysis of Food and Drug Administration (FDA) summary basis of approval reports. *Biol Psychiatry* 62: 345–354. http://dx.doi.org/0.1016/j.biopsych.2006.09.023

Austin JK, Dunn DW, Johnson CS, Perkins SM (2004) Behavioral issues involving children and adolescents with epilepsy and the impact of their families: recent research data. *Epilepsy Behav* 5: S33–S41. http://dx.doi.org/10.1016/j.yebeh.2004.06.014

*Barry JJ, Ettinger AB, Friel P, et al (2008) Consensus statement: the evaluation and treatment of people with epilepsy and affective disorders. *Epilepsy Behav* 13: S1–S29. http://dx.doi.org/10.1016/j.yebeh.2008.04.005

Birch SH, Ladd GW (1996) Interpersonal relationships in the school environment and children's early school adjustment: the role of teachers and peers. In: Juvonen J, Wentzel KR, editors. *Social Motivation: Understanding Children's School Adjustment*. New York: Cambridge University Press, pp. 199–255.

Breslau N (1985) Psychiatric disorder in children with physical disabilities. *J Am Acad Child Adolesc Psychiatry* 24: 87–94. http://dx.doi.org/10.1016/S0002-7138(09)60415-5

Bridge JA, Iyengar S, Salary CB, et al (2007) Clinical response and risk for reported suicidal ideation and suicide attempts in pediatric antidepressant treatment: a meta-analysis of randomized controlled trials. *JAMA* 297: 1683–1696. http://dx.doi.org/10.1001/jama.297.15.1683

Burden KA, Burns TG, O'Leary SD (2006) A comparison of children with epilepsy to an age- and IQ-matched control group on the Children's Memory Scale. *Child Neuropsychology* 12: 165–172.

Caplan R, Siddarth P, Gurbani S, et al (2005a) Depression and anxiety in pediatric epilepsy. *Epilepsia* 46: 720–730. http://dx.doi.org/10.1111/j.1528-1167.2005.43604.x

Caplan R, Sagun J, Siddarth P, et al (2005b) Social competence in pediatric epilepsy: insights into underlying mechanisms. *Epilepsy Behav* 6: 218–228. http://dx.doi.org/10.1016/j.yebeh.2004.11.020

Chin RFM, Cumberland PM, Pujar SS, et al (2011) Outcomes of childhood epilepsy at age 33 years: a population-based birth-cohort study. *Epilepsia* 52: 1513–1521. http://dx.doi.org/10.1111/j.1528-1167.2011.03170.x

Cunningham SD, Thomas PD, Warschausky S (2007) Gender differences in peer relations of children with neurodevelopmental conditions. *Rehab Psych* 52: 331–337. http://dx.doi.org/10.1037/0090-5550.52.3.331

Davies S, Heyman I, Goodman R (2003) A population survey of mental health problems in children with epilepsy. *Dev Med Child Neurol* 45: 292–295. http://dx.doi.org/10.1111/j.1469-8749.2003.tb00398.x

Dekker MC, Koot HM (2003) DSM-IV disorders in children with borderline to moderate intellectual disability. I: prevalence and impact. *J Am Acad Child Adolesc Psychiatry* 42: 915–922. http://dx.doi.org/10.1097/01. CHI.0000046892.27264.1A

Drewel EH, Bell DJ, Austin JK (2008) Peer difficulties in children with epilepsy: association with seizure, neurological, academic, and behavioral variables. *Child Neuropsychol* 15: 305–320. http://dx.doi. org/10.1080/09297040802537646

Dunn DW, Austin JK (2004) Social aspects. In: Wallace SJ, Farrell K, editors. *Epilepsy in Children*, 2nd edition. London: Arnold, pp. 363–473.

Dunn DW, Austin JK, Perkins SM (2009) Prevalence of psychopathology in children with epilepsy: categorical and dimensional measures. *Dev Med Child Neurol* 51: 364–372. http://dx.doi. org/10.1111/j.1469-8749.2008.03172.x

Dunn DW, Johnson CS, Perkins SM, et al (2010) Academic problems in children with seizures: relationships with neuropsychological functioning and family variables during the 3 years after onset. *Epilepsy Behav* 19: 455–461. http://dx.doi.org/10.1016/j.yebeh.2010.08.023

Dunn DW, Kronenberger WG, Sherman E (2011) Autistic spectrum disorder and attention deficit hyperactivity disorder in childhood epilepsy. In: Helmstaedter C, Hermann B, Lassonde M, Kahane P, Arzimanoglou A, editors. *Neuropsychology in the Care of People with Epilepsy*. Esher, UK: John Libbey Eurotext, pp. 273–284.

Dykens EM (2007) Psychiatric and behavioral disorders in persons with Down syndrome. *MRDD Res Rev* 13: 272–278.

*Fastenau PS, Shen J, Dunn DW, Austin JK (2008) Academic underachievement among children with epilepsy: proportion exceeding psychometric criteria for learning disability and associated risk factors. *J Learn Disabil* 41: 195–207. http://dx.doi.org/10.1177/0022219408317548

Fastenau PS, Johnson CS, Perkins SM, et al (2009) Neuropsychological status at seizure onset in children: risk factors for early cognitive deficits. *Neurology* 73: 526–534. http://dx.doi.org/10.1212/WNL.0b013e3181b23551

Ferro MA, Avison WR, Campbell MK, Speechley KN (2011) The impact of maternal depressive symptoms on health-related quality of life in children with epilepsy: a prospective study of family environment as mediators and moderators. *Epilepsia* 52: 316–325.

Gathercole SE, Alloway TP (2006) Practitioner review: short-term and working memory impairments in neurodevelopmental disorders: diagnosis and remedial support. *J Child Psychol Psychiatry* 47: 4–15. http://dx.doi.org/10.1111/j.1469-7610.2005.01446.x

Glauser T, Cnaan A, Shinnar S, et al (2010) Ethosuximide, valproic acid, and lamotrigine in childhood absence epilepsy *N Engl J Med* 362: 790–799.

Gonzalez-Heydrich J, Whitney J, Waber D, et al (2010) Adaptive phase I study of OROS methylphenidate treatment of attention deficit hyperactivity disorder with epilepsy. *Epilepsy Behav* 18: 229–237. http://dx.doi.org/10.1016/j.yebeh.2010.02.022

Gross-Tsur V, Manor O, van der Meere J, Joseph A, Shalev RS (1997) Epilepsy and attention deficit hyperactivity disorder: is methylphenidate safe and effective? *J Pediatr* 130: 670–674. http://dx.doi.org/10.1016/S0022-3476(97)70258-0

Gucuyener K, Erdemoglu AK, Senol S, Serdaroglu A, Soysal S, Kockar AI (2003) Use of methylphenidate for attention-deficit hyperactivity disorder in patients with epilepsy of electroencephalographic abnormalities. *J Child Neurol* 18: 109–112. http://dx.doi.org/10.1177/08830738030180020601

Hamiwka LD, Yu CG, Hamiwka LA, et al (2009) Are children with epilepsy at greater risk of bullying than their peers? *Epilepsy Behav* 15: 500–505. http://dx.doi.org/10.1016/j.yebeh.2009.06.015

Hamiwka L, Jones JE, Salpekar J, Caplan R (2011) Child psychiatry. *Epilepsy Behav* 22: 38–46. http://dx.doi.org/10.1016/j.yebeh.2011.02.013

Harris JC (2006) *Intellectual Disability: Understanding its Development, Causes, Classification, Evaluation, and Treatment*. New York: Oxford University Press.

Hermann B, Jones J, Sheth R, et al (2006) Children with new-onset epilepsy: neuropsychological status and brain structure. *Brain* 129: 2609–2619. http://dx.doi.org/10.1093/brain/awl196

Hermann B, Jones J, Sheth R, et al (2008) Growing up with epilepsy: a two-year investigation of cognitive development in children with new onset epilepsy. *Epilepsia* 49: 1847–1858. http://dx.doi.org/10.1111/j.1528-1167.2008.01735.x

Hernández AJC, Barragán PEJ (2005) Efficacy of atomoxetine treatment in children with ADHD and epilepsy. *Epilepsia* 46(Suppl. 6): 241.

Hoyme HE, May PA, Kalberg WO, et al (2005) A practical clinical approach to diagnosis of fetal alcohol spectrum disorders: clarification of the 1996 Institute of Medicine criteria. *Pediatrics* 115: 39–47. http://dx.doi.org/10.1542/peds.2005-0702

Jalava M, Sillanpää M (1996) Concurrent illnesses in adults with childhood-onset epilepsy: a population-based 35-year follow-up study. *Epilepsia* 37: 1155–1163. http://dx.doi.org/10.1111/j.1528-1157.1996.tb00547.x

Kledzik AM, Dunn D (2010) Treatment of attention deficit hyperactivity disorder in children with medical conditions. *Psychopharm Rev* 45: 49–55.

Lavigne JV, Faier-Routman J (1993) Correlates of psychological adjustment to pediatric physical disorders: a meta-analytic review and comparison with existing models. *J Dev Behav Pediatr* 14: 117–123.

Loring DW, Meador KJ (2004) Cognitive side effects of antiepileptic drugs in children. *Neurology* 62: 872–877. http://dx.doi.org/10.1212/01.WNL.0000115653.82763.07

*Moldavsky M, Lev D, Lerman-Sagie T (2001) Behavioral phenotypes of genetic syndromes: a reference guide for psychiatrists. *J Am Acad Child Adolesc Psychiatry* 40: 749–761. http://dx.doi.org/10.1097/00004583-200107000-00009

Moore PM, Baker GA (2002) The neuropsychological and emotional consequences of living with intractable temporal lobe epilepsy: implications for clinical management. *Seizure* 11: 224–230. http://dx.doi.org/10.1053/seiz.2001.0668

Newcomb AF, Bagwell CL (1998) The developmental significance of children's friendship relations. In: Bukowski WM, Newcomb AF, Hartup WW, editors. *Company They Keep: Friendship in Childhood and Adolescence*. New York: Cambridge University Press, pp. 289–321.

Nilson L, Ahlom A, Bahman Y, et al (2002) Risk factors for suicide in epilepsy: a case control study. *Epilepsia* 43: 644–651. http://dx.doi.org/10.1046/j.1528-1157.2002.40001.x

Parker JG, Asher SR (1993) Friendship and friendship quality in middle childhood: links with peer group acceptance and feelings of loneliness and social dissatisfaction. *Dev Psychol* 29: 611–621. http://dx.doi.org/10.1037/0012-1649.29.4.611

Parkes J, White-Konig M, Dickinson HO, et al (2008) Psychological problems in children with cerebral palsy: a cross-sectional European study. *J Child Psychol Psychiatry* 49: 405–413. http://dx.doi.org/10.1111/j.1469-7610.2007.01845.x

Research Units on Pediatric Psychopharmacology Autism Network (2005) Randomized, controlled, crossover trial of methylphenidate in pervasive developmental disorders with hyperactivity. *Arch Gen Psychiatry* 62: 1266–1274. http://dx.doi.org/10.1001/archpsyc.62.11.1266

*Rodenburg R, Stams JG, Meijer AM, Aldenkamp AP, Deković M (2005) Psychopathology in children with epilepsy: a meta-analysis. *J Pediatr Psychol* 30: 453–468. http://dx.doi.org/10.1093/jpepsy/jsi071

Rodenburg R, Meijer AM, Deković M, Aldenkamp AP (2006) Family predictors of psychopathology in children with epilepsy. *Epilepsia* 47: 601–614. http://dx.doi.org/10.1111/j.1528-1167.2006.00475.x

Rodenburg R, Wagner JL, Austin JK, Kerr M, Dunn DW (2011) Psychosocial issues for children with epilepsy. *Epilepsy Behav* 22: 47–54. http://dx.doi.org/10.1016/j.yebeh.2011.04.063

Rutter M, Graham P, Yule W (1970) *A Neuropsychiatric Study in Childhood*. Philadelphia, PA: Lippincott Williams & Wilkins.

Salpekar JA, Dunn DW (2007) Psychiatric and psychosocial consequences of pediatric epilepsy. *Semin Pediatr Neurol* 14: 181–188. http://dx.doi.org/10.1016/j.spen.2007.08.004

Semrud-Clikeman M, Wical B (1999) Components of attention in children with complex partial seizures with and without ADHD. *Epilepsia* 40: 211–215. http://dx.doi.org/10.1111/j.1528-1157.1999.tb02077.x

Sherman EMS, Slick DJ, Connolly MB, Eyrl KL (2007) ADHD, neurological correlates, and health-related quality of life in severe pediatric epilepsy. *Epilepsia* 48: 1083–1091.

Sigurdardottir S, Indredavik MS, Eiriksdottir A, Einarsdottir K, Gudmundsson HS, Vik T (2010) Behavioural and emotional symptoms of preschool children with cerebral palsy: a population-based study. *Dev Med Child Neurol* 52: 1056–1061. http://dx.doi.org/10.1111/j.1469-8749.2010.03698.x

Smith ML, Elliott IM, Lach L (2002) Cognitive skills in children with intractable epilepsy: comparison of surgical and nonsurgical candidates. *Epilepsia* 43: 632–637. http://dx.doi.org/10.1046/j.1528-1157.2002.26101.x

Stevanovic D, Jancic J, Lakic A (2011) The impact of depression and anxiety disorder symptoms on the health-related quality of life of children and adolescents with epilepsy. *Epilepsia* 52: e75–e78. http://dx.doi.org/10.1111/j.1528-1167.2011.03133.x

Torres A, Whitney J, Rao S, Tilley C, Lobel R, Gonzalez-Heydrich J (2011) Tolerability of atomoxetine for treatment of pediatric attention-deficit/hyperactivity disorder in the context of epilepsy. *Epilepsy Behav* 20: 95–102. http://dx.doi.org/10.1016/j.yebeh.2010.11.002

Turky A, Beavis JM, Thapar AK, Kerr MP (2008) Psychopathology in children and adolescents with epilepsy: an investigation of predictive variables. *Epilepsy Behav* 12: 136–144. http://dx.doi.org/10.1016/j.yebeh.2007.08.003

de Vries PJ, Bolton PF (2010) Tuberous sclerosis. In: Howlin P, Udwin O, editors. *Outcomes in Neurodevelopmental and Genetic Disorders*. New York: Cambridge University Press, pp. 272–298.

Wagner JL, Smith G, Ferguson PL, van Bakergem K, Hrisko S (2010) Pilot study of an integrated cognitive–behavioral and self-management intervention for youth with epilepsy and caregivers: Coping Openly and Personally with Epilepsy (COPE). *Epilepsy Behav* 18: 280–285. http://dx.doi.org/10.1016/j.yebeh.2010.04.019

Warchausky SA, Argento AG, Hurvitz E, Berg M (2003) Neuropsychological status and social problem solving in children with congenital or acquired brain dysfunction. *Rehab Psych* 48: 250–254. http://dx.doi.org/10.1037/0090-5550.48.4.250

Wernicke JF, Holdridge KC, Jin L, et al (2007) Seizure risk in patients with attention-deficit–hyperactivity disorder treated with atomoxetine. *Dev Med Child Neurol* 49: 498–502.

Williams J, Griebel ML, Dykman RA (1998) Neuropsychological patterns in pediatric epilepsy. *Seizure* 7: 223–228. http://dx.doi.org/10.1016/S1059-1311(98)80040-X

Williams J, Phillips T, Griebel ML, et al (2001) Factors associated with academic achievement in children with controlled epilepsy. *Epilepsy Behav* 2: 217–223.

Zadeh AY, Im-Bolter N, Cohen NJ (2007) Social cognition and externalizing psychopathology: an investigation of the mediating role of language. *J Abnorm Child Psychol* 35: 141–152. http://dx.doi.org/10.1007/s10802-006-9052-9

8
PEER RELATIONS AMONG CHILDREN WITH NEUROLOGICAL AND DEVELOPMENTAL CONDITIONS

Tracy Vaillancourt, Jennifer Hepditch, Irene Vitoroulis, Amanda Krygsman, Christine Blain-Arcaro, and Patricia McDougall

Overview

The focus of this chapter is on the peer relations of school-aged children (aged 5–18) with neurological and developmental conditions. We have chosen to focus on physical impairments involving vision and hearing, learning, intellectual function, and autism spectrum disorder (ASD) given their higher prevalence rates and because there are enough published studies from which to draw some conclusions. This review highlights the fact that children with neurological and developmental conditions have the same need as do typically developing children to form healthy relationships with peers. However, children with neurological and developmental conditions often need the support of adults to help promote these relationships.

> The desire for interpersonal attachment may well be one of the most far-reaching and integrative constructs currently available to understand human nature. If psychology has erred with regard to the need to belong, in our view, the error has not been to deny the existence of such a motive so much as to underappreciate it.
>
> (Baumeister and Leary 1995: 522).

Introduction

We were once seemingly prepared to treat the social world of childhood as dispensable when juxtaposed against the importance of family. After many decades of research, however, compelling evidence concerning the importance of peer relations demands that we recognize that peers exert an enormous influence on children (Harris 1995). It is in the context of peer relations that children become skilled at the 'politics of the playground' – learning vital social skills such as perspective taking, negotiating, conflict resolution, and fair play (Parker et al 1995, Bierman 2004). The fact that peers play an important role in healthy cognitive, emotional, and social development should not be surprising given evidence that humans are wired to affiliate socially (Vaillancourt et al 2010a) and that the need to belong is a fundamental human motivator (Baumeister and Leary 1995). When children do not belong, healthy development is derailed. Indeed, many children who are rejected, ignored, and/or abused by their peers do not thrive. They tend to have significantly more mental health issues, poorer physical health, and lower academic achievement than their more socially accepted peers (Vaillancourt et al 2010a,b). Furthermore, longitudinal research points to the fact that these associations represent causal outcomes of poor treatment by peers (Vaillancourt et al 2010a,b).

Compounding the issues associated with poor peer treatment is the fact that children who do not belong often fall further and further behind their peers in terms of age-appropriate social skills development. Because they are not included in their peers' interactions they are not privileged to the important developmental information being conveyed. In turn, the opportunities to practise their social skills are severely limited. This type of social neglect carries the significant risk of being translated into cognitive deficits as cognition has been shown to be socially mediated (e.g. Piaget 1959, Vygotsky 1962). The tasks of initiating, maintaining, and promoting positive peer relations are difficult even for the most skilled individuals. For children with developmental difficulties, the challenge can become almost insurmountable given that: (1) some do not have the physical, sensory, and/or intellectual capacities to acquire the social skills needed to maintain positive peer affiliations (King et al 1997); and (2) those who do have the necessary prerequisite social skills are often not included in the peer group, which in turn places them at risk for future underdevelopment of social skills (Frostad and Pijl 2007).

Physical impairments
Estimates of the prevalence of physical impairments vary depending on the types of impairments assessed. In the USA, 5% of children aged 5 to 15 years are estimated to have a hearing, visual, cognitive, ambulatory, self-care, or independent living impairment (Erickson et al 2010). Approximately 2% of 6- to 21-year-old children and young people have some form of physical impairment (e.g. hearing/visual or orthopaedic; US Department of Education, 2005). Other forms of physical impairments, such as spina bifida and cerebral palsy are estimated at about 3 cases every 10 000 and 4 cases every 1000, respectively (Shin et al 2010, Yeargin-Allsopp et al 2010). In Canada, 14% of 5- to 14-year-old young people have a mobility-related impairment (Statistics Canada 2001) and, according to the National Participation and Activity Limitation Survey, 19% of children with impairments, and specifically a physical impairment, live with parents (Statistics Canada 2006a).

Physical impairments probably limit children in certain areas of development; however, they do not reduce a child's desire to be accepted and valued by peers. Indeed, achieving a sense of belonging and approval is an important aspect of feeling successful in life for young people with and without physical impairments (King et al 2000). Research on the peer relationships of children with physical impairments indicates that, compared with their typically developing peers, these children have smaller social networks of friends and schoolmates (Skär and Tamm 2002) and they often report difficulty in communicating or forming relationships (Stevens et al 1996). According to parent and child reports, being included and having friends enhance the quality of life of children with poor functioning (Davis et al 2008).

However, children with physical impairments may become disabled once they experience social isolation or exclusion owing to constraints or lack of access to facilities, which prohibit them from participating in recreational activities (e.g. sports and games in the playground). In addition, peer perceptions that children with physical impairments are 'different' (e.g. Nadeau and Tessier 2006) may contribute to negative social experiences and thus create disability.

Disabled children report that their physical impairment does restrict them from social interactions (Skär 2003), and when they feel that peers perceive them as disabled they experience lower self-esteem (Wolman and Basco 1994). In addition, disabled children with physical impairments report having more negative experiences in the school context, such as social exclusion (e.g. Lindsay and McPherson 2012), and are at higher risk for being bullied and isolated relative to physically able peers (e.g. Sweeting and West 2001, Mihaylov et al 2004, Saylor and Leach 2009, Essner and Holmbeck 2010, Sentenac et al 2011). Bourke and Burgman (2010) conducted interviews with children with physical, hearing, and visual impairments and found that most of them reported being bullied at school and considered it important to have friends that help them both with respect to their impairment as well as with bullying. Turner and colleagues (2011) found that 36% of participants with a physical impairment reported experiencing peer assault or bullying. Students with hemiplegia experience more peer victimization than their classmates and receive fewer reciprocated friendship nominations (Yude et al 1998). Disabled students in general are more prone to feeling anxious about school safety and peer harassment and they are more concerned about being physically injured than typically developing peers (Saylor and Leach 2009).

Despite these bleak facts, there is some research that shows no differences in peer victimization among physically impaired and typically developing children (Piek et al 2005, Twyman et al 2010, Turner et al 2011), leading these researchers to suggest that sociodemographic characteristics such as family background (e.g. parental mental health) are related to peer victimization and other forms of victimization among disabled children. In addition, externalizing problems and lack of social competence appear to be related to bullying and peer victimization in children with attention-deficit–hyperactivity disorder (ADHD) and specific learning impairments, but not in children with physical impairments, suggesting that children's behaviour, and not their physical impairment per se, might place them at higher risk for peer victimization (Twyman et al 2010, Turner et al 2011). There is also evidence that young people with physical impairments are able to form and maintain healthy, supportive friendships with peers either with or without impairments.

The social networks of children with physical impairments are characterized by the presence of at least one best friend, who is usually also a child with a physical impairment, and membership within a social network consisting of 2 to 10 children with whom the focal child engages in social activities such as playing chess or watching television (Blum et al 1991, Skär and Tamm 2002, Shikako-Thomas et al 2008, Asbjørnslett et al 2012). Stevens et al (1996) found that the majority of adolescents with physical impairments had as many friends as non-impaired peers and reported similar levels of loneliness. However, their friendships tended to involve either younger or older peers (Skär 2003).

It is clear from research on the peer relations of children with physical impairments that friendships have a positive influence on their development and that perceived support from classmates and friends is associated with better mental health outcomes, such as fewer symptoms of depression (Appleton et al 1997, Antle 2004). Children with physical impairments also benefit from online communication with peers. For example, Lidström et al (2010) found that Internet use predicted meeting friends outside of school, and Asbjørnslett et al (2012) reported that Internet friendships contribute to children's confidence and social activities, such as reading and discussing shared interests. Lastly, in settings in which they are able to participate and to be included in physical activities, children with physical impairments report feeling a greater sense of belonging and similarity to peers (Taub and Greer 2000). In addition, perceived social acceptance and peer intimacy increase as children with physical impairments participate in more leisure activities and attend regular classes (Wendelborg and Kvello 2010).

Visual and hearing impairments

In the USA, the percentage of children with visual and hearing impairments served under the Individuals with Disabilities Education Act is relatively low (<1% and 1%, respectively); however, the number of children with visual/hearing and comorbid conditions is thought to be much higher (US Department of Education 2002). In Canada, 13% of children under 15 years of age have a hearing impairment and 9% have a visual impairment (Statistics Canada 2001). The peer relationships of children with visual or hearing impairments are similar to those of children with other physical impairments, and the severity of the impairment (e.g. deaf/blind vs visual/hearing impaired) plays an important role in the quality and quantity of social interactions.

Children with visual or hearing impairments have poorer social skills and more difficulties with communication (e.g. Wolters et al 2011), and may be unable to recognize emotions in others (e.g. Dyck et al 2004). In addition, they are less likely to participate in physical activities, although children with hearing impairments are more active than those with visual impairments (Longmuir and Bar-Or 2000). In one study, visually impaired and blind adolescents were found to have four friends on average, and 65% of them had fewer than five friends (Kef et al 2000). Deaf children report having fewer friends in the classroom than their hearing peers and they experience more peer rejection (Nunes et al 2010), social withdrawal, and depression (Wauters and Knoors 2007, Theunissen et al 2011). Lastly, children with visual impairment may experience more peer victimization than typically developing peers (Pinquart and Pfeiffer 2011), and self-identification as hearing impairment is associated with higher frequency of self-reported peer victimization (Kent 2003).

The social networks and activities of children with visual/hearing impairments may be limited; however, there is evidence supporting the notion that they also do have positive social experiences. Recent findings indicate that children with hearing impairments or those who have cochlear implants are similar to their peers with normal hearing in terms of being confident, social, and happy, and they do not differ from their hearing peers on peer acceptance and victimization, social status, and number of mutual friendships (Wauters and Knoors 2007, Percy-Smith et al 2008, Bauman and Pero 2011). Children with visual impairments are also capable of establishing friendships, commonly with those who have similar past life experiences (Rosenblum 1998), and report equal levels of social support and companionship with hearing peers (Kef and Decović 2004). Although visual impairment has a negative impact on the range of activities in which children engage, they are still able to share common interests (e.g. music) or participate in activities not requiring high physical demands. Deaf or blind children may have limited contact with non-impaired peers; however, those attending mainstream schools have more opportunities for peer interaction. Leigh et al (2009) found that children who attend only deaf schools were less acculturated to hearing peers, whereas children with cochlear implants attending integrated schools were more acculturated and integrated with hearing peers. Finally, children with hearing impairments who receive cochlear implants show an improvement in oral communication skills (Bat-Chava and Deigman 2001) and report higher quality of life (Loy et al 2010, Edwards et al 2012). Therefore, with advances in technology and medical procedures, children with hearing disabilities may be in a position to experience significant improvements in the social domain.

Specific learning impairments

Specific learning impairments are defined as a heterogeneous grouping of disorders 'characterized by academic functioning that is substantially below that expected given the person's chronological age, measured intelligence, and age-appropriate education' (American Psychiatric Association 2000: 39). Specific learning impairments include disorders of reading, mathematics, written expression, and learning disorders not otherwise specified which range in severity and result from impairments in processes such as language processing, phonological processing, visual–spatial processing, processing speed, memory and attention, and executive functions (e.g. planning and decision making; Learning Disabilities Association of Canada 2002). Specific learning impairments are the most common form of impairments facing Canadian children, with a 3% prevalence rate for those between the ages of 5 and 14. In fact, more children have a specific learning impairment than all other impairment types combined; and of all children with impairments, 69% have a specific learning condition (Statistics Canada 2006b). In the USA, for the school year 2008–09, 5% of children and young people enrolled in state school between the ages of 3 and 21 years were identified as having specific learning impairments (US Department of Education 2011).

Many children with specific learning impairments are engaged and included in the peer group, although many still demonstrate an elevated risk of peer problems when compared with children without learning impairments (Estell et al 2008). For example, Vaughn and colleagues (1996) found that, over the course of the school year, children with specific learning impairments faced more social alienation and lower levels of peer liking than their typically developing peers and were actually liked less by the end of the school year. Importantly, this low peer regard occurred within the context of inclusive classrooms (i.e. when these students were educated in the same classroom as their non-impaired peers). In another study in which students were followed from third to sixth grade, Estell and colleagues (2008) found that, compared with typically developing children, those with specific learning impairments consistently achieved lower popularity and much lower social preference (i.e. peer liking).

In addition to not being as well liked by their peers, children with specific learning impairments are far more likely to experience peer abuse than their typically developing peers (Luciano and Savage 2007, Mepham 2010, Rose et al 2011a; see also Rose et al 2011b for a review). In particular, more children with specific learning impairments report being bullied by their peers than do children without learning impairments, and when they do experience abuse students with specific learning impairments report more frequent victimization (Luciano and Savage 2007, Rose et al 2011b). Teachers confirm that students with impairments are bullied more than their typically developing or gifted classmates (Estell et al 2008). Compared with their typically developing peers, students with specific learning impairments suffer a higher rate of verbal, social, and physical aggression (Rose et al 2011b). Although prevalence rates of victimization are inconsistent across studies owing to a variety of factors (e.g. demographics, educational contexts, and types of impairment), there is consistent evidence that students with specific learning impairments face an increased risk (Rose et al 2011b). In one study their elevated risk was three times greater than the rates of peer victimization experienced by typically developing peers (36% vs 12%; Conti-Ramsden and Botting 2004).

Not only are children with specific learning impairments at risk of being bullied but they also place their peers at risk for poor treatment. These children demonstrate significantly elevated rates of inflicting harm on other children through bullying, both verbal and physical aggression, and fighting (Rose et al 2011a,b). In their recent review of the literature on bullying and victimization among students with impairments, Rose and colleagues (2011b) highlighted that, across several studies, children with learning and emotional–behavioural conditions perpetrated bullying at twice the rate of their non-impaired peers, a phenomenon that has been confirmed using peer and teacher reports (Estell et al 2008). Rose and colleagues (2011b) suggested that this greater incidence of aggression towards peers may be secondary to the chronic victimization experienced by some children with specific learning impairments; an alternate possibility is that these young people misinterpret, and/or over-react to, certain social situations consequent of having a specific learning impairment.

The friendships and friendship quality of children with specific learning impairments are also problematic. According to parents, teachers, and peers, these children have fewer reciprocal friendships than their typically developing peers, despite their own reports of similar numbers of friendships (Estell et al 2008; see also Wiener 2004 for a review). A paucity of friendships may partially account for the elevated risk of peer victimization among this group as reciprocal friendships can be protective (Rose et al 2011b). The friendships that do exist for children with specific learning disorders are also relatively less stable and of poorer quality, characterized by less contact, intimacy, and validation and more conflict and difficulty in resolving conflicts (Wiener and Schneider 2002, Wiener 2004, Rose et al 2011b). Compared with children without learning impairments, their friendships are more likely to involve children two or more years younger than themselves, children with teacher-reported learning impairments themselves, and/or children who do not attend the same school (Wiener and Schneider 2002).

Deficits in social cognitive abilities, communication/language skills, social skills, and emotion regulation may account for the peer difficulties that children with specific learning impairments tend to face (see Kavale and Forness 1996 and Wiener 2004 for a review; McLaughlin et al 2010). For example, such children struggle with social problem-solving tasks such as identifying or coming up with solutions to social problems in stories (Wiener 2004). They also tend to have compromised non-verbal communication, including difficulties interpreting facial expressions, fewer non-verbal initiations of play, and fewer responses to the initiations of others (Weiner 2004, Agaliotis and Kalyva 2008). Pragmatic and expressive language difficulties have been linked to peer problems for children with specific learning impairments, and controlling for differences in receptive vocabulary has been shown to eliminate the differences in peer victimization between children with and without learning impairments (Conti-Ramsden and Botting 2004, Luciano and Savage 2007). Social skills can also be a problem, with such children being less cooperative and assertive and more competitive and possessive over objects than non-impaired peers (see Wiener 2004 for a review). In fact, in a meta-analysis on social skill deficits in children with specific learning impairments, Kavale and Forness (1996) found that across teacher-, parent-, and self-reports as many as 75% of children with a specific learning impairment had significant social skill deficits compared with their typically developing peers. Deficits in emotion regulation and sustained attention, both associated with social problems, may also be due to the higher incidence of ADHD in these children (Wiener 2004, Andrade et al 2009).

The peer difficulties faced by children with specific learning impairments, such as poorer quality friendships, peer rejection, victimization, and bullying, have been demonstrated to have devastating consequences for children's mental health, school performance, self-esteem, and perceptions of loneliness (Bear et al 1993, Margalit and Al-Yagon 2002, Pijl and Frostad 2010, Rose et al 2011b). In particular, peer difficulties are associated with anxiety, depression, less classroom participation, school avoidance, and poor academic achievement (Buhs and Ladd 2001, Rose et al 2011b). Students with specific learning impairments who are not accepted by the peer group often have negative self-perceptions (Bear et al 1993, Pijl and Frostad 2010). Higher rates of loneliness are consistently found among these children than in their peers and are no doubt a consequence of their peer relations challenges (see Margalit and Al-Yagon 2002 for a review).

Notwithstanding challenges within the peer group, there are circumstances that *foster* the social development of children with specific learning impairments and personal characteristics that then *improve* their level of peer acceptance. For example, inclusion in regular classrooms rather than segregation into special education classrooms has been associated with more positive outcomes for some aspects of peer relationships, such as having more reciprocal friendships and being more socially accepted (Vaughn et al 1996, Wiener and Tardif 2004). In a study of the peer relationships of children with specific learning impairments in an inclusive setting, Estell and colleagues (2008) found that across middle childhood these children were similar to their typically developing peers in terms of their likelihood of participating in a friendship group, their level of centrality in that group (usually secondary or nuclear vs peripheral), and having friendship groups of comparable size and centrality in the classroom social network. The authors suggested that proximity to typically developing peers may provide positive social experiences and prevent children with specific learning impairments from developing a larger gap in social skills over time. Furthermore, those children who are viewed by peers as smart, athletic, or physically attractive tend to be popular (Siperstein et al 1978).

Other personal characteristics such as being more cooperative and less disruptive, aggressive, or dependent have been associated with more peer acceptance among these children (Wiener et al 1990). When children with specific learning impairments have a few close friendships they experience better outcomes, including better self-perceptions of their own social acceptance (Bear et al 1993). For educators and parents of children with specific learning impairments, nurturing the development of friendships with compatible peers for these children may help buffer against the effects of peer rejection and may be more realistic, and perhaps more effective, than other interventions such as social skills training (Wiener and Schneider 2002). Also, Margalit and Al-Yagon (2002) found that positive coping skills, such as actively seeking friends or engaging in solitary activities (e.g. exercising, reading, listening to music) helped such children avoid feelings of loneliness or manage them more effectively when they arose.

Intellectual impairments
The current definition of intellectual impairment or disability (also known as learning disability in the UK, see Chapter 2 for the discussion on impairment and disability) typically includes three elements: (1) limitations in intellectual functioning; (2) limitations in adaptive behaviour; and (3) onset prior to 18 years of age (Schalock et al 2007, Parmenter 2011, American Association on Intellectual and Developmental Disabilities 2012). Intellectual impairment can be categorized as mild, moderate, severe, or profound (Katz and Lazcano-Ponce 2007). As a result of the shift in conceptualizing impairment from a person-centred characteristic to a multidimensional human phenomenon stemming from biological and social factors, the terms intellectual impairment or disability have increasingly become accepted in place of the term mental retardation (Schalock et al 2007, Parmenter 2011). Individuals who meet diagnostic criteria for mental retardation also meet criteria for intellectual impairment (Schalock et al 2007). The prevalence of intellectual impairments varies depending on the definition and cut-off criteria used. One Canadian study of children and adolescents aged 14 to 20 found an overall prevalence rate of <1% for intellectual impairment (Bradley et al 2002; see also Winzer 2008). Boyle et al (2008) also found a rate of <1% for intellectual impairment in children aged 3 to 17 years in the USA from 1997 to 2008 (see also American Psychiatric Association 2000).

Children with intellectual impairment are at greater risk for mental health problems than their typically developing peers. Approximately 40% of these children also meet diagnostic criteria for at least one psychiatric disorder (Einfeld and Tonge 1996, Dekker and Koot 2003, Emerson 2003). Disruptive behaviour disorders are more prevalent in children with mild to moderate intellectual impairment (Einfeld and Tonge 1996, Dekker and Koot 2003). These children also show elevated scores on social problems and attention problems compared with their typically developing peers (Dekker et al 2002).

Children with intellectual impairments are at particular risk for peer interaction difficulties given the nature of their impairment. Many children with intellectual impairments have communication skills deficits and difficulty with social information processing that makes the tasks of being understood and understanding others that much more difficult. For example, Leffert and Siperstein (1996) found that although children with a mild intellectual impairment performed at the same level as typically developing peers on interpreting hostile intention in peer conflict situations, they nevertheless had greater difficulty interpreting more benign intention cues. Difficulty in processing social information and deficits in communication skills also have an impact on the rate at which these children have the opportunity to interact with peers. Initiating appropriate interactions with peers occurs much less frequently in adolescents with intellectual impairments (5% of observations) compared with typically developing students in general education (18% of observations; Hughes et al 1999). When these young people do interact with others, they have more frequent interactions with other young people with intellectual impairments than with typically developing peers (Cutts and Sigafoos 2001).

Despite infrequent interaction with peers, children with intellectual impairments in early primary school have been found to have average confidence in their abilities to interact with peers (Zic and Igric 2001). In fact, their confidence level has been shown to be similar to that of typically developing children. However, despite this confidence, children with intellectual impairments experience less peer acceptance and more peer rejection than their classmates (Zic and Igric 2001). Children with intellectual impairments also get bullied and teased more often by children at school than their typically developing peers (Guralnick et al 1996, Mishna 2003). As in peers without intellectual impairments, being a victim of bullying relates to emotional and interpersonal problems (Reiter and Lapidot-Lefler 2007). An important qualifier, however, is that although it appears that children with intellectual impairments are inaccurate in their appraisal of their peer relations at school (tending to think that they are better than observations would suggest), their reported satisfaction may relate to successful neighbourhood relationships (Zic and Igric 2001). These neighbourhood relationships tend to occur with younger peers who may be at a similar developmental level, thus allowing for more successful interpersonal exchanges. Children with intellectual impairments also interact more frequently with each other, which may further enhance feelings of competence (Cutts and Sigafoos 2001).

A child's level of social skill appears to be particularly important in terms of adaptation to the environment. For example, McIntyre and colleagues (2006) found that, after controlling for developmental and adaptive functioning in children with and without intellectual impairments, social skills predicted positive school adaptation. This finding suggests that it may be the lower social skills and greater behavioural problems that have an impact on positive adaptation to peers rather than the intellectual impairments per se. In another study, Siperstein and Leffert (1997) found that some children with intellectual impairments (16%) were indeed accepted by their peers. Similar to typically developing peers, socially accepted children with intellectual impairments were seen as more sociable, friendly, and helpful. In contrast, socially rejected children had more difficulty making friends and more often appeared sad or upset. Observational studies have shown that, although children with intellectual impairments interacted less frequently with peers, when they did interact the exchanges were mostly positive (Hughes et al 1999, Cutts and Sigafoos 2001). Taken together, research suggests that positive social interaction may still be occurring, although at lower rates than in typically developing peers. Some individuals with intellectual impairments do develop sufficient social skills to be accepted by the peer group. These social skills appear to be important in adapting to the school environment.

Autism spectrum disorders
ASDs are neurodevelopmental conditions of undetermined aetiology that affect roughly 1 in 88 American children (Centers for Disease Control and Prevention 2012) and 1 in 147 Canadian children (Fombonne 2003, Lazoff et al 2010). The defining impairments of ASD include impairments in socialization and communication, inflexibility, and stereotyped

behaviour, which manifest in varying degrees across individuals (American Psychiatric Association 2000).

Weiss and Harris' (2001) review article highlights certain key features identified among children diagnosed with ASD that contribute to their deficit in social skills. These include lack of orientation towards a social stimulus and inadequate use of eye contact, difficulties in initiating social interactions and using appropriate greetings, difficulty interpreting verbal and non-verbal cues, and inappropriate affect, as well as lack of empathy to the distress of others. Social reciprocity, including skills and strategies that promote meaningful friendships, is a central feature of peer relations and friendships (Denham et al 2001). Unfortunately, many children diagnosed with ASD have been found to have difficulties sharing affective experiences or understanding the perspective of others (Gutstein and Whitney 2002), and these difficulties persist over time (Sigman and Ruskin 1999). Not surprisingly, findings from a study examining quality of friendship among children diagnosed with ASD indicate that these individuals report poorer quality in their best friendships than their typically develop-ing peers (Whitehouse et al 2009). Although these children are able to identify friendship, they have difficulties in identifying affective characteristics when presented with pictures depicting social scenes (Bauminger et al 2004). Children diagnosed with ASD (vs typically developing peers) also reported lower, yet not absent, self-determined motivation to develop friendships. Although they are motivated to have friends, children with ASD report that it is difficult for them to make friends and these friendships are harder to maintain without help from parents and teachers (Bauminger and Shulman 2003, Knott et al 2006). Children with ASD also report feeling lonelier than typically developing peers (Bauminger and Kasari 2000, White and Robertson-Nay 2009, Lasgaard et al 2010), providing evidence that children with ASD do have a need for positive peer affiliation (Causton-Theoharis et al 2009). Moreover, when they do report having friends, children with ASD also report higher general self-worth and lower loneliness (Bauminger et al 2004).

Research examining the social networks of children with ASD who were enrolled in regu-lar classrooms suggests that they are not well integrated within the peer group. For example, Chamberlain and colleagues (2007) found that children with ASD were lower on peer group centrality, peer group acceptance, companionship, and friendship reciprocity. These charac-teristics are consistent with typically developing children who are considered 'neglected' by the peer group. Neglected children are ignored by peers, tend to be less social and aggressive, and tend to have few friends (Newcomb et al 1993), and because they have fewer friends they also report being more lonely than their more accepted peers (Asher et al 1984). The 'silver lining' of this type of social experience is that neglected children get bullied less than their peers who are rejected (Knack et al 2012). In fact, neglected students are bullied at rates similar to their accepted peers. Unfortunately, the same cannot be said for children with ASD. Little (2001) found that as many as 75% of children with ASD reported being victimized by their peers. Moreover, high-functioning children with ASD have good insight about bullying; in fact, their ability to correctly identify bullying situations was the same as their typically developing peers (van Roekel et al 2010). However, children with ASD who experienced increased rates of peer victimization were more likely to misinterpret non-bullying situations as bullying than children without ASD.

Despite the identified difficulties faced by children diagnosed with ASD in regard to developing friendships, being accepted by peers, and being integrated in the peer group, there are studies suggesting that some children with ASD do learn the necessary social skills that facilitate the development and maintenance of friendships. An empirical review of a cognitive behavioural intervention for children diagnosed with ASD aimed at developing social–emotional understanding and social interactions demonstrated growth in overall positive social interactions among children with ASD, highlighting the fact that emotion can be taught and that social understanding can be improved through specialized training (Bauminger 2002). In a more recent study by Bauminger and colleagues (2008) several similarities between friendships among children with ASD and typically developing peers were found, such as durability of friendships and the sharing of leadership roles within the relationship, as well as sharing experiences, emotions, and attention. These findings suggest that meaningful friendships are possible for children with ASD. In fact, there is evidence that mixed friendships between children diagnosed with ASD and typically developing peers are more durable and stable, with higher levels of positive social orientation and cohesion, and more complex levels of coordinated play than in non-mixed dyad friendships (Bauminger et al 2008). One caveat to note, however, is that studies reporting positive peer experiences for children with ASD tend to apply to individuals at the higher end of functioning.

Implications for clinical and education practice
It is clear from the research literature that belonging is a fundamental human motivator that extends to children with impairments. Unfortunately, until recently, the social relationships of children with neurological and developmental conditions have been all but ignored and the focus has been on the physical and mental health aspects of the impairment and what they mean for educational attainment. This paucity of attention to the social world of children with impairments is curious given the strong body of literature pointing to the negative sequelae that result from not belonging. Given the fundamental need to belong, it behoves healthcare providers and educators to prioritize the peer relationships of children and young people with and without impairments. How can this prioritization be achieved? Regrettably, there are currently no established guidelines on how this should be accomplished. Nevertheless, we offer the following suggestions for consideration, extending from the extensive review of the literature provided here.

CLINICAL
1   Children who are under the care of healthcare practitioners must be defined by more than the circumstances of their impairment. Children with impairments want to have friends and they want to be included, and those who do not have their need to belong met fare poorly. The current state of knowledge is that comorbid physical and mental health conditions are part, or an extension, of the impairment. It is important to consider that comorbidity may be due to poor peer integration. Accordingly, healthcare practitioners need to screen for peer difficulties and work in partnership with the school and family to help promote positive social relationships (see Lamb et al 2009).

2   When the parents of children with impairments seek health services, the children may present with a number of health-related difficulties. It would be helpful for healthcare providers to validate the notion that concerns about social development, specifically those tied to challenging peer relationships, are legitimate, significant, and worthy of as much careful attention and necessary intervention as the biomedical impairments.

3   Like other children, children with impairments benefit from and need positive social relationships with peers of the same age within the context of the school environment. If success within this realm is not possible, however, emphasis should be placed on building and maintaining positive peer relationships outside of school with peers of different ages. The key is to find the context in which children will have the chance to fulfil their fundamental need to belong.

EDUCATIONAL

1   Children with impairments, even more than typically developing children, depend on adults to help facilitate inclusion within the peer group (Diamond et al 2011). For example, a child with a mobility impairment needs to be in a classroom in which consideration has been paid to how the physical environment can help promote easy movement and hence access to peers. Educators need to consider carefully the child's physical environment as a way of promoting peer group integration.

2   Programmes promoting social interaction among individuals with intellectual impairments and their peers in general education are encouraged (Carter et al 2005). This suggestion is based on research demonstrating the importance of social interaction on cognitive, emotional, and social development (see above review) and research indicating that when individuals with intellectual impairments were paired with a typically developing peer: (1) the frequency of social interactions significantly increased; (2) social interactions were of higher quality; and (3) individuals with intellectual impairments experienced more positive affect (e.g. Carter et al 2005).

3   An examination of children's attitudes towards intellectual impairment (i.e. Down syndrome) after being educated on the impairment and disability showed increased positive attitudes and greater friendship intentions than those who were not given the educational material (Laws and Kelly 2005). Furthermore, the most negative attitudes were found to be for children with aggressive and disruptive behaviours, followed by those with intellectual impairments and those with physical impairments (Laws and Kelly 2005, Nowicki 2006). Because children with impairments are stigmatized at a far greater rate than typically developing children, teachers need to reduce stigma by promoting inclusion and by debunking myths concerning differences.

4   Peer attitudes and perceptions of impairment and disability are important factors to consider in children's interactions with impaired students. Not all impairments share the same peer risk factors. Experimental research suggests that students hold positive intentions and attitudes towards children with physical impairments (as one example) and would be willing to include children in a wheelchair in their play activities (Morgan et al 1998, Tamm and Prellwitz 1999). In contrast, children with neurological and developmental conditions who display atypical behaviours, such as low social competence or

externalizing problems, are more likely to experience peer victimization (Twyman et al 2010, Turner et al 2011). Therefore, children with physical impairments or less severe intellectual and learning impairments may have more positive socialization and integration experiences than children with more severe impairments or disruptive behaviour.

5   Children need to learn the social script that is appropriate to their age group. If they are paired with an educational assistant who becomes their primary social support person in the school, they are less likely to be integrated within the peer group and thus less likely to learn the social norms. Educational assistants who are working with children with neurological and developmental conditions need to be mindful of how their presence has an impact on the child's peer relations and respond in a way that maximizes the child's success with peers. For example, having a child spend all of his or her time with the educational assistant does little to promote friendships.

Conclusion

The fact that some research fails to find differences between children with and without neurological and developmental conditions within elements of the social world is a reason for hope. It is certainly clear that not all children with impairments will experience the same degree of deprivation of positive socialization experiences or end up with the same negative outcomes. For example, we know that, as in other circumstances, the presence of a solid friendship can buffer a child against the challenges of the social world (e.g. Bourke and Burgman 2010). Accordingly, it would be particularly useful for future research to identify additional 'protective' factors and strategies that may be particularly relevant for children with neurological and developmental conditions (or perhaps subgroups of children with different types of impairments). This information could inform the development and implementation of individualized interventions.

REFERENCES

Key references

Agaliotis I, Kalyva E (2008) Nonverbal social interaction skills of children with learning disabilities. *Res Dev Disabil* 29: 1–10. http://dx.doi.org/10.1016/j.ridd.2006.09.002

American Association on Intellectual and Developmental Disabilities (2012) Definition of an intellectual disability. Available at: www.aaidd.org/content_100.cfm?navID=21 (accessed 23 March 2012).

American Psychiatric Association (2000) *Diagnostic and Statistical Manual of Mental Disorders, Text Revision* (DSM-IV-TR). Washington, DC: American Psychiatric Association.

Andrade BF, Brodeur DA, Waschbusch DA, Stewart SH, McGee R (2009) Selective and sustained attention as predictors of social problems in children with typical and disordered attention abilities. *J Attention Disord* 12: 341–352. doi:10.1177/1087054708320440.

Antle BJ (2004) Factors associated with self-worth in young people with physical disabilities. *Health Social Work* 29: 167–175. http://dx.doi.org/10.1093/hsw/29.3.167

Appleton PL, Ellis NC, Minchom PE, Lawson V, Boll V, Jones P (1997) Depressive symptoms and self-concept in young people with spina bifida. *J Pediatr Psychol* 22: 702–722. http://dx.doi.org/10.1093/jpepsy/22.5.707

Asbjørnslett M, Engelsrud GH, Helseth S (2012) 'Friendship in all directions': Norwegian children with physical disabilities experiencing friendship. *Childhood* 19: 481–494. http://dx.doi.org/10.1177/0907568211428093

*Asher SR, Hymel S, Renshaw PD (1984) Loneliness in children. *Child Dev* 55: 1456–1464. http://dx.doi.org/0009–3920/84/5504–0005$01.00

Bat-Chava Y, Deigman E (2001) Peer relationships of children with cochlear implants. *J Deaf Stud Deaf Educ* 6: 186–199. http://dx.doi.org/10.1093/deafed/6.3.186

Bauman S, Pero H (2011) Bullying and cyberbullying among deaf students and their hearing peers: an exploratory study. *J Deaf Stud Deaf Educ* 16: 236–253. http://dx.doi.org/10.1093/deafed/enq043

*Baumeister RL, Leary MR (1995) The need to belong: desire for interpersonal attachments as a fundamental human motivation. *Psychol Bull* 117: 497–529. http://dx.doi.org/10.1037/0033–2909.117.3.497

Bauminger N (2002) The facilitation of social–emotional understanding and social interaction in high-functioning children with autism: intervention outcomes. *J Autism Dev Disord* 32: 283–298. http://dx.doi.org/0162–3257/02/0800–0283/0

Bauminger N, Kasari C (2000) Loneliness and friendship in high-functioning children with autism. *Child Dev* 71: 447–456. http://dx.doi.org/0009–3920/2000/7102–0014

*Bauminger N, Shulman C (2003) The development and maintenance of friendship in high-functioning children with autism. *Autism* 7: 81–97. http://dx.doi.org/10.1177/1362361303007001007

Bauminger N, Shulman C, Agam G (2004) The link between perceptions of self and of social relationships in high-functioning children with autism. *J Dev Physical Disabil* 16: 193–214. http://dx.doi.org/1056–263X/04/0600–0193/0

Bauminger N, Solomon M, Aviezer A, et al (2008) Children with autism and their friends: a multidimensional study of friendship in high-functioning autism spectrum disorder. *J Abnorm Child Psychol* 36: 135–150. http://dx.doi.org/10.1007/s10802-007-9156-x

Bear GG, Juvonen J, McInerney F (1993) Self-perceptions and peer relations of boys with and boys without learning disabilities in an integrated setting: a longitudinal study. *Learning Disability Quarterly* 16: 127–136. http://dx.doi.org/10.2307/1511135

*Bierman KL (2004) *Peer Rejection: Developmental Processes and Intervention Strategies*. New York: Guilford Press.

Blum R, Resnick MD, Nelson R, St Germaine A (1991) Family and peer issues among adolescents with spina bifida and cerebral palsy. *Pediatrics* 88: 280–285.

Bourke S, Burgman I (2010) Coping with bullying in Australian schools: how children with disabilities experience more support from friends, parents and teachers. *Disabil Soc* 25: 359–371. http://dx.doi.org/10.1080/09687591003701264

Boyle CA, Boulet S, Schieve LA, et al (2008) Trends in the prevalence of the developmental disabilities in US children, 1997–2008. *Pediatrics* 127: 1034–1042. http://dx.doi.org/10.1542/peds.2010–2989.

Bradley EA, Thompson A, Bryson SE (2002) Mental retardation in teenagers: prevalence data from the Niagara region, Ontario. *Can J Psychiatry* 47: 652–659.

Buhs E, Ladd G (2001) Peer rejection as antecedent of young children's school adjustment: an examination of mediating processes. *Dev Psychol* 37: 550–560. http://dx.doi.org/10.1037/0012–1649.37.4.550

Carter EW, Hughes C, Guth CB, Copeland SR (2005) Factors influencing social interaction among high school students with intellectual disabilities and their general education peers. *Am J Ment Retard* 110: 366–377. http://dx.doi.org/10.1352/0895–8017%282005%2911%5B366:FISIAH%5D2.0.CO;2

Causton-Theoharis J, Ashby C, Cosier M (2009) Islands of loneliness: exploring social interaction through the autobiographies of individuals with autism. *Intellectual Dev Disabil* 47: 84–96. http://dx.doi.org/10.1352/1934-9556-47.2.84

Centers for Disease Control and Prevention (2012) Prevalence of autism spectrum disorders – autism and developmental disabilities monitoring network, 14 sites, United States, 2008. Surveillance Summaries, 61(SS03), 1–19. Available at: www.cdc.gov/mmwr/preview/mmwrhtml/ss6103a1.htm?s_cid=ss6103a1_w (accessed 30 May 2012).

Chamberlain B, Kasari C, Rotheram-Fuller E (2007) Involvement or isolation? The social networks of children with autism in regular classrooms. *J Autism Dev Disord* 37: 230–242. http://dx.doi.org/10.1007/s10803-006-0164-4

Conti-Ramsden G, Botting N (2004) Social difficulties and victimization in children with SLI at 11 years of age. *J Speech Lang Hearing Res* 47: 145–161. http://dx.doi.org/10.1044/1092–4388(2004/013)

Cutts S, Sigafoos J (2001) Social competence and peer interactions of students with intellectual disability in an inclusive high school. *J Intellect Dev Disabil* 26: 127–141. http://dx.doi.org/10.1080/13668250020054444-0

Davis E, Shelly A, Waters E, et al (2008) Quality of life of adolescents with cerebral palsy: perspectives of adolescents and parents. *Dev Med Child Neurol* 51: 193–199. http://dx.doi.org/10.1111/j.1469-8749.2008.03194.x

Dekker MC, Koot HK (2003) DSM-IV disorders in children with borderline to moderate intellectual disability. I: Prevalence and impact. *J Am Acad Child Adolesc Psychiatry* 42: 915–922. http://dx.doi.org/10.1097/01. CHI.0000046892.27264.1A

Dekker MC, Koot HM, van der Ende J, Verhulst FC (2002) Emotional and behavioural problems in children with and without intellectual disability. *J Child Psychol Psychiatr* 43: 1087–1098. http://dx.doi. org/10.1111/1469-7610.00235

Denham S, Mason T, Caverly S, et al (2001) Preschoolers at play: co-socialisers of emotional and social competence. *Int J Behav Dev* 4: 290–301. http://dx.doi.org/10.1080/016502501143000067

*Diamond KE, Huang H-H, Steed EA (2011) The developmental of social competence in children with disabilities. In: Smith PK, Hart CH, editors. *The Wiley-Blackwell Handbook of Childhood Social Development*, 2nd edition. Oxford: Wiley-Blackwell, pp. 627–645. http://dx.doi.org/10.1002/9781444390933.ch33

Dyck MJ, Farrugia C, Shochet IM, Holmes-Brown M (2004) Emotion recognition/understanding ability in hearing or vision impaired children: do sounds or words make a difference? *J Child Psychol Psychiatry* 45: 789–800. http://dx.doi.org/10.1111/j.1469–7610.2004.00272.x

Edwards L, Hill T, Mahon M (2012) Quality of life in children and adolescents with cochlear implants and additional needs. *Int J Pediatr Otorhinolaryngol* 76: 851–857. http://dx.doi.org/10.1016/j.ijporl.2012.02.057

Einfeld SL, Tonge BJ (1996) Population prevalence of psychopathology in children and adolescents with intellectual disability: II epidemiological findings. *J Intellect Disabil Res* 40: 99–109. http://dx.doi. org/10.1046/j.1365-2788.1996.767767.x

Emerson E (2003) Prevalence of psychiatric disorders in children and adolescents with and without intellectual disability. *J Intellect Disabil Res* 47: 51–58. http://dx.doi.org/10.1046/j.1365–2788.2003.00464.x

Erickson W, Lee C, von Schrader S (2010) Disability Statistics from the 2008 American Community Survey (ACS). Ithaca, NY: Cornell University Rehabilitation Research and Training Center on Disability Demographics and Statistics (StatsRRTC). Available at: www.disabilitystatistics.org (accessed January 2012).

Essner BS, Holmbeck GN (2010) The impact of family, peer, and school contexts on depressive symptoms in adolescents with spina bifida. *Rehabil Psychol* 55: 340–350. http://dx.doi.org/10.1037/a0021664

*Estell DB, Farmer TW, Irvin MJ, Crowther A, Akos P, Boudah DJ (2008) Students with exceptionalities and the peer group context of bullying and victimization in late elementary school. *J Child Fam Studies* 18: 136–150. http://dx.doi.org/10.1007/s10826-008-9214-1

Fombonne E (2003) Epidemiological surveys of autism and other pervasive developmental disorders: an update. *J Autism Dev Disord* 33: 365–382. http://dx.doi.org/0162–3257/03/0800–0365/0

*Frostad P, Pijl SP (2007) Does being friendly help in making friends? The relation between the social position and social skills of pupils with special needs in mainstream education. *Eur J Spec Needs Educ* 22: 15–30. http://dx.doi.org/10.1080/08856250601082224

Guralnick MJ, Connor RT, Hammond MA, Gottman JM, Kinnish K (1996) The peer relations of preschool children with communication disorders. *Child Dev* 67: 471–489. http://dx.doi.org/10.1111/1467–8624. ep9605280322

Gutstein SE, Whitney T (2002) Asperger syndrome and the development of social competence. *Focus on Autism and Other Developmental Disabilities* 17: 161–171. http://dx.doi.org/10.1177/10883576020170030601

*Harris JR (1995) Where is the child's environment? A group socialization theory of development. *Psychol Rev* 102: 458–489. http://dx.doi.org/10.1037/0033–295X.102.3.458

Hughes C, Rodi MS, Lorden SW, et al (1999) Social interaction of high school students with mental retardation and their general education peers. *Am J Ment Retard* 104: 533–544. http://dx.doi. org/10.1352/0895-8017(1999)104<0533:SIOHSS>2.0.CO;2

Katz G, Lazcano-Ponce E (2007) Intellectual disability: definition, etiological factors, classification, diagnosis, treatment and prognosis. *Salud Publica Mex* 50(Suppl. 2): S132–S141.

Kavale KA, Forness SR (1996) Social skill deficits and learning disabilities: a meta-analysis. *J Learn Disabil* 29: 226–227. http://dx.doi.org/10.1177/002221949602900301

Kef S, Decović M (2004) The role of parental and peer support in adolescents well-being: a comparison of adolescents with and without a visual impairment. *J Adolescence* 27: 453–466. http://dx.doi.org/10.1016/j.adolescence.2003.12.005

Kef S, Hox JJ, Habekothé HT (2000) Social networks of visually impaired and blind adolescents. Structure and effect on well-being. *Social Networks* 2: 73–91. http://dx.doi.org/10.1016/S0378–8733(00)00022–8

Kent BA (2003) Identity issues for hard-of-hearing adolescents aged 11, 13, and 15 in mainstream setting. *J Deaf Stud Deaf Educ* 8: 315–324. http://dx.doi.org/10.1093/deafed/eng017

King GA, Specht JA, Schultz I, Warr-Leeper G, Redekop W, Risebrough N (1997) Social skills training for withdrawn, unpopular children with physical disabilities: a preliminary evaluartion. *Rehabil Psychol* 42: 47–60. http://dx.doi.org/10.1037/0090–5550.42.1.47

King GA, Cathers T, Polgar MJ, MacKinnon E, Havens L (2000) Success in life for older adolescents with cerebral palsy. *Qualitative Health Research* 10: 734–749. http://dx.doi.org/10.1177/104973200129118796

Knack JM, Tsar V, Vaillancourt T, Hymel S, McDougall P (2012) What protects rejected adolescents from also being bullied by their peers? The moderating role of peer-valued characteristics. *J Research Adolesc* 22: 467–479. http://dx.doi.org/10.111/j.1532–7795.2012.00792.x

Knott F, Dunlop AW, Mackay T (2006) Living with ASD: how do children and their parents assess their difficulties with social interaction and understanding? *Autistic Soc* 10: 609–617. http://dx.doi.org/10.1177/1362361306068510

Lamb J, Pepler DJ, Craig W (2009) Approach to bullying and victimization. *Can Fam Physician* 55: 356–360.

Lasgaard M, Nielson A, Eriksen ME, Goossens L (2010) Loneliness and social support in adolescent boys with autism spectrum disorders. *J Autism Dev Disord* 40: 218–226. http://dx.doi.org/10.1007/s10803–009–0851-z

Laws G, Kelly E (2005) The attitudes and friendship intentions of children in United Kingdom mainstream schools towards peers with physical or intellectual disabilities. *Int J Disabil Dev Educ* 52: 79–99. http://dx.doi.org/10.1080/10349120500086298

Lazoff T, Zhong L, Piperni T, Fombonne E (2010) Prevalence of pervasive developmental disorders among children at the English Montreal School Board. *Can J Psychiatry* 55: 715–720.

Learning Disabilities Association of Canada (2002) Official definition of learning disabilities. Available at: www.ldac-acta.ca/en/learn-more/ld-defined.html (accessed 28 November 2012).

Leffert JS, Siperstein GN (1996) Assessment of social–cognitive processes in children with mental retardation. *Am J Ment Retard* 100: 441–455.

Leigh IW, Bat-Chava Y, Maxwell-McCaw D, Christiansen JB (2009) Correlates of psychosocial adjustment in deaf adolescents with and without cochlear implants: a preliminary investigation. *J Deaf Stud Deaf Educ* 14: 244–259. http://dx.doi.org/10.1093/deafed/enn038

Lidström H, Ahlsten G, Hemmingsson H (2010) The influence of ICT on the activity patterns of children with physical disabilities outside of school. *Child Care Health Dev* 37: 313–321. http://dx.doi.org/10.1111/j.1365–2214.2010.01168.x

Lindsay S, McPherson AC (2012) Experiences of social exclusion and bullying at school among children and youth with cerebral palsy. *Disabil Rehabil* 34: 101–109. http://dx.doi.org/10.3109/09638288.2011.587086

Little L (2001) Peer victimization of children with Asperger spectrum disorders. *J Am Acad Child Adolesc Psychiatry* 40: 995–996. http://dx.doi.org/10.1097/00004583–200109000–00007

Longmuir PE, Bar-Or O (2000) Factors influencing the physical activity levels of youth with physical and sensory disabilities. *Adapted Physical Activity Q* 17: 40–53.

Loy B, Warner-Czyz AD, Tong L, Tobbey EA, Roland PS (2010) The children speak: an examination of the quality of life of pediatric cochlear implant users. *Otolaryngol Head Neck Surg* 142: 247–253. http://dx.doi.org/10.1016/j.otohns.2009.10.045

Luciano S, Savage RS (2007) Bullying risk in children with inclusive educational settings. *Can J School Psychol* 22: 14–31. http://dx.doi.org/10.1177/0829573507301039

McIntyre LL, Blacher J, Baker BL (2006) The transition to school: adaptation in young children with and without intellectual disability. *J Intellect Disabil Res* 50: 349–361. http://dx.doi.org/10.1111/j.1365–2788.2006.00783.x

McLaughlin C, Byers R, Vaughn RP (2010) Responding to bullying among children with special educational needs and/or disabilities. London: Anti-Bullying Alliance. Available at: www.anti-bullyingalliance.org.uk/research/sen-and-disabilities.aspx (accessed 28 November 2012).

Margalit M, Al-Yagon M (2002) The loneliness experiences of children with learning disabilities. In: Wong BYL, Donahue M, editors. *The Social Dimensions of Learning Disabilities.* Mahwah, NJ: Lawrence Erlbaum Associates, pp. 53–75.

Mepham S (2010) Disabled children: the right to feel safe. *Child Care Pract* 16: 19–34. http://dx.doi.org/10.1080/13575270903368667

Mihaylov SI, Jarvis SJ, Colver AF, Beresford B (2004) Identification and description of environmental factors that influence participation of children with cerebral palsy. *Dev Med Child Neurol* 46: 299–304. http://dx.doi.org/10.1017/S0012162204000490

Mishna F (2003) Learning disabilities and bullying: double jeopardy. *J Learn Disabil* 36: 336–347. http://dx.doi.org/10.1177/00222194030360040501

Morgan SB, Bieberich AA, Walker M, Schwerdtfeger H (1998) Children's willingness to share activities with a physically handicapped peer: am I more willing than my classmates? *J Pediatr Psychol* 23: 367–375. http://dx.doi.org/10.1037/0090–5550.44.2.131

Nadeau L, Tessier R (2006) Social adjustment of children with cerebral palsy in mainstream classes: peer perception. *Dev Med Child Neurol* 48: 331–336. http://dx.doi.org/10.1017/S0012162206000739

Newcomb AF, Bukowski WM, Pattee L (1993) Children's peer relations: a meta-analytic review of popular, rejected, neglected, controversial, and average sociometric status. *Psychol Bull* 113: 99–128. http://dx.doi.org/10.1037/0033–2909.113.1.99

Nowicki EA (2006) A cross-sectional multivariate analysis of children's attitudes towards disabilities. *J Intellect Disabil Res* 50: 335–348. http://dx.doi.org/10.1111/j.1365–2788.2005.00781.x

Nunes T, Pretzlik U, Olsson J (2010) Deaf children's social relationships in mainstream schools. *J Deaf Education Int* 3: 123–136. http://dx.doi.org/10.1179/146431501790560972

*Parker JG, Rubin KH, Price JM, DeRosier ME (1995) Peer relationships, child developmental and adjustment: a developmental psychopathological perspective. In: Cicchetti D, Cohen D, editors. *Developmental Psychopathology*, Vol. 2. *Risk, Disorder, and Adaptation*. New York: Wiley, pp. 96–161.

Parmenter TR (2011) What is intellectual disability? How is it assessed and classified? *Int J Disabil Dev Education* 58: 303–319. http://dx.doi.org/10.1080/1034912X.2011.598675

Percy-Smith L, Cayé-Thomasen P, Gudman M, Jensen JH, Thomsen J (2008) Self-esteem and social well-being of children with cochlear implant compared to normal hearing children. *Int J Pediatr Otorhinolaryngol* 72: 1113–1120. http://dx.doi.org/10.1016/j.ijporl.2008.03.028

Piaget J (1959) *The Language and Thought of the Child*, 3rd edition. London: Routledge and Kegan Paul. (Original work published in 1923 and 1948.)

Piek JP, Barrett NC, Jones AA, Louise M (2005) The relationship between bullying and self-worth in children with movement coordination problems. *Br J Educ Psychol* 75: 453–463. http://dx.doi.org/10.1348/000709904X24573

Pijl SJ, Frostad P (2010) Peer acceptance and self-concept of students with disabilities in regular education. *Eur J Special Needs Educ* 25: 93–105. http://dx.doi.org/10.1080/08856250903450947

Reiter S, Lapidot-Lefler N (2007) Bullying among special education students with intellectual disabilities: differences in social adjustment and social skills. *Intellect Dev Disabil* 45: 174–181. http://dx.doi.org/10.1352/1934–9556(2007)45[174:BASESW]2.0.CO;2

van Roekel E, Scholte RHJ, Didden R (2010) Bullying among adolescents with autism spectrum disorders: prevalence and perception. *J Autism Dev Disord* 40: 63–73. http://dx.doi.org/10.1007/s10803-009-0832-2

*Rose CA, Espelage DL, Aragon SR, Elliott J (2011a) Bullying and victimization among students in special education and general education curricula. *Exceptionality Educ Int* 21: 2–14. Available at: http://ejournals. library.ualberta.ca/index.php/eei/article/view/12229 (accessed 28 November 2012).

*Rose CA, Monda-Amaya LE, Espelage DL (2011b) Bullying perpetration and victimization in special education: a review of the literature. *Remedial Special Educ* 32: 114–130. http://dx.doi.org/10.1177/0741932510361247

Rosenblum P (1998) Best friendships of adolescents with visual impairments: a descriptive study. *J Visual Impair Blindness* 92: 593–608.

Saylor CF, Leach JB (2009) Perceived bullying and social support in students accessing special inclusion programming. *J Dev Phys Disabil* 21: 69–80. http://dx.doi.org/10.1007/s10882-008-9126-4

Schalock RL, Luckasson RA, Shogren KA, et al (2007) The renaming of mental retardation: understanding the change to the term intellectual disability. *Intellect Dev Disabil* 45: 116–124. http://dx.doi. org/10.1352/1934-9556%282007%2945%5B116:TROMRU%5D2.0.CO;2

Sentenac M, Gavin A, Arnaud C, Molcho M, Godeau E, Gabhainn SN (2011) Victims of bullying among students with a disability or chronic illness and their peers: a cross-national study between Ireland and France. *J Adolesc Health* 48: 461–466. http://dx.doi.org/10.1016/j.jadohealth.2010.07.031

Shikako-Thomas K, Majnemer A, Law M, Lach L (2008) Determinants of participation in leisure activities in children and youth with cerebral palsy: systematic review. *Phys Occupat Ther Pediatr* 28: 155–169. http:// dx.doi.org/10.1080/01942630802031834

Shin M, Besser LM, Siffel C, et al (2010) Prevalence of spina bifida among children and adolescents in 10 regions in the United States. *Pediatrics* 136: 274–279. http://dx.doi.org/10.1542/peds.2009–2084

Sigman M, Ruskin E (1999) Continuity and change in social competence of children with autism, Down syndrome, and developmental delays. *Monographs of the Society for Research in Child Development* 64(1, Serial No. 256).

Siperstien GN, Leffert JS (1997) Comparison of socially accepted and rejected children with mental retardation. *Am J Ment Retard* 101: 339–351. Available at: http://ovidsp.ovid.com/ovidweb.cgi?T=JS&PAGE=referen ce&D=psyc3&NEWS=N&AN=1997-02425-001 (accessed 26 March 2012).

Siperstein G, Bopp MJ, Bak JJ (1978) Social status of learning disabled children. *J Learn Disabil* 11: 98–102. http://dx.doi.org/10.1177/002221947801100206

Skär LRN (2003) Peer and adult relationships of adolescents with disabilities. *J Adolesc* 26: 635–649. http:// dx.doi.org/10.1016/S0140-1971(03)00061-7

Skär L, Tamm M (2002) Disability and social network. A comparison between children and adolescents with and without restricted mobility. *Scandinavian J Disabil Res* 4: 118–137. http://dx.doi. org/10.1080/15017410209510788

Statistics Canada (2001) Profile of disability among children. 89–577-XIE. Available at: www.statcan.gc.ca/ pub/89–577-x/4065023-eng.htm (accessed January 2012).

Statistics Canada (2006a) Living with disabilities series. Social participation of children with disabilities. 11–008-X No. 88 2009002. Available at: www.statcan.gc.ca/pub/11–008-x/2009002/article/11021-eng. htm (accessed January 2012).

Statistics Canada (2006b) Participation and Activity Limitation Survey (PALS): facts on learning limitations. Available at: www.statcan.gc.ca/pub/89-628-x/89-628-x2009014-eng.pdf (accessed January 2012).

Stevens ES, Steel CA, Jutai JW, Kalnins IV, Bortolussi JA, Biggar DW (1996) Adolescents with physical disabilities: some psychosocial aspects of health. *J Adolesc Health* 19: 157–164. http://dx.doi. org/10.1016/1054-139X(96)00027-4

Sweeting H, West P (2001) Being different: correlates of the experience of teasing and bullying at age 11. *Res Papers Educ* 16: 225–246. http://dx.doi.org/10.1080/02671520110058679

Tamm M, Prellwitz M (1999) 'If I had a friend in a wheelchair': children's thoughts on disabilities. *Child Care Health Dev* 27: 223–240. http://dx.doi.org/10.1046/j.1365–2214.2001.00156.x

Taub DE, Greer KR (2000) Physical activity as a normalizing experience for school-age children with physical disabilities: implications for legitimation of social identity and enhancement of social ties. *J Sport Soc Issues* 24: 395–414. http://dx.doi.org/10.1177/0193723500244007

Theunissen SCPM, Rieffe C, Kouwenberg M, Soede W, Briaire JJ, Frijns JHM (2011) Depression in hearing-impaired children. *Int J Pediatr Otorhinolaryngol* 75: 1313–1317. http://dx.doi.org/10.1016/j.ijporl.2011.07.023

Turner HA, Vanderminden J, Finkelhor D, Hamby S, Shattuck A (2011) Disability and victimization in a national sample of children and youth. *Child Maltreatment* 16: 275–286. http://dx.doi.org/10.1177/1077559511427178

Twyman KA, Saylor CF, Saia D, Macias MM, Taylor LA, Spratt E (2010) Bullying and ostracism experiences in children with special health care needs. *J Dev Behav Pediatr* 31: 1–8. http://dx.doi.org/10.1097/DBP.0b013e3181c828c8

US Department of Education (2002) Twenty-fourth annual report to Congress on the implementation of the Individuals with Disabilities Education Act. Available at: www2.ed.gov/about/reports/annual/osep/2002/index.html (accessed January 2012).

US Department of Education, National Center for Education Statistics (2011) Digest of Education Statistics, 2010 (NCES 2011-015), Chapter 2. Available at: http://nces.ed.gov/fastfacts/display.asp?id=64 (accessed 28 November 2012).

US Department of Education, Office of Special Education and Rehabilitative Services, Office of Special Education Programs (2005) Twenty-Sixth Annual (2004) Report to Congress on the Implementation of the Individuals with Disabilities Education Act, vol. 1. Washington, DC: US Department of Education.

*Vaillancourt T, Hymel S, McDougall P (2010a) Why does being bullied hurt so much? Insights from neuroscience. In: Espelage D, Swearer S, editors. *Bullying in North American Schools*. New York: Taylor & Francis Group, Inc., pp. 23–33.

*Vaillancourt T, Clinton J, McDougall P, Schmidt L, Hymel S (2010b) The neurobiology of peer victimization and rejection. In: Jimerson SR, Swearer SM, Espelage DL, editors. *The Handbook of Bullying in Schools: An International Perspective*. New York: Routledge, pp. 293–327.

Vaughn S, Elbaum BE, Schumm JS (1996) The effects of inclusion on the social functioning of students with learning dis-abilities. *J Learn Disabil* 29: 598–608. http://dx.doi.org/10.1177/002221949602900604

Vygotsky LS (1962) *Thought and Language*. Cambridge, MA: MIT Press. http://dx.doi.org/10.1037/11193-000

Wauters LN, Knoors H (2007) Social integration of deaf children in inclusive settings. *J Deaf Stud Deaf Educ* 13: 21–36. http://dx.doi.org/10.1093/deafed/enm028

*Weiss MJ, Harris SL (2001) Teaching social skills to people with autism. *Behav Modification* 25: 785–802. http://dx.doi.org/10.1177/0145445501255007

Wendelborg C, Kvello Ø (2010) Perceived social acceptance and peer intimacy among children with disabilities in regular schools in Norway. *J Applied Res Intellect Disabil* 23: 143–153. http://dx.doi.org/10.1111/j.1468-3148.2009.00515.x

White SW, Robertson-Nay R (2009) Anxiety, social deficits, and loneliness in youth with autism spectrum disorders. *J Autism Dev Disord* 39: 1006–1013. http://dx.doi.org/10.1007/s10803-009-0713-8

Whitehouse AJO, Durkin K, Jaquet E, Ziatas K (2009) Friendship, loneliness and depression in adolescents with Asperger's syndrome. *J Adolesc* 32: 309–322. http://dx.doi.org/10.1010/j.adolescence.2008.03.004

*Wiener J (2004) Do peer relationships foster behavioral adjustment in children with learning disabilities? *Learn Disabil Quarterly* 27: 21–30. http://dx.doi.org/10.2307/1593629

Wiener JR, Schneider BH (2002) A multi-source exploration of the friendship patterns of children with and without learning disabilities. *J Abnorm Child Psychol* 30: 127–141. http://dx.doi.org/10.1023/A:1014701215315

Wiener J, Tardif CY (2004) Social and emotional functioning of children with learning disabilities: does special education placement make a difference? *Learn Disabil Res Pract* 19: 20–32. http://dx.doi.org/10.1111/j.1540-5826.2004.00086.x

Wiener J, Harris PJ, Shirer C (1990) Achievement and social behavioral correlates of peer status in children with learning disabilities. *Learn Disabil Quarterly* 13: 114–127. http://dx.doi.org/10.2307/1510655

Winzer M (2008) *Children with Exceptionalities in Canadian Classrooms*, 8th edition. Toronto, ON: Pearson Prentice Hall.

Wolman C, Basco DE (1994) Factors influencing self-esteem and self-consciousness in adolescents with spina bifida. *J Adolesc Health* 15: 543–548. http://dx.doi.org/10.1016/1054-139X(94)90137-R

Wolters N, Knoors HET, Cillessen AHN, Verhoeven L (2011) Predicting acceptance and popularity in early adolescence as a function of hearing status, gender, and educational setting. *Res Dev Disabil* 32: 2553–2565. http://dx.doi.org/10.1016/j.ridd.2011.07.003

Yeargin-Allsopp M, Van Naarden Braun K, Doernberg NS, Benedict RE, Kirby RS, Durkin MS (2010) Prevalence of cerebral palsy in 8-year-old children in three areas of the United States in 2002: a multisite collaboration. *Pediatrics* 121: 547–554. http://dx.doi.org/10.1542/peds.2007-1270

Yude C, Goodman R, McConachie H (1998) Peer problems of children with hemiplegia in mainstream primary schools. *J Child Psychol Psychiatry* 39: 533–541. http://dx.doi.org/10.1017/S002196309800239X

Zic A, Igric L (2001) Self-assessment of relationships with peers in children with intellectual disability. *J Intellect Disabil Res* 45: 202–211. http://dx.doi.org/10.1046/j.1365-2788.2001.00311.x

9

ROMANTIC RELATIONSHIPS AND SEXUAL EXPERIENCES IN YOUNG PEOPLE WITH NEURODEVELOPMENTAL CONDITIONS

Diana Wiegerink and Marij Roebroeck

Overview

All humans, including children, are sexual beings, so it must be recognized that children and young adults with neurodevelopmental conditions also seek to develop romantic and sexual relationships. This chapter describes the development of romantic and sexual relationships in adolescents with physical disabilities and the phases that can be discerned. Using empirical data from young adults with cerebral palsy (CP) and spina bifida the chapter will elaborate on the emergence of romantic relationships and sexual interest and the attainment of sexual milestones over time. It is important for healthcare professionals to be aware of potential facilitators of and barriers to romantic relationships and sexual experience. It is also noteworthy that physical, social, attitudinal, and emotional limitations can hinder young adults with neurodevelopmental conditions in their sexual behaviour.

Introduction

Sexuality is a dimension of human life that is poorly addressed and inadequately taught as far as it concerns young people with impairments. Young people with neurological and developmental conditions have a specific need for information regarding the impact of their condition on sexuality, and they can legitimately expect healthcare professionals to bring up this subject during their clinic visits. This chapter presents several approaches, methods, and materials that are available to support this process. These can help professionals, during their regular contacts with patients, to raise the topic and pay attention to romantic relationships and sexuality.

Emergence of romantic relationships and sexual development

Children are born as sexual beings. Different aspects of their sexuality develop at different stages, which are linked to the child's development (World Health Organization and German Federal Center of Health Education 2010). Specific developmental explorations emerge at different ages or stages of development. Young children, for example, discover the physical differences between male and female, discover their own body, play with their genitals, examine the bodies of their friends in 'playing doctor', and become curious about the origin of babies. At the age of 6 to 9 years, children learn to differentiate emotions, express their own wishes, and manage disappointments. Feelings of friendship, love, and jealousy are a natural part of this development. The period between 12 and 25 years of age is essential for human sexual development: key aspects of this period of life include physical changes, masturbation, dating, sexual identity, starting romantic relationships, and sexual experiences. This applies equally to people with physical impairments or chronic conditions.

Manning and colleagues (2005) found that 60% of sexually active American teenagers have experienced sex in both romantic and non-romantic contexts. Sexual experiences are not static over time. Adolescence is a time for exploration and seizing opportunities. Having casual sex in a non-romantic context can also involve taking advantage of a well-timed opportunity. As the underlying developmental processes for establishing romantic relationships and actual sexual activities can be different, we distinguish between these two aspects, referring separately to the *development of romantic relationships* and *sexual development*.

In *developing romantic relationships* it is important that young people participate in social activities with friends. In adolescence there is a shift away from family-centred activities towards peer-centred activities. The opinions of friends and their advice acquire more weight than the viewpoint of parents (see Chapter 8). Within the context of peer relationships, contacts develop with opposite-sex counterparts including mutual social activities as well as romantic and sexual relationships (Connolly et al 1999, 2000, Zimmer-Gembeck 2002, Zimmer-Gembeck et al 2004). From their same-sex peers teenagers learn flirting etiquette and sexual conduct. The opinions of others are important and young people develop a sexual self-image. Within a mixed-sex peer group the first romantic and sexual relationships will develop. These tend to begin first with holding hands and kissing during activities with peers and are followed by dating activities as a couple, experimenting with their relationship.

Sexual development in puberty (12–15 years) starts with sexual fantasies, searching for sex in the media, and masturbation. Between the ages of 12 and 20 young people gradually develop their sexual orientation and start gaining sexual experience (World Health Organization and German Federal Center of Health Education 2010). They experience kissing and caressing. The sexual development of young people typically proceeds as follow: kissing, touching and caressing under clothes, naked petting, sexual intercourse (heterosexuals), and finally, perhaps, oral sex and sometimes anal sex. In adolescence young people also start negotiating their wishes and boundaries in sexual relationships.

In a review of the literature on *young people with physical disabilities* (impairments) Lock (1998) notes three developmental stages of adolescence, each of which can bring about specific problems related to relationships and sexuality. In the early phase (about 11–13 years), adolescents are concerned about physical (pubescent) development, such as development of secondary sexual characteristics and a changing outward appearance. Almost all youngsters of this age share these concerns, but adolescents with physical impairments are also likely to feel uncertain about differences in their body and/or their physical appearance.

In the middle stage (about 14–16 years), contacts with peers become central in their lives. Especially in peer groups, there is a lot to gain and share when it comes to dating and sexual experiences. Social activities undertaken with peers are important for the development of romantic relationships (Wiegerink et al 2010a). It is essential to support young people with physical impairments as they seek contact with peers without the presence of parents. Exchanges of opinion about 'the other', and discussing flirting and dating experiences, happen within the intimacy of peer contacts. Young people with impairments often experience challenges regarding access to transport that can certainly hinder these contacts.

In the third stage (about 17–19 years), the development of long-term romantic relationships becomes central and, with that, questions about fertility and genetics become more prominent. Many young adults with neurodevelopmental conditions have little information about their biomedical diagnosis, its potential genetic implications, and the consequences for fertility, pregnancy, and bringing up children.

For some young people dependence on parents can make it difficult to develop into the adult roles that are so important for building the relationships required for experiencing intimacy. The uncomfortable but at times realistic possibility that they will be dependent on a potential partner for their personal care worries young adults with any impairment.

This chapter focuses specifically on young adults without severe intellectual impairments. This is because sexual development is even more complex for young adults with severe intellectual impairment, whether or not they have additional physical impairments. For many young people with significant intellectual challenges, cognitive development, emotional level, and social functioning may be at significantly different levels. In addition, they are often dependent on adults or professional caregivers for many aspects of their social functioning (participation). In discussing sexuality or feelings of love and lust parents or professional caregivers have to consider these different levels of functioning. For example, a 16-year-old boy with severe intellectual impairment has to learn that masturbation is a private activity that is not socially appropriate in the classroom or in public. A further description of these aspects is beyond the scope of this chapter.

Development over time in young adults with neurodevelopment impairments

Indicators of the development of romantic relationships in young adults with impairments include their experiences with dating and with steady romantic relationships. Sexual development includes sexual interest and sexual milestones from French kissing to sexual intercourse. Based on our own research, we describe the course of these indicators over a 4-year period for young adults with CP between 16 and 24 years of age. Descriptions relate to a cohort of young adults with CP without severe intellectual disabilities of whom 82% functioned at Gross Motor Function Classification System (GMFCS) level I to II (meaning that they had relatively good independent mobility) (Wiegerink et al 2010b).

DATING AND ROMANTIC RELATIONSHIPS

The dating activity of young adults with CP increased from 52% to 76% over a 4-year period. In the same period their experience with romantic relationships did not increase (73–79%). Moreover, much lower numbers of young people had a current romantic relationship (Fig. 9.1). At the age of 20 to 24 years, 30% of the young adults with CP had a romantic relationship, compared with 63% of an age-appropriate comparison group.

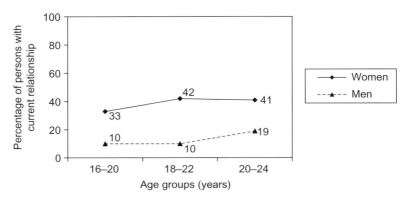

Fig. 9.1 Development over time of having a current romantic relationship for women and men with cerebral palsy (Wiegerink et al 2010b).

Similarly, only 25% of young adults with spina bifida had a partner (Verhoef et al 2005). Significantly more women than men with CP were in a current romantic relationship (Fig. 9.1) (Wiegerink et al 2010b).

SEXUAL INTEREST

Young adults with CP displayed similar levels of sexual interest, in the form of sexual fantasies (66% of the men and 33% of the women), as an age-matched comparison group. The percentage of people having experience with masturbating increased over 4 years from 53% to 80%, similar to the comparison population. More men than women with CP had experience with sexual fantasies and masturbating. It is important for parents and professionals to recognize these manifestations as part of normal psychosexual development. Despite their normal interest, young people with CP had fewer sexual encounters than a comparison population.

SEXUAL MILESTONES

In contrast to romantic relationships, the sexual experience of young adults with CP did increase over a 4-year period (Fig. 9.2). At 20 to 24 years of age, 83% had experience with French kissing, and 60% with sexual intercourse. Among young people with spina bifida (16–25 years) 64% had been sexually active, including sexual contact and masturbating, and 22% had experience of sexual intercourse in the previous year (Verhoef et al 2005). Among young adults with CP, those at GMFCS levels III to V had a slower increase and less experience of sexual intercourse (from 6% to 33%). On average, young people with CP reached their sexual milestones significantly later than the comparison population (de Graaf et al 2005), see Table 9.1 (Wiegerink et al 2010b).

Facilitators of and barriers to romantic relationships and sexual experience

In a similar way to that in typically developing young people, participation in peer interactions and social activities may facilitate young adults with CP in developing a romantic relationship (Wiegerink et al 2010a). Having more friends and venturing out socially, for example to

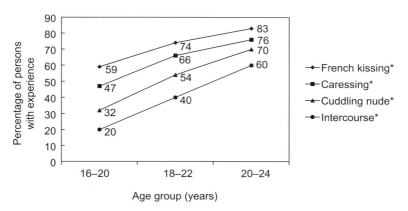

Fig. 9.2 Development over time of sexual activity in young adults with cerebral palsy (Wiegerink et al 2010b).*Significant increases over 4 years.

TABLE 9.1
Mean age (years:months) at time of first experience of sexual milestones

	Young people with cerebral palsy (*n*=103)	Comparison population (*n*=1813)	*p*-Value
French kissing	16:3 (2:4)	14:0	<0.001
Caressing	16:5 (2:2)	15:4	0.001
Cuddling nude	17:5 (2:2)	16:3	0.001
Intercourse	18:4 (2:3)	16:7	<0.001

The comparison population is a Dutch population of the same age, 912 males and 901 females (de Graaf et al 2005). The age given in parenthesis is the SD.

birthday parties or for nightlife entertainment, are factors that facilitate dating. Not surprisingly, dating is an important activity through which romantic relationships and sexual activity are developed (Wiegerink et al 2010a). Young people with spina bifida may experience challenges with transport in visiting family and friends and pursuing leisure activities (Verhoef et al 2005, Barf et al 2009). These restrictions may put them at a disadvantage in terms of creating opportunities for mixed-sex peer contact and dating. Personal and environmental factors may facilitate young adults with CP in having a current romantic relationship and sexual experience. These issues are further elaborated below.

FACTORS OF IMPORTANCE FOR A CURRENT ROMANTIC RELATIONSHIP
Being female and having good psychological adjustment, positive self-esteem, a positive sense of one's sexual self, and feelings of competence regarding self-efficacy may all be important contributors to having a current romantic relationship (Wiegerink et al 2006, 2012). An

overprotective style of parenting and other people's unhelpful attitudes may negatively influence the self-efficacy of young people with CP (Wiegerink et al 2006). Note that the level of gross motor functioning and educational level did not correlate with the likelihood of having a romantic relationship (Wiegerink et al 2012).

FACTORS OF IMPORTANCE FOR SEXUAL EXPERIENCE

Being a few years older and having better gross motor functioning seem to facilitate experience of intercourse. Positive sexual self-esteem and the ability to take the initiative also contributed significantly to a person's intercourse experience. It appears that attending a mainstream school may also facilitate sexual experience (Wiegerink et al 2012). Of a sample of 55 young adults with CP who had a sexual partner, only seven had a sexual partner with physical impairment (Wiegerink et al 2012). Although this finding includes only a small number of people, having a disabled partner may be a limiting factor in terms of sexual experience.

Problems in sexuality experienced by people with impairments

> People with disabilities (impairments) have the same emotional and physical needs and desires as people that are not disabled [but] ... social isolation as well as functional limitations can often impact social/sexual development.
>
> (Tepper et al 2001)

These findings were confirmed in a sample of 74 young adults aged 20 to 24 years (Wiegerink et al 2011). Significantly more men (86%) than women with CP (56%) fantasized about the opposite sex. The majority (78%) reported experiencing feelings of sexual arousal, and two-thirds of the sample had experienced an orgasm. Twenty per cent experienced anorgasmia. Young people with CP may experience a variety of problems or challenges with sexuality. Four out of five reported physical limitations with sex related to CP, notwithstanding few restrictions in gross motor functioning. Table 9.2 shows the difficulties most frequently reported as physical obstacles to having sex. These vary from spasticity (41%) or stiffness (28%) to lack of energy, loss of muscle strength (18%), or trembling (13%). On the other hand, having sex may also have beneficial effects on spasticity or stiffness: 12% of the young adults with CP experienced relaxation as a positive effect.

Young people with spina bifida also reported several problems with sexual functioning, mostly related to impaired genital sensitivity or sexual excitement, incontinence, and problems with erection, orgasm, and ejaculation (Verhoef et al 2005).

Emotional limitations are also common. Forty-five per cent of the young people with CP experienced emotional inhibition to initiate sexual contact. Young people with CP may lack self-confidence (19%) or may be ashamed of their own body (15%) or of their limitations (11%) or of scars (9%). Twenty per cent experienced their body differently from typically developing young people. This may partly be explained by having so often had their bodies viewed in a very functional way by healthcare providers. Young people with spina bifida experienced similar emotional obstacles, and it was their perception that others treat them differently (Verhoef et al 2005).

TABLE 9.2
The top 10 difficulties cited by young adults with CP as physical obstacles to having sex

Ranking	Difficulty	Percentage *n*=59
1	Spasticity	41
2	Difficulty spreading legs	31
3	Difficulties with pelvic tilt	29
4	Stiffness of joints and muscles	28
5	Fatigue	25
6	Balance problems	22
7	Impaired manual ability	20
8	Lack of energy	18
8	Loss of muscle strength	18
10	Trembling	13

Source: Wiegerink et al (2011).

Interventions

NEED FOR SPECIFIC INFORMATION
In the Netherlands almost all young people with CP (Wiegerink et al 2011) or spina bifida (Verhoef et al 2005) have received general sex education about reproduction, birth control, and sexually transmitted diseases as part of the regular school sex educational curriculum. Parents also appeared to be important sources of sex information. Sexual harassment had been discussed with half to three-quarters of the young people with impairments. Of course, covering all aspects of sex information is paramount. If young people hear only about the risks and dangers, they have no benchmark against which to judge present sexual experiences.

However, although young adults do have many specific questions on sexuality, topics specific to impairment and sexuality are rarely discussed. There are many issues regarding sexuality about which young adults with CP or spina bifida would like information, including the heritability of their condition and the impact of CP or spina bifida on sexuality and fertility (Cho et al 2004). Practical issues mentioned included treatment options, (medical) devices and medication, and how to deal with sexuality if one has an impairment. Sometimes there are questions about latex allergy and condom use, concerns regarding loss of genital sensitivity and incontinence and sexuality, and requests for information about sexual aids and alternatives. Satisfaction with one's body is an important topic, as are issues relating to the social aspects of relationships and impairment, such as how to discuss sexual problems with a partner, and homosexuality.

DISCUSSING SEXUALITY ISSUES
Most young adults indicated that the topic of sexuality had not come up at appointments for habilitative care. For many people sexuality is a difficult topic to approach, and thus many

prefer to have others raise the subject. Young adults with CP or spina bifida recommend that the physician or other healthcare professional take an active role in initiating communication on sexuality and providing the necessary information (Verhoef et al 2005, Wiegerink et al 2011).

WHOSE RESPONSIBILITY IS IT? THE PLISSIT MODEL
Most healthcare providers feel uncomfortable discussing sexuality and avoid initiating a conversation on this topic. In a multidisciplinary team it is also convenient to fall back on other team members ('It is not necessarily my job, my colleague would be a much better person to talk about sexuality issues' or 'I wouldn't know the answers to specific questions'). The PLISSIT model (Madorsky and Dixon 1983) shows that there are different levels of conversation and engagement when discussing sexuality: Permission, Limited Information, Specific Suggestions, Intensive Therapy. At the first level, a professional gives the patient permission to start talking openly about sexuality issues, simply by identifying sexuality as a permissible topic during the history-taking or during the conversation with the patient. At the level of limited information, the professional can give the patient diagnosis-specific information on sexuality: for example, 'We know that for some people with spina bifida incontinence can be an obstacle to having sex …' This kind of limited (introductory) information can be discussed during a clinic visit, or be prompted by information on a leaflet, by playing a specific game, or watching a video with a group of adolescents. Once a person has a specific question about his or her individual situation (e.g. positioning during sex, incontinence, starting a discussion with a partner) then specific suggestions and advice are warranted. Occasionally sexuality issues can be so complex that intensive therapy is recommended. In most cases a referral to a specialist such as a sexologist or psychotherapist might be necessary.

DISCUSSING WITH PARENTS OR YOUNG PEOPLE?
Sexual development starts at birth and is a normal part of the overall development of a child. During childhood the parents are the first people to discuss these issues. There are, of course, also opportunities during individual contact the child has with healthcare professionals for age-appropriate discussions on topics such as having friends, falling in love, and leisure activities. It is important to be sensitive during medical examinations or when teaching clean intermittent catheterization to adolescents. This includes issues such as requesting permission to examine or touch 'private parts' and asking if the person needs assistance. This helps to give the individual permission to have control and to understand the concept of modesty. Teaching bowel and bladder programmes and other activities of daily living should be done as early as possible to avoid potential abuse by others and to encourage independence.

At puberty and during adolescence young people will usually not discuss their personal issues with their parents. In clinical contacts with professionals the presence of parents usually hampers open discussion of sexual topics. Thus, in general, by around the age of 12 years it is appropriate to promote independence and self-efficacy in young adolescents in all domains of participation and self-responsibility for the consequences of their condition, as they learn to talk about all important topics with their healthcare providers. This can start with a 5-minute private discussion without the parents, and, by the time adolescents are about 16 years old, they can discuss most questions and issues alone, without their parents. In these private moments permission can be given to ask questions about sexuality or to give general diagnosis-specific limited information (the first and second level of the PLISSIT model).

TOPICS

For children with neurodevelopmental conditions there is no natural moment during the prolonged treatment period to talk about sexual development and intimate relationships. During childhood and puberty it is important to discuss topics in line with the stage of development of the children or young people. Table 9.3 summarizes important topics that are relevant to young people with neurodevelopmental conditions.

TABLE 9.3
Age-related specific sexual topics for children, adolescents, and young adults with neurodevelopmental conditions (considering their development and ability to understand)

ICF domains	9–12 years	12–15 years	16–21 years
Physical functioning • The human body • Fertility and reproduction	Early puberty: body changes, menstruation, breast development, wet dreams	Condom use and latex allergy (non-latex condoms) Fertility and heritability, folic acid Knowing the personal sexual body: challenges for erection or orgasm, sexual options for problems with physical disabilities	(Medical) devices and medicines Alternatives to a sexual partner, safe ways of meeting others
Activities and participation • Relationships and lifestyle • Peers • Media	Social participation: friends, recreation, activities outside the house Learning to negotiate in social situations (builds on past) Building on decision-making skills Social media	Going out with friends without parents Healthy relationships Expressing personal borders and wishes in intimate contacts (a trusted adult or someone with the same disability to talk with) Images in the media versus personal body image (activities to amplify self-esteem)	Learning about talking with a partner about sexual intimacy: expectations, possibilities, positions, alternatives Safe sex
Environmental factors • Privacy	Privacy and social behaviour Privacy vs public behaviour How to avoid sexual abuse or sexually transmitted diseases	Privacy in personal care: independence from parents	
Personal factors • Sexuality • Emotions • Health and well-being	Self-management of bladder and bowel programmes Hygiene: self-care skills to avoid odours and prevent accidents Managing emotion regulation (for CP) Identifing with another person (for spina bifida)	Body image (physical presentation as well as the naked body): scars, deviations	

ICF, International Classification of Functioning, Disability and Health.
Source: Labhard et al (2010).

POSSIBILITIES, MATERIALS, AND PROGRAMMES

Permission
In 'giving permission' to talk about romantic relationships and sexuality, it can be helpful to name sexuality as one of the topics for management or counselling. Examples of ways this can be done include:

- In the Rotterdam Transition Profile (Donkervoort et al 2009) sexuality and romantic relationships are domains of 'participation' additional to work, housing, etc.
- The abbreviation HEADSS can be used as a sequence of questions about Home, Education, Activities, Drugs, Sex, and Suicide (Ehrman and Matson 1998, Van Amstel et al 2004, Yeo et al 2005).
- Just add a question to the standard history-taking. For example:
  – 'Do you have experience of courtship?'
  – 'Are you content with your body and physical appearance?'
  – 'Do you know if your physical limitations can influence your sexual activities?'

Limited information
Under limited information (level two of the PLISSIT model) general aspects of sexuality regarding a specific diagnosis can be discussed. It is useful to inform adolescents and young adults about relevant websites that can help them to find the information they need for their general orientation on this topic. For groups of adolescents or young adults with neurode-velopmental conditions discussions about romantic relationships and sexuality can also be facilitated by using board games and special videos. In the Netherlands the board game 'SexTalk' has been developed specifically for young people with chronic diseases or physical impairments (van der Stege et al 2010). For a list of books, videos, and websites, see Appendix.

Specific suggestions
Before thinking about romantic relationships and sexual activities, the first stage in the development of adolescents and young adults with neurodevelopmental conditions is social participation (see also Chapter 5). Having friends, participating in peer groups, taking advantage of opportunities for going out – these topics need specific individual suggestions to fit in with the personal wishes and possibilities of young people. In the peer group flirting, dating, kissing, and intimate relationships will develop. It can be helpful for adolescents with neurodevelopmental conditions to get advice and to engage in role-playing regarding these skills. In the Netherlands a group module has been developed regarding friends, courtship, and sex (Hilberink et al 2013).

Concerning sexuality, specific suggestions include personal advice on positioning, support devices, and bed mobility. Medical mechanical methods can also be discussed: vacuum devices, injections, MUSE (medicated urethral systems for erections, implants, vibrators). It can be helpful to make a clinical toolkit with sample materials. A useful website is www.intimaterider.com.

Intensive therapy

For complex issues regarding sexuality, intensive therapy is recommended. This is the work of a specialist. It can be helpful to recommend this in the right circumstances, and to refer young adults to a suitable specialist in the area who can help them.

Future directions

In our prospective study we followed young adults with CP up to the age of 20 to 24 years. However, experience indicates that their sexual development is not yet complete at this age. The present results do not indicate whether young adults with CP are delayed in terms of their sexual development and developing romantic relationships or whether some will continue to experience reduced sexual activity. Ideally, follow-up studies on the development of sexuality in young people with CP should continue further into adulthood, for example into the late twenties and beyond (see Chapter 24).

At present we lack evidence on effective coaching methods or available tools or insight about which subgroups of adolescents and young adults need treatment or assistance. Based on our present knowledge, restrictions in gross motor function are not the primary obstacles to initiating romantic relationships and sexual activity among adolescents with CP. Personal factors such as self-esteem, self-efficacy, and sexual self-esteem are better indicators of success or problems in romantic relationships and sexual activities than physical barriers. Even for young people without physical impairments, sexuality is a process of experimentation and trial and error and most will eventually succeed. This is also true for young people with CP, making it important to follow their sexual development and to discuss sexual issues with these adolescents and young adults as an ongoing process in order to gain insight into their questions and unsolved problems. Coaching programmes or other tools may increase their successful experiences of romantic relationships and sexuality. We expect that evaluation studies of these interventions may add to our insight into these processes of change and identify key elements that may improve the professional coaching of young people with neurodevelopmental conditions during their regular care.

Further resources

Books

Labhard S, Laird C, Linroth R, et al (2010) *Sexuality and Spina Bifida*. Washington, DC: Spina Bifida Association.

Kroll K, Klein EL (2001) *Enabling Romance: A Guide to Love, Sex, and Relationships for People with Disabilities (And the People who Care About Them)*. Horsham, PA: No Limits Communications.

McLaughlin K, Topper K, Lindert J. *Sexuality Education for Adults with Developmental Disabilities*. Burlington, VT: Planned Parenthood of Northern New England and Green Mountain Self-Advocates. Available at: http://www.plannedparenthood.org/ppnne/development-disabilities-sexuality-31307.htm (accessed 5 December 2012).

Maurer LT (1999) *Talking Sex: Practical Approaches and Strategies for Working with People Who Have Developmental Disabilities When the Topic is Sex*. Ithaca, NY: Planned Parenthood of Tompkins County.

National Coalition to Support Sexuality Education (NCSSE). Available from: www.ncsse.org

Sexuality across the Lifespan for Children and Adolescents with Developmental Disabilities: An Instructional Guide for Educators, 2005. Tallahassee, FL: Florida Developmental Disabilities Council.

Sexuality across the Lifespan for Children and Adolescents with Developmental Disabilities: Instructional Guide for Parents/Caregivers, 2005. Tallahassee, FL: Florida Developmental Disabilities Council.

WEBSITES

www.SexualHealth.com

www.sexualityandu.com

www.disabilityresources.org/SEX

www.mypleasure.com

http://goaskalice.columbia.edu

VIDEOS AND DVDS

A Boy's Guide to Puberty and Personal Safety. Accession Number: H3009, Marsh Media, 2006.

A Girl's Guide to Puberty and Personal Safety. Accession Number: H3009, Marsh Media, 2006.

REFERENCES

Key references

*Barf HA, Post MW, Verhoef M, Jennekens-Schinkel A, Gooskens RH, Prevo AJ (2009) Restrictions in social participation of young adults with spina bifida. *Disabil Rehabil* 31: 921–927. http://dx.doi.org/10.1080/09638280802358282

*Cho SR, Park ES, Park CI, Na SI (2004) Characteristics of psychosexual functioning in adults with cerebral palsy. *Clin Rehabil* 18: 423–429. http://dx.doi.org/10.1191/0269215504cr739oa

Connolly J, Craig W, Goldberg A, Pepler D (1999) Conceptions of cross-sex friendships and romantic relationships in early adolescence. *J Youth Adolesc* 28: 481–494. http://dx.doi.org/10.1023/A:1021669024820

Connolly J, Furman W, Konarski R (2000) The role of peers in the emergence of heterosexual romantic relationships in adolescence. *Child Dev* 71: 1395–408. http://dx.doi.org/10.1111/1467-8624.00235

*Donkervoort M, Wiegerink DJ, Van Meeteren J, Stam HJ, Roebroeck ME (2009) Transition to adulthood: validation of the Rotterdam Transition Profile for young adults with cerebral palsy and normal intelligence. *Dev Med Child Neurol* 51: 53–62. http://dx.doi.org/10.1111/j.1469-8749.2008.03115.x

Ehrman WG, Matson SC (1998) Approach to assessing adolescents on serious or sensitive issues. *Pediatr Clin North Am* 45: 189–204. http://dx.doi.org/10.1016/S0031-3955(05)70589-7

de Graaf H, Meijer S, Poelman J, Vanwesenbeeck I (2005) *Seks Onder Je 25e. Seksuele Gezondheid van Jongeren in Nederland Anno 2005.* [*Sex Under the Age of 25. Sexual Health of Youth in the Netherlands in the Year 2005.*] Delft: Eburon.

Hilberink SR, Kruijver E, Wiegerink DJHG, Vliet Vlieland TPM (2013) A pilot implementation of an intervention to promote sexual health in adolescents and young adults in rehabilitation. *Sex Disabil* (epub ahead of print, 19 January 2013). http://dx.doi.org/10.1007/ss11195-013-9288-6

*Labhard S, Laird C, Linroth R, et al (2010) *Sexuality and Spina Bifida.* Washington, DC: Spina Bifida Association.

*Lock J (1998) Psychosexual development in adolescents with chronic medical illnesses. *Psychosomatics* 39: 340–349. http://dx.doi.org/10.1016/S0033-3182(98)71322-2

*Madorsky JG, Dixon TP (1983) Rehabilitation aspects of human sexuality. *West J Med* 139: 174–176.

Manning WD, Monica A, Longmore MA, Giordano PC (2005) Adolescents' involvement in non-romantic sexual activity. *Soc Sci Res* 34: 384–407. http://dx.doi.org/10.1016/j.ssresearch.2004.03.001

van der Stege HA, Van Staa A, Hilberink SR, Visser AP (2010) Using the new board game SeCZ TaLK to stimulate the communication on sexual health for adolescents with chronic conditions. *Patient Educ Couns* 81: 324–331. http://dx.doi.org/10.1016/j.pec.2010.09.011

Tepper MS, Whipple B, Richards E, Komisaruk BR (2001) Women with complete spinal cord injury: a phenomenological study of sexual experiences. *J Sex Marital Ther* 27: 615–623. http://dx.doi.org/10.1080/713846817

Van Amstel LL, Lafleur DL, Blake K (2004) Raising our HEADSS: adolescent psychosocial documentation in the emergency department. *Acad Emerg Med* 11: 648–655. http://dx.doi.org/10.1197/j.aem.2003.12.022

*Verhoef M, Barf HA, Vroege J, et al (2005) Sex education, relationships, and sexuality in young adults with spina bifida. *Arch Phys Med Rehabil* 86: 979–987. http://dx.doi.org/10.1016/j.apmr.2004.10.042

*Wiegerink DJ, Roebroeck ME, Donkervoort M, Stam HJ, Cohen-Kettenis PT (2006) Social and sexual relationships of adolescents and young adults with cerebral palsy: a review. *Clin Rehabil* 20: 1023–1031. http://dx.doi.org/10.1177/0269215506071275

*Wiegerink DJ, Roebroeck ME, Van Der Slot WM, Stam HJ, Cohen-Kettenis PT (2010a) Importance of peers and dating in the development of romantic relationships and sexual activity of young adults with cerebral palsy. *Dev Med Child Neurol* 52: 576–582. http://dx.doi.org/10.1111/j.1469-8749.2010.03620.x

*Wiegerink DJ, Stam HJ, Gorter JW, Cohen-Kettenis PT, Roebroeck ME (2010b) Development of romantic relationships and sexual activity in young adults with cerebral palsy: a longitudinal study. *Arch Phys Med Rehabil* 91: 1423–1428. http://dx.doi.org/10.1016/j.apmr.2010.06.011

*Wiegerink D, Roebroeck M, Bender J, Stam H, Cohen-Kettenis P (2011) Sexuality of young adults with cerebral palsy: experienced limitations and needs. *Sex Disabil* 29: 119–128. http://dx.doi.org/10.1007/s11195-010-9180-6

*Wiegerink DJ, Stam HJ, Ketelaar M, Cohen-Kettenis PT, Roebroeck ME (2012) Personal and environmental factors contributing to participation in romantic relationships and sexual activity of young adults with cerebral palsy. *Disabil Rehabil* 34: 1481–1487. http://dx.doi.org/10.3109/09638288.2011.648002

*World Health Organization Regional Office for Europe and the German Federal Centre of Health Education (2010) *Standards for Sexuality Education in Europe. A framework for policy makers, educational and health authorities and specialists*. Geneva: WHO.

Yeo MS, Bond LM, Sawyer SM (2005) Health risk screening in adolescents: room for improvement in a tertiary inpatient setting. *Med J Aust* 183: 427–429.

Zimmer-Gembeck MJ (2002) The development of romantic relationships and adaptations in the system of peer relationships. *J Adolesc Health* 31: 216–225. http://dx.doi.org/10.1016/S1054-139X(02)00504-9

Zimmer-Gembeck MJ, Siebenbruner J, Collins WA (2004) A prospective study of intraindividual and peer influences on adolescents' heterosexual romantic and sexual behavior. *Arch Sex Behav* 33: 381–394. http://dx.doi.org/10.1023/B:ASEB.0000028891.16654.2c

10
CONTEXTUAL FACILITATORS: RESILIENCE, SENSE OF COHERENCE, AND HOPE

Veronica Smith and Kim Schonert-Reichl

Overview

Understanding the factors that children and adolescents need to be successful in life has long been an important objective for parents as well as professionals across a variety of disciplines interested in promoting competence and preventing unfavourable long-term outcomes. This is especially important when a neurological or developmental condition compounds the challenge. Often difficult to determine and assess when overshadowed by early developmental risks or impairments, strengths are mostly eclipsed by the families' circumstances, distress, or conflict. Furthermore, strengths may be overlooked by health professionals who are usually trained to focus on describing and treating impairments, deficits, parenting difficulties, or mental health conditions. This chapter discusses a positive orientation to health, one that focuses on the processes and mechanisms that facilitate resistance to what seem inevitable yet often unpredictable stressors associated with having or parenting a child with a neurological or developmental condition.

Introduction

Drawing on the rich interdisciplinary research in the area of a strengths-based approach to health, three interrelated constructs will be discussed: resilience, sense of coherence, and hope. By describing the usefulness of these frameworks for addressing the individual and parenting needs that are compounded by neurological or developmental conditions, we hope to provide evidence that makes the case for taking a positive perspective – one in which the primary focus is on recognizing strengths rather than simply reducing risks associated with the disabling conditions. The frames of reference of resilience, sense of coherence, and hope provide a lens for addressing the International Classification of Functioning, Disability and Health (ICF) dynamic processes and interconnected components of functioning, context, and experience (World Health Organization 2001; see also Chapter 4). This chapter delineates and summarizes some key research findings that have recently emerged that support these frameworks and discusses the important roles of development and context in promoting competence for individuals and families.

Throughout this chapter, we take what Aaron Antonovsky (1979) coined as a 'salutogenic' perspective, an orientation to understanding human functioning that identifies factors that contribute to the dynamic developmental 'ease/dis-ease' continuum. It is important to note that Antonovsky borrowed from Latin *salus*, the word for health and well-being, to emphasize that this orientation focuses more on health than on pathology. Using Antonovsky's framework, we hope to address some new approaches and alternative practices that facilitate the environments for individuals with neurological or developmental conditions.

The impact of impairment: a focus on stress

Until recently, there has been scant attention paid to the positive manifestations of having a neurological or developmental condition, especially among studies examining development. In a review of over 20 years of studies on families of children with impairments, Helff and Glidden (1998) found that '… investigators still emphasized predominantly negative response' when reporting on findings regarding the impact of raising a child with an impairment. Since the late 1990s, we find that the most recent decade of research has been dominated by studies exploring the causes of the negative impacts of neurological and developmental conditions, particularly parenting stress. These explanations include poorly met informational needs (Hawley et al 2003), negative responses from others regarding diagnoses (Lawson 2004), associations of increased stress with demanding intervention programmes (Warfield 2005), and a decreased sense of parenting competence (Hassall et al 2005). While these findings have provided useful guidance to orienting support, the thrust of many outcome investigations is on the impact on deficits, which further entrenches the discourse to one in which either having or parenting a child with impairment is stressful, negative, and accomplished with few rewards. Missing in these investigations is the notion that impairment, although present, may not be limiting, may only partially impair interaction, or may, in fact, be transformative in one or more life domain (Scorgie and Sobsey 2000, Morris 2009).

A new focus: resilience

The construct of resilience – the ability to withstand and rebound from crisis and adversity – has valuable potential for framing interventions and prevention services aimed at strengthening and supporting individuals with neurological and developmental conditions and their families. Resilience was originally conceptualized as residing within the individual (Walsh 1996) but has been broadened to include family, community, and cultural or societal assets (Wright and Masten 2006). Discerning how children's early experiences pave the road for later adjustment was spurred, in part, by research that indicated that childhood risk is generally a strong predictor of poor adult outcomes (e.g. Werner and Smith 1982, 1992, 2001). Indeed, many children and young people with developmental issues confront obstacles that compromise both their present and their future adjustment. For many of these children, their early experiences follow a predictable course – one filled with uncertainty and struggle in a society that views impairments as a stigma or 'undesired difference' (see Chapter 12 on stigma) and often fails to provide adequate services to meet their developmental needs. Predictable risks among children with identified impairments are too often the focus of treatments and services for children with neurological and developmental conditions to the exclusion of an examination of strengths that might better predict outcomes and adjustment in society.

The study of *resilience* goes back 50 years when a handful of pioneers in the field, such as Norman Garmezy, Michael Rutter, and Emmy Werner, began to discover that there were some children who succeeded in the face of great risk (Schonert-Reichl and LaRose 2008). Norman Garmezy, for instance, in his early research on the children of mothers with schizophrenia, found that a subset of the children identified as at high risk for psychopathology had surprisingly healthy adaptation. Rather than dismiss these children as 'atypical cases', Garmezy and his colleagues sought to discover the factors that might account for their success. This change from a focus on risk to one of resiliency represented a paradigm shift from a focus on pathology or disorder to one of strength and success (Garmezy and Rutter 1983).

Early on in the history of resiliency research, children who succeeded despite extreme adversity were characterized as 'invulnerable' or 'invincible'. Accordingly, invulnerable or invincible children were considered to be 'untouched' by the stresses they encountered. It quickly became apparent, however, that this terminology was erroneous – these children were not 'made of steel' whereby all of the risks thrown at them were deflected or averted. Few children, it was found, exhibited such complete immunity to disorder in the presence of risk factors. It was surmised that neither vulnerability nor invulnerability was an all-or-none phenomenon.

Today, the term invulnerability has been replaced by resilience – a term that is preferred because it refers to the capacity of children and young people to face stress without being incapacitated; it does not mean that they never experience distress or that they cannot be wounded, as the term invulnerability had implied. Since its inception the resiliency construct has been defined in multiple ways, with some researchers using the term to refer to the maintenance of healthy development despite the presence of threat (e.g. poverty, impairments) and other researchers using the term to refer to the speed of recovery from trauma (e.g. death of a parent, diagnosis of disabling condition). Although a single definition of resiliency may not capture the complexities inherent in the term, an assortment of definitions does create problems for research and policy and may hinder progress in the field. However, what remains consistent despite the varied terminology is that resilience is a multidimensional phenomenon that is context specific and involves developmental change.

One definition of resiliency, put forth by Garmezy and Masten, captures the essence of many of the current definitions:

> ... a process of, or a capacity for, or the outcome of successful adaptation despite challenging and threatening circumstances
>
> (Garmezy and Masten 1991)

Almost all definitions include the following four components: (1) the characteristics of the individual; (2) the nature of the context; (3) the risk factors – that is, the presence of adversity; and (4) the counteracting, protective, and compensatory factors.

According to Rutter (1979), resistance to stress or *resilience* is: (1) *not a monolithic construct* that, once achieved, will always be present – it is relative and not absolute; (2)

the result of environmental as well as individual factors; (3) not a fixed attribute or quality of the individual; and (4) dependent on context. That is, *resiliency is not a universal construct that applies to all life domains* – children and adolescents may be resilient to specific risk conditions but quite vulnerable to others. Take, for example, the child of a parent with intellectual impairment. This child may demonstrate high levels of competence at home, as evidenced by taking care of younger siblings, making meals, organizing laundry, and grocery shopping. However, this same child in other contexts, such as in school and in peer relationships, may demonstrate poor competence and may experience school failure and poor peer relationships.

A discussion of the way that researchers have conceptualized factors that lead to resilience is useful. Arnold Sameroff (1999) provides a description of three factors that take into account the many ecological influences of development: *risk*, *promotive*, and *protective* factors. The term *risk* comes originally from the epidemiological literature and was adopted by developmental scientists as it is predicated on the notion that deleterious outcomes are usually not of a single origin – generally there are multiple factors that when combined put one 'at risk'. *Promotive* factors are on the opposite, but positive, extreme of the variable that is seen as having the potential for risk (e.g. parenting). Promotive factors are conceptualized to have the same effect for low- and high-risk populations. For example, responsive parenting (a promotive factor) is seen as positive for both children at high risk (i.e. as in children with neurodevelopmental conditions such as autism; Siller and Sigman 2008) and children at low risk (i.e. as in children with typical development; Hart and Risley 1995). In contrast, a *protective* factor interacts with the group's level of risk. In a low-risk group, a protective factor makes no or little difference (e.g. a universal programme to prevent reading failure has little or no effect on children who are not at risk for reading failure; Smith 2004), whereas in a high-risk group (e.g. those at risk for reading failure) a protective factor (e.g. programme to prevent reading failure) has a high impact (Smith 2004). Another example of this can be seen in a programme to encourage peer interaction. For those children with neurodevelopmental conditions with very few friends it may be very helpful, but for those who have good peer relationships it may have little or no effect (Locke et al 2012).

The importance of taking a developmental perspective (see also Chapter 6)
Early on in resilience research, it became apparent that children and adolescents might have different risk, promotive, and protective factors during different developmental phases. For instance, during the earliest stage of development, because of the total dependence on caregivers, infants are highly vulnerable to the consequences of loss of their parents or mistreatment by caregivers. In contrast, infants are more protected from the impact of a critical stressful event, such as war or natural disaster, because they lack understanding of what is happening. As children grow and move beyond the family into the larger spheres of school and community, they can be exposed to a wider array of risk and protective factors such as unsupervised activities and involvement with peers. This exposure may lead to increased risk but also may provide the opportunity for children to encounter others in their social networks, such as neighbours or teachers, who provide support. Adolescents may be confronted with other risk or protection as they develop, such as increased cognitive abilities to think and plan for

the future. Moreover, some factors might have 'sleeper' effects across development. Werner (1993) found that positive temperament in a group of children with learning challenges did not buffer negative outcomes for 18-year-olds but, by the time these individuals were 32 years old, early measures of temperament did predict positive adjustment, including vocational and marital satisfaction.

Considering context and process in resiliency

Emmy Werner's landmark Kauai study (Werner 1992), which was followed by other large-scale, longitudinal risk studies (e.g. Garmezy and Rutter 1983, Cicchetti and Tucker 1994, Cowen et al 1997, Masten 2001), clarified that resilient children differ from children with less positive outcomes in multiple factors, some individual but others family and systemic. Among the individual factors are positive self-esteem, a sense of self-efficacy or mastery, and a core sense of security that promotes autonomy, as well as prosocial competencies including empathy and the ability to seek and accept help from others. Importantly, we also see intellectual capacities that are marked by curiosity, exploration, and problem-solving abilities (Wright and Masten 2006).

The longitudinal studies tell us that many individual attributes are already present in infancy. During infancy, resilient children demonstrate temperaments that are predictable, adaptable, and active, and have greater emotionality and sociability. In general, they have qualities that make them more 'easy to care for' and more likely to elicit attention, warmth, and social support (Laucht et al 1997). However, this does not mean that they are also the strongest, the most assertive, or the most aggressive children (Papousek 2011). Importantly, beyond their own qualities, children who are described as 'resilient' also tend to rely on at least one stable and secure attachment relationship in or outside the family (e.g. teacher, relative, friend, or neighbour), along with other family, community, and systemic supports (Werner 2001). Wright and Masten (2006: 24) identified a 'short list' of these supports (Table 10.1) and posited that they 'reflect the fundamental adaptive systems supporting human development'.

Case scenario 1

Ten-year-old Gemma attends her local elementary school in an inner city neighbourhood where a large majority of the students live below the poverty line. Gemma is the first born of four children and lives with her now single mother in subsidized housing close to the school. The school has additional 'inner city' funding but is struggling to meet the needs of the many children who have difficulties. Gemma turns up at school early every morning on her own, without breakfast, and the school secretary, June, who lives in the neighbourhood and is the first to arrive, lets her come in, provides her with some nutrition, and then gives her small jobs around the office. In the past year, Gemma has discovered where June lives and makes a point of playing in front of her house or sitting on her front porch. June now invites her in and will offer to make her dinner and has made arrangements with her mother to let her stay over when her granddaughter, who is roughly the same age, is over for the weekend. Gemma now spends

---

a lot of time at June's house. Gemma has a severe speech impairment and is often difficult to understand. Despite the challenges of being understood, June, Gemma's teachers, and other school staff find her charming and amusing and have gone out of their way to obtain the additional resources of a speech and language pathologist. Her grade 1 teacher continues to provide her with extra tuition in reading after school despite the fact that Gemma is included in a grade 4 classroom. The school counsellor regularly visits Gemma's home to provide supports for her mother who struggles with depression and managing her household. Despite her impairments, during her tenure at the school, Gemma has slowly learned to read, and her speech is gradually becoming clearer. Gemma has Down syndrome.

For some children and adolescents identified as 'at risk', their developmental trajectory is redirected – pushed off course by other forces – more positive forces, as illustrated by Gemma's story. Much less is known about this atypical path – especially the path of children and young people with neurological and developmental conditions who, in the face of adversity and against the odds, develop into well functioning and relatively healthy adults. This is Gemma's story. People like her survive their risky environments with their self-confidence, their coping skills, and their success in school and other contexts relatively intact. These individuals demonstrate competence and success despite the odds against them. They demonstrate resilience. The story of Gemma serves to illustrate the construct of resiliency. Consider her story – a young girl who, despite her intellectual impairments, when confronted with possible parental neglect and a generally disorganized household, decides to seek places where and adults with whom she can flourish and succeed. Her ingenuity, tenacity, and perseverance are evident, as illustrated by the tactics she uses to find supports for herself – she simply waits on the front steps every day for the school secretary who she has identified as a suitable mentor. At school, she charms and endears herself to her teachers and therapists; they become attached to her and take over the advocacy role missing in her home environment.

Longitudinal research also provides information about caregivers. Caregivers of resilient children are more likely to provide sensitive care, warmth, physical safety, acceptance, and respect and to follow an educational style fostering self-esteem, self-efficacy, independence, and autonomy. According to Bayat (2007), a growing field of interest concerns family resilience and the factors that contribute to a family becoming stronger in spite of dealing with adversity. Despite this interest, the topic is only beginning to be explored in families of children with impairments.

In an effort to better understand how resilience is realized in families of children with autism, Bayat (2007) examined family connectedness and closeness, making positive meaning of the impairment, and spiritual and personal growth in a group of 175 families of children with autism between the ages of 2 and 18 years. She found evidence that 40% of the participating families displayed factors of resilience, notably becoming closer as a family and finding a greater appreciation of life generally and other people specifically. Like Scorgie and Sobsey (2000), who investigated the transformational experiences of parenting a child with intellectual

125

TABLE 10.1
Examples of factors associated with resilience

Child factors	Social and adaptable temperament in infancy
	Good natured; affectionate disposition (resilient temperament)
	Good cognitive abilities and problem-solving skills
	Effective emotional and behavioural regulation strategies
	Positive view of self (self-confidence, high self-esteem)
	Positive outlook on life, trusting
	Sense of self-efficacy; sense of control over 'fate'
	Accurate processing of interpersonal cues
	Effective in work, play, and love
	Asks for help; assertive
	Above average in social intelligence
	Ability to have close relationships
	Healthy expectations and needs
	Uses talents to personal advantage
	Delays gratification
	Has future orientation (plans for the future)
	Has faith and a sense of meaning in life
	Has characteristics valued by society and self (talents, sense of humour, attractiveness to others)
Family factors	Stable and supportive home environment
	Low level of parental discord
	Parental warmth
	Close relationship to responsive caregiver
	Authoritative parenting style (high on warmth, structure/monitoring, and expectations)
	Positive sibling relationships
	Supportive connections with extended family members
	Parents involved in child's education
	Parents have individual qualities listed above as protective for child
	Socio-economic advantages
	Postsecondary education of parent
Community factors	High neighbourhood quality
	Safe neighbourhood
	Low level of community violence
	Affordable housing
	Access to recreational centres
	Clean air and water
	Effective schools
	Well-trained and well-compensated teachers
	After-school programmes
	School recreation resources (sports, music, art)
	Employment opportunities for parents and teenagers
	Good public health care
	Access to emergency services (police, fire, medical)
	Sense of school belonging
	Connections to significant and caring adults (e.g. teachers, coaches)
	Connections to pro-social peers
Cultural or societal factors	Protective child policies (child labour, child health, and welfare)
	Value and resources directed at education
	Prevention of and protection from oppression or political violence
	Low acceptance of physical violence

impairment, Bayat (2007) found that families became stronger as a result of an impairment in the family. These findings tell us that not all aspects of family identity and functioning are automatically negatively affected by having a child with an impairment. This awareness is important for health professionals, as it may serve to trigger discussion among struggling families to examine aspects of their functioning that have been enhanced or enriched rather than less productive discussions that focus on negative aspects of their new parenting challenges.

Increasingly, resilience research is providing guidance on how to foster hidden sources of strength in families in need of additional supports. Such factors as providing more predictable structure and enhanced parental responsivity have become ubiquitous with the core components of many parenting programmes for typically developing children (e.g. Triple P Positive Parenting Program; Sanders 1999), children at risk for behaviour disorders (e.g. Incredible Years; Webster-Stratton 2001), and children with neurological and developmental conditions (e.g. More Than Words, a programme designed for parents of children with autism; Sussman 2008). For example, Papousek (2011) describes work at the Munich Intervention Program for Fussy Babies that capitalizes on the dynamic interactions that begin early in the child's development and are rooted in regulatory processes involved in the caregiver–infant system (Cicchetti and Tucker 1994). In this system, infants express intrinsic and intuitive capacities to draw their parents towards them and the parent responds in competent ways that are also intuitive. By understanding this system of interaction, Papousek makes a case for applying a strengths-based approach to counselling families of infants with developmental impairments. For example, in the Munich programme, clinicians use carefully planned video recordings of parent–infant interaction to capture positive examples of parent responsivity. While reviewing the recordings with the parents, the clinicians are able to help the parent 're-experience' the positive interaction, thereby reinforcing the mother's experience of her intuitive competence (Papousek 2011). Thus, the programme builds on existing strengths rather than addressing parent or child deficits within these caregiver–infant interactions.

It is important to note, however, that research on resilience tells us that 'being resilient' is not a matter of innate personality characteristics but evolves from dynamic interactions between positive constitutional attributes and particular care-receiving experiences, such as those illustrated in Papousek's work. Competence or resilience ensues from complex interactions between a child and the environments in which he or she resides; as a result, competence will change as a child changes and as his or her environment changes. Accordingly, a child's capabilities along with the contexts or environments experienced will influence competence. What is critical to note here is that, while a child must act to demonstrate competence, the environments in which a child finds him- or herself can impart competence. It is the proficient adults or peers in that environment that can lead a child to perform at a more advanced level and reach his or her highest potential by providing the child with structure and support.

As implied by the work of Bayat (2007), Scorgie and Sobsey (2000), and others (e.g. King et al 2006, Papousek 2011), parents of children with impairments are not immune to the bidirectional effects of development: just as impairment impacts the way they parent, so does their child's impairment influence who they are and the sense that they make of the world. The ways in which parents make sense of the world and impart competence is our next focus.

Meaning making: sense of coherence

The way families approach new challenges, adversity, and unfamiliar territory is fundamental to resilience. According to Froma Walsh, who has investigated family resilience in families who have children with developmental impairments, families approach new challenges with a 'we shall overcome' attitude (Walsh 2003: 6). Aaron Antonovsky provides a useful framework for describing the process of acquiring this general orientation to life, the sense of coherence (SOC). Antonovsky defines the SOC as follows:

> … a global orientation that expresses the extent to which one has a pervasive, endur-
> ing though dynamic feeling of confidence that (1) the stimuli deriving from one's
> internal and external environments in the course of living are structured, predictable,
> and explicable; (2) the resources are available to one to meet the demands posed
> by these stimuli; and (3) these demands are challenges, worthy of investment and
> engagement.

(Antonovsky 1987: 19)

The three components of SOC have come to be known as: (1) *comprehensibility* (the person's ability to make sense of what is happening); (2) *manageability* (the assessment and confidence that resources available are adequate); and (3) *meaningfulness* (the sense that this is worthwhile engaging with).

Antonovsky (1987: 150) stated that the strong SOC individual '… is more likely to be aware of his or her emotions, can more easily describe them, feels less threatened by them. They are more likely to be personally and culturally acceptable; hence there is less need to disregard their existence. They are more appropriately responsive to the reality of the situation one is in.'

Case scenario 2

After a long-awaited pregnancy Marci gives birth early to a girl who, she is told, will probably have severe impairments. She takes time to listen to the paediatrician, who recommends several tests and careful monitoring to better ascertain the nature of the impairments. Marci has difficulty taking it all in but listens carefully and then spends time talking about the news with her husband and extended family who come to visit her in the hospital. She finds she has more questions and asks to see the paediatrician again.

Marci shows signs of trying to make sense of this news in the few behaviours described above. By sharing the news with her family and then seeking more information she is simultaneously checking out her resources and trying to make sense of the news about her daughter's health. If a mother is high in SOC, she ultimately believes that she has the capacity to deal with this new situation. She views her situation as a challenge and is confident that she needs to better understand more about what this will mean for her family. Through this process she gradually accesses resources that are available to her in her community. Her strong SOC facilitates her move towards the better-health end of the good health–bad health continuum and moderates her overall stress. A mother low in SOC may feel overwhelmed and adopt an avoidance coping mechanism. By not processing the information, and making meaning of it, she becomes more challenged in garnering the resources that she needs to help facilitate her child's development.

To examine the utility of SOC, Antonovsky identified characteristics that address how people view life in stressful situations, which he used to construct a scale (Orientation to Life Questionnaire). It includes questions such as 'Do you have the feeling that you're being treated unfairly?', 'Do you have the feeling that you are in an unfamiliar situation and don't know what to do?', and 'When something has happened do you generally feel that you saw things in the right proportion or under-/overestimated its importance?' This scale has found utility among health professionals in many countries and has been translated into over 30 languages. In 2006, Erikkson and Lindstrom reviewed 453 studies using the SOC, published up to 2003. They found that the SOC measure had been utilized in healthy populations from children to adults, in individuals with acute and chronic impairments, and in many contexts such as health services, learning situations, and care of relatives. In each of these populations SOC was strongly related to health, particularly mental health. Erikkson and Lindstrom (2006) concluded that the construct of SOC seems to be a health-promoting resource, which strengthens resilience and brings about a positive state of health.

Research led by Malka Margalit has helped us to better understand SOC in parents of children with developmental impairments (e.g. Margalit et al 1991, 1992). She found that parents of children who have impairments reported lower SOC than those in the general population but, similar to the general population, parents' SOC scores varied, indicating that some parents of children with impairments show strength in this area. Although the research examining SOC in families with neurological and developmental conditions is primarily descriptive and exploratory, it appears that SOC is lower in families of children with developmental impairments and is associated with parental stress, avoidance, and depression (Margalit et al 1991, King et al 2006, Oelofsen and Richardson 2006).

In an effort to address whether SOC can be enhanced among parents of children with developmental impairments, Margalit and Kleitman (2006) examined whether it could be altered in a group of parents of children with developmental impairments who participated in an early intervention programme. Interestingly, of the 70 mothers who participated, 24 showed a higher SOC at the start of the intervention. When the programme was completed, these mothers showed lower stress and greater satisfaction with the programme. In contrast, the mothers who had lower levels of SOC at the beginning of the programme had, by the end of the programme, even lower SOC and higher stress. The results provide a possible explanation for why some families do better in some interventions than others. This has implications for the planning of effective intervention programmes and indicates that addressing family needs prior to embarking on interventions might serve some families better.

Finding solutions: hope
Hope is another framework that helps us understand the resiliency process. Interestingly, despite a preponderance of autobiographical and biographical accounts that document personal

accounts of hope among individuals with neurological and developmental conditions and their families (see, as an example, people's accounts of living with autism), experimental examinations of hope have received very little attention (Lloyd and Hastings 2009). As a psychological construct, hope is not analogous to 'optimistic wishing' (as in 'I hope he gets better') or 'positive affect' (as in 'they are hopeful'), as in lay usage. Hope theory is distinguished from optimism and positive affect, as it describes a psychological process, and relies on the premise that human behaviour is essentially goal driven. In contrast, optimism or wishing is a generalized expectancy that good, rather than bad, things will happen. To be 'optimistic', like its opposite, 'pessimistic', is thought of as a 'dispositional' trait (Seligman and Csikszentmihalyi 2000). Similarly, 'positive affect', although often associated with hope (and optimism), refers to positive attitudes, emotions, and moods and is more commonly accepted as a basic aspect of happiness (Lyubormirsky et al 2005). Hope theory was initially introduced by Charles Snyder in 1991 who conceptualized hope as a state of focusing on goals and the perceived ability to reach those goals. Hope, as a psychological construct, includes both the perception that the goals can be met (agency) and the ability to plan ways of meeting those goals (pathways) (Snyder et al 2002). In Snyder's view, 'agency' describes the ability of individuals in initiating and maintaining the actions to maintain the goals and 'pathways' refers to the perception that individuals have the ability to develop workable routes to attain these goals (Snyder et al 1991, 1996).

In order to test hope, Snyder developed the Hope Scale (Snyder et al 1991), which has subsequently been used in countless studies. The scale consists of 12 items: four each are used to measure agency with such items as 'I energetically pursue my goals' and pathways with such items as 'I can think of many ways to get out of a jam'. Babyak and colleagues (1993) conducted a confirmatory factor analysis of the Hope Scale and found that the agency and pathways items were independent of each other. Further research has demonstrated that higher agency and pathways thinking are associated with higher hope (Snyder 2002). However, the components are not always dependent, as persons high in agency may be able to initiate goal-directed action but may be low in pathways thinking. Thus, when goals are not met these people are unable to find new ways of meeting goals and may not continue to pursue them, resulting in a reduction in hope. An example of this might be a parent who begins an intervention with her child but, upon seeing few changes, gives up and decides that the intervention will not help her child, rather than seeking other interventions or making modifications to the first intervention to better accommodate her child's needs.

With the additional demands of parenting, such as obtaining appropriate medical and educational interventions as well, in many cases, as financing the expenses of such care (Baker-Ericzen et al 2005, DuPont 2009), parents of children with neurological and developmental conditions must demonstrate considerable agency and planning to find ways of meeting their child's additional needs. These behaviours are fundamental to hope's characteristics (Snyder et al 1991).

The few studies that have investigated the presence and nature of hope in parents of children with neurological and developmental conditions have some noteworthy findings. Kausar and colleagues (2003) asked 19 parents of children with developmental conditions to comment on their feelings of hope. Although they did not define hope in the same manner as Snyder and colleagues (1991), instead describing hope as a 'positive transformation and dynamic process' and helpful for parents to 'reframe their lives', they found that hope, as a phenomenon, was something that parents had considered. Eight themes emerged from their analyses, including positive attitudes and spirituality as sources of hope, hope as a consequence of the realistic acceptance of the child and his or her impairment, and hope as an outcome of parenting a child with an intellectual impairment. Kearney and Griffin (2001), in a qualitative investigation of parents' experiences of raising a child with a developmental impairment, found that both mothers and fathers felt that hope was an important notion; however, the parents' comments did not reflect positively on professionals. That is, in some instances, parents revealed that they felt that professionals imposed messages of 'no hope' on them, even when the parents felt optimistic and hopeful about the future. In addition, when parents expressed their feelings of hope, professionals interpreted this as behaviour that was maladaptive in their situation. Both studies demonstrate that hope as a construct resonates for parents who have a child with a neurological or developmental condition.

In a study that used Snyder's conception of hope, Lloyd and Hastings (2009) explored the relationship between levels of hope, child behavioural problems, and parental well-being in 138 families of children with intellectual impairment. They found that for mothers, lower levels of hope (agency and pathways) and more child behaviour problems predicted maternal depression. Positive affect was predicted by less problematic child behaviour and by higher levels of hope agency. For fathers, anxiety and depression were predicted by low hope agency, and positive affect was predicted by high hope agency. Hope pathways, or the ability to plan ways of meeting goals, were not a significant predictor of paternal well-being. Hope agency and pathways interacted in the prediction of maternal depression such that mothers reporting high levels of both hope dimensions reported the lowest levels of depressive symptoms. Their findings reveal that hope was highly associated with family well-being and is worthy of further investigation.

What these studies on hope indicate is not simply that 'more hope is better'; rather, they indicate that hope is a complex construct that is related to positive family functioning. The research has the potential to offer health providers a framework for helping families accurately frame and explore more hopeful cognitions. Accurate and appropriate goal-setting and clarity about how to achieve goals are important processes for families to engage in. Family-centred practices (e.g Rosenbaum et al 1998, Dunst and Trivette 2005) that actively engage families in the goal-setting process have the potential to enhance long-term outcomes related to family resiliency behaviours that will be beneficial for family functioning beyond discrete intervention regimes.

Summary and future directions

Many factors facilitate overall well-being in individuals with neurological and developmental conditions, including their unique characteristics, their family structure and support, their cultural and societal supports, and the systemic supports available in their community. Frameworks with a resilience perspective are useful to understand the many positive interactions that influence development and provide a more holistic outlook on health that addresses the dynamic processes and interconnected components of functioning, context, and experience implied by the ICF. Most current researchers in the resilience field agree that resilience is tied in with demonstrating competence in the face of serious current or past adversity. Positive frameworks direct our gaze to processes and mechanisms that might otherwise be overlooked when the focus on patient care addresses only the disabling aspects of these conditions.

It is no surprise that some researchers who study impairment and disability have been quick to take up strength-based models (e.g. Margalit and Kleitman 2006) as a lens to better understand development and the effectiveness of interventions. Donahue and Pearl (2003) cite several reasons for the usefulness of the resilience lens, the primary ones being that it allows researchers to conceptualize variation in outcomes and provides better multilayered guides for prevention and intervention efforts. When our lens is too narrowly focused on individual outcomes that obscure how these individuals and their families view their own lives, our interventions, and the healthcare management they receive, we may fail to discern why some children and families are resistant to interventions and why some others blossom. The resilience framework suggests that there are multiple and interactive characteristics at play in development – individual, family, and community – that create risks or protective and promotive influences – and it helps us to clarify and make sense of this complexity.

Psychological processes such as SOC and hope allow us to reconceptualize how families of children with neurological and developmental conditions develop coping strategies or ways to make sense of the world, engage in positive planning, and impart competence. Such positive frameworks are also useful in policy and practice as they potentially offer guidance on approaches to intervention that expand existing or ineffective procedures (Seccombe 2002).

Although a great deal needs to be learned about the manner in which strength-based approaches and interventions may promote the healthy development of children with neurological or developmental conditions, the present review of resilience and positively oriented cognitive frameworks, such as SOC and hope, support the notion that this area of research has the potential to shed light on the underlying processes and mechanisms. This orientation to supporting children and families may also provide much-needed direction for improving the implementation of intervention programmes aimed at promoting protective factors. There is probably no single route or 'magic bullet' that will address the unique families and children who present with neurodevelopmental conditions. This review suggests that by considering the many facets that contribute to development, including the strengths, we can realize new insights into the ways we understand and address this complex phenomenon.

REFERENCES

*Key references

Babyak MA, Snyder CR, Yoshinobu L (1993) Psychometric propertis of the Hope Scale: a confirmatory factor analysis. *J Res Pers* 27: 154–169. http://dx.doi.org/10.1006/jrpe.1993.1011

Antonovsky A (1979) *Health, Stress, and Coping: New Perspectives on Mental and Physical Well-being*. San Francisco, CA: Jossey-Bass.

Antonovsky A (1987) *Unraveling the Mystery of Health. How People Manage Stress and Stay Well*. San Francisco, CA: Jossey-Bass.

Baker-Ericzen MJ, Brookman-Frazee L, Stahmer A (2005) Stress levels and adaptability in parents of toddlers with and without autism spectrum disorders. *Res Pract Persons Severe Disabil* 30: 194–204. http://dx.doi.org/10.2511/rpsd.30.4.194

*Bayat M (2007) Evidence of resilience in families of children with autism. *J Intellect Disabil Res* 51: 702–714. http://dx.doi.org/10.1111/j.1365-2788.2007.00960.x

Cicchetti D, Tucker D (1994) Development and self-regulatory structures of the mind. *Dev Psychopathol* 6: 533–549. http://dx.doi.org/10.1017/S0954579400004673

Cowen EL, Wyman PA, Work WC, Kim JY, Fagen DB, Magnus KB (1997) Follow-up study of young stress-affected and stress-resilient urban children. *Dev Psychopathol* 9: 565–577. http://dx.doi.org/10.1017/S0954579497001326

Donahue ML, Pearl R (2003) Studying social development and learning disabilities is not for the faint hearted: comments on the risk/resilience framework. *Learn Disabil Res Pract* 18: 90–93. http://dx.doi.org/10.1111/1540-5826.00064

*Dunst CJ, Trivette CM (2005) Characteristics and consequences of family-centred helpgiving practices. *CASEmakers* 1: 6, 1–4. Available at: www.fippcase.org/casemakers/casemakers_vol1_no6.pdf (accessed 10 March 2012).

DuPont MR (2009) An exploration of resilience in families with a child diagnosed with an autism spectrum disorder. PhD dissertation, Texas Woman's University, Houston, TX. Retrieved from Dissertations & Theses: Full Text (Publication No. AAT 3399069) 9 March 2012.

Eriksson M, Lindstrom B (2006) Antonovsky's sense of coherence scale and the relation with health: a systematic review. *J Epidemiol Health* 60: 376–381. http://dx.doi.org/10.1136/jech.2005.041616

*Garmezy N, Masten AS (1991) The protective role of competence indicators in children at risk. In: Cummings EM, Greene AL, Karraker KH, editors. *Life-span Developmental Psychology: Perspectives on Stress and Coping*. Mahwah, NJ: Lawrence Erlbaum Publishers, pp. 151–174.

*Garmezy N, Rutter M, editors (1983) *Stress, Coping, and Development*. New York: McGraw-Hill.

*Hart B, Risley T (1995) *Meaningful Differences in the Everyday Lives of Children*. New York: Brookes Publishing.

*Hassall R, Rose J, McDonald J (2005) Parenting stress in mothers of children with an intellectual disability: the effects of parental cognitions in relation to child characteristics and family support. *J Intellect Disabil Res* 49: 405–418. http://dx.doi.org/10.1111/j.1365-2788.2005.00673.x

Hawley CA, Ward AB, Magnay AR, Long J (2003) Parental stress and burden following traumatic brain injury amongst children and adolescents. *Brain Injury* 17: 1–23. http://dx.doi.org/10.1080/0269905021000010096

Helff CM, Glidden LM (1998) More positive or less negative? Trends in research on adjustment of families rearing children with developmental disabilities. *Ment Retard* 36: 457–464. http://dx.doi.org/10.1352/0047-6765(1998)036<0457:MPOLNT>2.0.CO;2

Kausar S, Jevne RF, Sobsey D (2003) Hope in families of children with developmental disabilities. *J Dev Disabil* 10: 35–46.

Kearney PM, Griffin T (2001) Between joy and sorrow: being a parent of a child with developmental disability. *J Adv Nurs* 34: 582–592. http://dx.doi.org/10.1046/j.1365-2648.2001.01787.x

King GA, Zwaigenbaum L, King S, Baxter D, Rosenbaum P, Bates A (2006) A qualitative investigation of changes in the belief systems of families of children with autism or Down syndrome. *Child Care Health Dev* 32: 353–369. http://dx.doi.org/10.1111/j.1365-2214.2006.00571.x

*Laucht M, Esser G, Schmidt MH (1997) Developmental outcome of infants born with biological and psychosocial risks. *J Child Psychol Psychiatry* 38: 843–854. http://dx.doi.org/10.1111/j.1469-7610.1997.tb01602.x

Lawson J (2004) Disclosing childhood impairment and the consequences for professional relationships. *Practice* 16: 273–281. http://dx.doi.org/10.1080/09503150500046095

*Lloyd TJ, Hastings R (2009) Hope as a psychological resilience factor in mothers and fathers of children with intellectual disabilities. *J Intellect Disabil Res* 53: 957–968. http://dx.doi.org/10.1111/j.1365-2788.2009.01206.x

Locke J, Rotheram-Fuller E, Kasari C (2012) Exploring the social impact of being a typical peer model for included children with autism spectrum disorder. *J Autism Dev Disabil* 42: 1895–1905. doi:10.1007/s10803-011-1437-0.

*Luthar SS, Zigler E (1991) Vulnerability and competence: a review of research on resilience in childhood. *Am J Orthopsychiatry* 61: 6–22. http://dx.doi.org/10.1037/h0079218

Lyubomirsky S, King L, Diener E (2005) The benefits of frequent positive affect: does happiness lead to success? *Psychol Bull* 131: 803–855. http://dx.doi.org/10.1037/0033-2909.131.6.803

Margalit M, Kleitman T (2006) Mothers' stress, resilience, and early intervention. *Eur J Spec Needs Educ* 21: 269–283. http://dx.doi.org/10.1080/08856250600810682

Margalit M, Raviv A, Ankonina DB (1992) Coping and coherence among parents with disabled children. *J Clin Child Psychol* 21: 202–209. http://dx.doi.org/10.1207/s15374424jccp2103_1

Margalit M, Leyser Y, Ankonina DB, Avraham Y (1991) Community support in Israeli kibbutz and city families of disabled children: family climate and parental coherence. *J Spec Educ* 24: 427–440. http://dx.doi.org/10.1177/002246699102400404

*Masten AS (2001) Ordinary magic: resilience processes in development. *Am Psychologist* 56: 227–238. http://dx.doi.org/10.1037/0003-066X.56.3.227

Morris C (2009) Measuring participation in childhood disability: does the capability approach improve our understanding? *Dev Med Child Neurol* 51: 92–102. http://dx.doi.org/10.1111/j.1469-8749.2008.03248.x

Oelofsen N, Richardson P (2006) Sense of coherence and parenting stress in mothers and fathers of preschool children with developmental disability. *J Intellect Dev Disabil* 31: 1–12. http://dx.doi.org/10.1080/13668250500349367

*Papousek M (2011) Resilience, strengths, and regulatory capacities: hidden resources in developmental disorders of infant mental health. *Infant Ment Health J* 32: 29–46. http://dx.doi.org/10.1002/imhj.20282

Rosenbaum P, King S, Law M, King G, Evans J (1998) Family-centred services: a conceptual framework and research review. *Physiother Occupat Ther Pediatr* 18: 1–20. http://dx.doi.org/10.1080/J006v18n01_01

Rutter M (1979) Protective factors in children's responses to stress and disadvantage. In: Kent MW, Rolf JE, editors. *Primary Prevention in Psychopathology, Vol. 8. Social Competence in Children*. Hanover, NY: University Press New England, pp. 49–74.

Sameroff A (1999) Ecological perspectives on developmental risk. In: Osofsky JD, Fitzgerald HE, editors. *WAIMH Handbook of Infant Mental Health, Vol. 4. Infant Mental Health Groups at Risk*. New York: Wiley, pp. 223–248.

Sanders MR (1999) Triple-P Positive Parenting Program: towards an empirically validated multilevel parenting and family support strategy for the prevention of behaviour and emotion problems in children. *Clin Child Fam Psychol Rev* 2: 71–89. http://dx.doi.org/10.1023/A:1021843613840.

Schonert-Reichl KA, LaRose M (2008) Considering resilience in children and youth: fostering positive adaptation and competence in schools, families, and communities. The National Dialogue on Resilience and Youth Conference, 17–19 November, Winnipeg, MN. Available at: www.thelearningpartnership.ca/page.aspx?pid=468 (accessed 2 March 2012).

*Scorgie K, Sobsey D (2000) Transformational outcomes associated with parenting children who have disabilities. *Ment Retard* 38: 195–206. http://dx.doi.org/10.1352/0047-6765(2000)038<0195:TOAWPC>2.0.CO;2

Seccombe K (2002) 'Beating the odds' versus 'changing the odds': poverty, resilience, and family policy. *J Marriage Fam* 64, 384–394. http://dx.doi.org/10.1111/j.1741-3737.2002.00384.x

Seligman MEP, Csikszentmihalyi M (2000) Positive psychology: an introduction. *Am Psychol* 55: 5–14. http://dx.doi.org/10.1037/0003-066X.55.1.5

Siller M, Sigman M (2008) Modeling longitudinal change in the language abilities of children with autism: parent behaviors and child characteristics as predictors of change. *Dev Psychol* 44: 1691–1704. http://dx.doi.org/10.1037/a0013771

Smith V (2004) Preventing Early Reading Failure. Unpublished dissertation, University of British Columbia, Vancouver, BC.

*Snyder CR (2002) Hope theory: rainbows in the mind. *Psychol Inquiry* 13: 249–275. http://dx.doi.org/10.1207/ S15327965PLI1304_01

Snyder CR, Harris C, Anderson JR, Holleran SA, Yoshinobu L, Gibb J, et al (1991) The will and the ways: development and validation of an individual – differences measure of hope. *J Pers and Soc Psychol* 60: 570–585. http://dx.doi.org/10.1037/0022-3514.60.4.570

Snyder CR, Sympson SC, Ybasco FC, Borders TF, Babyak MA, Higgins RL (1996) Development and validation of the State Hope scale. *J Pers Soc Psychol* 70: 321–335. http://dx.doi.org/10.1037/0022-3514.70.2.321

*Snyder CR, Rand KL, Sigmon DR (2002) Hope theory: a member of the positive psychology family. In: Snyder CR, Lopez SJ, editors. *Handbook of Positive Psychology.* New York: Oxford University Press, pp. 257–276.

Sussman F (2008) *More than Words: Helping Parents Promote Communication in Children with Autism Spectrum Disorders.* Toronto, ON: The Hanen Centre.

*Walsh F (2003) Family resilience: a framework for clinical practice. *Fam Process* 42: 1–8. http://dx.doi. org/10.1111/j.1545-5300.2003.00001.x

Warfield ME (2005) Family and work predictors of parenting role stress among two earner families of children with disabilities. *Infant Child Dev* 14: 155–176. http://dx.doi.org/10.1002/icd.386

Webster-Stratton C (2001) The Incredible Years: Parents, teachers, and children's training series. Seattle, WA: The Incredible Years.

Werner EE (1993) Risk, resilience, and recovery: perspectives from the Kauai Longitudinal Study. *Dev Psychopathol* 5: 503–515. http://dx.doi.org/10.1017/S095457940000612X

Werner EE, Smith RS (1982) *Vulnerable but Invincible: A Study of Resilient Children.* New York: McGraw-Hill.

Werner EE, Smith RS (1992) *Overcoming the Odds: High-risk Children from Birth to Adulthood.* New York: Cornell University Press.

*Werner EE, Smith RS (2001) *Journeys from Childhood to Midlife: Risk, Resilience and Recovery.* New York: Cornell University Press.

World Health Organization (2001) *International Classification of Functioning, Disability and Health.* Geneva: World Health Organization.

*Wright MO, Masten A (2006) Resilience processes in development: fostering positive adaptation in the context of adversity. In: Goldstein S, Brooks RB, editors. *Handbook of Resilience in Children.* New York: Springer, pp. 17–47.

11
THE FAMILY DOES MATTER!

Lucyna Lach

Overview

Almost all children and adolescents are raised in the context of some type of family; certainly, all children are born into one. Most practitioners would agree with the uncontroversial statement that the family is an important determinant of child well-being (an essential 'environmental' context, in World Health Organization terms). However, far more compelling yet complicated questions include: 'What aspects of family are important to the well-being of children and adolescents?' and 'To what extent are these characteristics important in comparison to other factors?' This chapter starts with the assumption that there are aspects of the family that are important to the well-being of all children; when a child has a neurological or a developmental condition, there are additional challenges that must be addressed by the family. This suggests that something more is required of the family unit than would otherwise be the case. Using theoretical depictions and empirical studies that address family function of children with neurological and developmental conditions, this chapter strives to unpack the various dimensions, both generic and extraordinary, that provide a substantive basis for our point of departure, which is that the family matters!

What counts as family in our contemporary and diverse society?

Prior to embarking on this important story about families of children with neurological and developmental conditions, it is incumbent on us to define what constitutes a family, as there are multiple definitions, each highly contingent on who is defining family and for what purpose. For example, family as defined by a geneticist refers to a group of individuals who are biologically connected. Such a definition is important for tracking intergenerational transmission of genetic information, a diagnostic procedure that is essential to understanding inheritance, probability of exposure to risk, and phenotypic expression of disease. A sociologist is more likely to refer to a family as a network of individuals who operate within a range of specified roles, share a past and a future, and are bound by a commitment to one another. Such a definition helps us to understand how the nature of family has been informed by historical, social, political, and economic circumstances. Alternatively, a psychologist or social worker may view the family as a group of individuals who are emotionally, behaviourally, and/or cognitively connected (Crosbie-Burnett and Klein 2009). For these professionals, meeting with the 'family' or reference to 'family' in a psychosocial assessment rarely connotes the consideration of every biologically or socially connected member. Instead, family for these professionals becomes a type of shorthand term used for those who are most affected by or implicated in the issue at hand.

In reviewing the theoretical and empirical literature about children with neurological and developmental conditions as a source for how 'family' is constructed in the social science literature, the meaning of 'family' is equally heterogeneous. Journal articles and chapter titles may use the word 'family' to refer to family characteristics such as the style of communication or extent of closeness or cohesion among family members (e.g. Hiemen and Berger 2008). Alternatively, it may be used to refer to parent stress (e.g. Glenn et al 2008), mental or physical health (e.g. Miodrag and Hodapp 2011), or parenting (e.g. Rodenburg 2006). The meaning of the term 'family' in the literature is therefore quite broad and multidimensional and is sometimes used somewhat indiscriminately, making the comparison of studies quite challenging. For this reason, this chapter will be broad in its coverage of what constitutes 'family matters', covering theoretical and empirical literature about the family, the parents (mothers and fathers), and parenting, as each brings us closer to understanding what it is about the family that matters.

Family matters

When thinking about and/or studying 'the family', one must decide whether to pay attention to documenting family pathology or family strengths or both. There is certainly a legacy for each of these perspectives in the literature; overall an emphasis on documenting pathology prevails. The first part of the story about families of children with neurological and developmental conditions asks the question: Are families of children with neurological and developmental conditions worse off than other families? Population-based studies are known for their rigour in sampling and generalizability. They have unequivocally established that families of children with neurological and developmental conditions are more distressed than those in which children do not have these chronic conditions, and that the risk for distress is higher when their children are also behaviourally dysregulated (Raina et al 2005, Brehaut et al 2009, 2011, Lach et al 2009). Clinical studies echo this same finding (e.g. Majnemer et al 2012).

There are, however, two caveats to this story. First, only a small proportion of the sample score in what would be considered the clinically distressed range, indicating that most are not clinically impaired. Second, we really know nothing from population-based studies about family characteristics that reflect a more positive valence about families, such as how engaged or close family members feel towards one another among families of children with neurological and developmental conditions and how they compare to those without. This kind of question lends itself more readily to smaller clinical studies that are typically not as rigorous in design but that allow for the use of much more specific and interesting measures of family function. For example, families of children with neurological and developmental conditions were asked to reflect on the positive and negative ways in which their child's disability had an impact on their family life (Trute and Heibert-Murphy 2002, Trute et al 2007). Qualitative studies also document how parents experience fatigue, loss of sleep, employment, and worry about their child's future, as well as simultaneously experiencing inspiration (Davis et al 2009).

ACCORDING TO FAMILY THEORY

Family systems theory has been used extensively to understand the way in which families respond and adapt to challenges, imposed both internally and externally. As an interactional system, the family comprises smaller subsystems (e.g. parental, marital, sibling groupings) and is embedded within larger systems (e.g. health, school, neighbourhood groupings). The structure of the family is rendered visible through the ways in which roles are assigned and negotiated and how boundaries are maintained (Cox and Paley 1997). The latter refers to the nature of relational lines dividing individual family members and family subsystems (e.g. parents, parent–child, spouses). One of the ways in which boundaries operate is to monitor the extent to which information is exchanged within and across systems. A family whose boundaries are closed would be one that does not easily permit external stimuli and information to influence its internal operations and that maintains an emotional distance from health professionals; a family whose boundaries are more open and permeable allows for the flow of information both in and out of the family system, providing members with an opportunity to process new information and to make changes accordingly (Minuchin et al 2007).

One can imagine how a newly immigrated family that does not yet understand the way in which Western health systems work may be worried about the extent to which health system information is made available to 'immigration officials' and so are wary of 'professionals'. As a result they disclose very little about their personal beliefs, attitudes, or understandings, thereby appearing to have more closed boundaries, and they engage only minimally with well-meaning healthcare providers. They may be viewed as disengaged or even hostile (Fadiman 1998). Alternatively, a family that easily discloses intimate details of family life and may expect professionals to be unconditionally available to them by email or telephone, and page or text professionals at inopportune times, is likely to have boundaries that are at the other end of the spectrum. Appreciating that boundaries are psychologically and socially informed allows professionals to address family matters in a way that demonstrates respect for the diverse ways in which family boundaries are constructed while taking responsibility for negotiating and maintaining how their own expectations of family boundaries intersect with these.

The example above describes how family systems theory serves as a metatheory for practice issues. It is beyond the scope of this chapter to cover all relevant family theories: a comprehensive overview is provided elsewhere (Boss et al 1993). However, two models that warrant individual attention are Olson's Circumplex Model of Family Functioning (Olson 2000) and models of family resilience (McCubbin et al 1996, Patterson 2002). Both types of models contain very important ideas about concepts that are relevant when considering what it is that matters about the family.

The matter of family adaptability and cohesion

In viewing the family as an interactional system, family *adaptability* is the degree to which a family is flexible and can regain equilibrium in an environment that challenges its core beliefs, values, traditions, and rules for behaviour. Among families whose child has a neurological or developmental condition, adaptability is particularly important as changes in the child's condition, new stage-related developmental challenges, or changes in the systems that provide care require the family to adapt its routines and familiar ways of operating to accommodate these extraordinary demands. For example, parents of children with epilepsy adapt their routines to accommodate seizures and ensure safety. The following excerpt[a] is taken from an interview with a mother of a 15-year-old female with epilepsy who is describing how she and her husband have had to adapt to their daughter's seizures:

> Yes, it's all part of who [she is], and we treat that like anything. It's all part of our lifestyle now. We don't stop everything when she's having a seizure. Life doesn't stop in the family. [For example], we're on our way to somewhere, I remember my mom, my mom and dad's anniversary mass. We're on our way to go to mass and she had a seizure. And I just [thought] 'well, we'll just be ten minutes behind everybody, you know' [laughs]. We just arrived in the church later, and she was tired, she just curled up next to me in the pew. We just carried on. We wouldn't just stop, never. Or, um, we never think 'we're not going to do this', you know. Now, there are some things that we used to do, downhill skiing, and we don't do that with Martha. So Martha doesn't take lessons. Teresa [her sister] and Robert [her father] do that. She's learned [that] there are things that are not safe for her to do. Like we went scuba diving and she didn't do that; and, we went snorkelling; she went snorkelling, but again, keeping her close to you. You just never know. She could have one [a seizure] out in the ocean. And teaching her things, like logical things, like when we're out on the dock, she walks in between Bob and I, just in case she has a seizure and went flying in, you know. Water is what scares us you know. In the pool, one of us has to say, 'OK, I'm watching'. Even at this age [laughing], you'd think by fifteen, but we can't sit and drink or socialize around the pool with friends. One of us has to pay attention to Martha.

What is particularly striking is how this family balanced its need to maintain the integrity of valued family routines but did so in a way that maximized the daughter's safety. The creative ways in which parents ensured participation while managing issues of safety was echoed by other parents of adolescents who had to weigh in on invitations for sleepovers and requests to join and participate in organized team sports, high school dances, and other typical peer group activities. The tension between safety and promotion of increased independence is typical in all families, including ones who have a child with a neurodevelopmental impairment. Adolescents with neurological and developmental conditions are no less likely to want to engage in developmentally typical activities than are other adolescents: families are not 'spared' these developmental crises. In fact, they may be amplified among those who have adolescents with neurological and developmental conditions.

---

a   Identifying data have been altered throughout this chapter to ensure anonymity.

Family *cohesion*, the second of the dimensions, refers to the degree of closeness and con-nectedness within a family. In 'typical' family function terms, cohesion is considered in the context of the family's stage of development. That is, the degree of closeness/proximity of family members to one another is a function of the developmental stage of the children in the family and what is required of family members in their 'coming of age'. When a family is in the stage of rearing school-aged or adolescent children with neurological and developmental conditions, the normative sense of family cohesion is necessarily altered as the opportunities related to 'coming of age' are altered. The degree of closeness and connectedness may be prolonged either temporarily or indefinitely depending on the child's level of impairment.

> … because everyone is so connected in our family in terms of relationships, because we need to be. And there is this tremendous sense of cooperation and everyone just knows it. It's like we need to work together here because if I'm not accessible to assist Henry when he gets, when he, um, goes down for a seizure, then someone else better step in, and there's just no question about it … Yeah he's the, like his sister, from a young age, when we were out, she would just do it, not because we expected her to or told her to. It was only just because of a matter of circumstance, you know it was. So I think I think the relationship and the things are, I guess that word 'intense' just keeps coming back. It's so much a part of it.

Family members may be willing and able to maintain higher levels of cohesion for a period of time. However, as siblings grow older and educational, vocational, or romantic partnerships call them away from the familial home, roles are reassigned and the family con-figuration that had contributed to a sense of cohesion is challenged. Sustaining these same levels over longer periods is clearly more challenging as siblings age and parents grow older (McMillan 2005). However, the story about families managing this transition is not always a negative one. When researchers enquire about the positive aspects of raising a child or living with a sibling who has a neurological or developmental condition, families describe how this has brought them closer together in a way that might otherwise not have been possible (Dykens 2005, Findler and Vardi 2009). Over time, siblings find ways of maintaining the expertise that they have gained throughout their lifetime and generate creative ways of remaining engaged in spite of other obligations (Kuo and Lach 2012).

The matter of family stress
The shift to enquiring about positive aspects of family life has been driven by family theorists Hamilton McCubbin and Joan Patterson. Starting with Hill's (1949) ABCX family crisis model, which articulated how a family's experience of stress was contingent on the type of stressor, the family's crisis-meeting resources, and the meaning that the crisis had for the fam-ily, they identified a more complex process towards adaptation to family stressors, referring to the model as the Double ABCX Model (McCubbin et al 1983). After this, it appears that McCubbin and Patterson parted ways. Patterson referred to her version of the model as the

Family Adjustment and Adaptation Model (Patterson 1988, 2002), while the McCubbins went on to develop the Typology Model of Family Adjustment and Adaptation (McCubbin et al 1987) and the Resiliency Model of Family Stress, Adjustment, and Adaptation (McCubbin and McCubbin 1996). This series of models was essentially driven by an attempt to unpack the process of family adjustment and adaptation in response to the question 'Why do some families who are faced with similar stressful circumstances fare better than others?' The following describes key concepts from this group of models and applies them to families of children with neurological and developmental conditions.

Stressor

There are events or experiences that occur at the individual, family, or community level (Patterson 1988) such as a parent learning about his or her child's diagnosis for the first time, the family's experience of the adolescent transitioning out of high school, or the sudden and unexpected reduction of support offered to the family by the school or social service agency. When grouped with strains such as demands placed on one's time and energy, and daily hassles such as getting children to school on time or ensuring that adequately nutritious meals are consumed, these factors represent demands placed on a family that require the deployment of resources.

Stress

This term refers to the state of the individual, family, or community in response to the stressor. Stress may be functional and experienced as a normal/typical part of daily living; when experienced in excess, it may be quite problematic. In the later version of McCubbin and Patterson's models, there was no variable called 'stress' per se. Instead, stress was treated as the process that the family went through in responding to various stressors in their lives, a definition similar to that of Lazarus (1999).

Appraisal

The experience of any particular stressor for one family is not the same as it is for another. This is partly mitigated by the way in which the stressor is evaluated or appraised; the meaning of the stressor for the individual and the family therefore varies. For some, the same stressor may represent an impediment, loss, or difference that they never anticipated, while for others that same stressor may be appraised as a challenge or even possibly a gift that has caused them and their family to re-evaluate their priorities. This means that parents raising a child with a neurological or developmental condition such as intellectual impairment, autism, or Down syndrome can generate, when asked, an appraisal of their experience as one of tremendous hardship and loss, while others may represent their experience as enriching individual family members as well as the family as a whole (King et al 2009). What is most interesting is that these experiences are rarely connoted as exclusively one or the other. Most often, family members can simultaneously articulate both positive and negative aspects of their experience (Frederickson and Losada 2005): when asked questions with a positive valence such as 'What are the kinds of ways in which raising your son/daughter has had a positive impact on your family?' family members are invited to reflect on aspects such as growth, insight, and enrichment; when asked questions with a negative valence, such as 'How has raising your son/daughter been hard on your family?', a different narrative is invited. Both perspectives are subjective, but both are highly relevant and are consistent with the complexity of how families experience raising a child with neurological and developmental conditions (Trute et al 2007, 2010).

Coping

This highly popularized term is used to reflect how a family as a whole, as well as its individual members, responds to stressors. The response may be physical, cognitive, emotional, and/or behavioural, and is directed at restoring a balance between demands on resources and the resources available to meet those demands. McCubbin et al (1987) grouped family coping strategies into five patterns: reducing the number and/or intensity of demands on resources, acquiring additional resources, maintaining existing resources, managing tension, and changing the meaning of a situation. Resources referred to individual characteristics such as physical health and time, to family resources such as support and communication, and to community resources such as health services.

The diagnosis of a neurological or developmental condition during adolescence requires families to adjust their routines to accommodate the increased need for independence and proximity to peers. This requires a shift in the rules and organization associated with the way in which family members spend time together. Expectations need to be adjusted regarding energy that is dedicated to doing activities together as a family versus energy expended facilitating activities with peers outside of the family. The challenge for all families is to maintain a sense of family connectedness and cohesion while creating opportunities for the adolescent to engage safely in activities with peers outside the family home (e.g. attending school dances, going to see a film). When there is a child with a neurological or developmental condition, that normative tension may be more difficult to navigate as adolescents may not have the same opportunities, or, if they exist, the opportunities require the mobilization of additional resources. For example, in our study regarding the quality of life of children with epilepsy, some parents described being quite active in creating, facilitating, and organizing opportunities for their adolescents to engage socially. In addition, they were 'on-call' in case seizures occurred outside the family home.

> … for some reason, the Sony Playstation would bring on seizures. I remember he said, 'Oh Mom, I just want to go to Gerry's [a friend's] place,' and I said, 'OK, OK, you can go.' I said, 'No problem,' and I said to Gerry, 'Here's the phone number and if something happens, phone me, I will come and get him.' And, he got there, fifteen minutes later the phone rang and it was his mother on the phone, 'Oh, I don't know what's wrong with Peter. He's passed right out. I can't get him to come out. Come, he's unconscious.' So I went over and I said … she knew, but she didn't know it would be this bad, right, so he never went back again.

In the above example, 15-year-old Peter asked for permission to be with his friend Gerry; however, ensuring the success and safety of this very typical social experience was much more complicated. It required his own mother to be 'on alert', ready to step up should the need arise, as well as an appropriate and not overexaggerated response by Gerry and his mother. Parents of children with neurological and developmental conditions may find that coping with the adolescent's desire for increased autonomy is a stressor and that one way of managing the tension that this provokes is to err on the side of permissiveness, hoping for the best. In the above example, this required Peter's mother to acknowledge the potential risk and to demonstrate a willingness to set it aside in order to support her son's desire for autonomy.

Family resilience

Theory and research related to resilience emerged from psychology (Garmezy 1996, Rutter 2006), and the concept was introduced into the lexicon of family stress theory with an equivalent level of variability in its understanding. Definitions and applications range from ones that treat resilience as a 'trait' (e.g. this family is 'resilient') to viewing it as a 'process' whereby risk and protective factors interact with one another to inform family outcome (also discussed in Chapter 10). In the former, resilience is a characteristic of the family that reflects high levels of bonding and flexibility among family members (McCubbin and McCubbin 1987); the latter treats resilience as an outcome of a process of risk and protective factors interacting with one another to produce a well-adjusted/-adapted family in spite of the stressors it has faced. Adjustment/adaptation would be evaluated by the degree to which the family has been able to sustain a sense of balance and harmony. Applied to families raising a child with neurological and developmental conditions, resilience is evident in families that are faced with significant stressors associated with their child's condition who manage to use their established ways of interacting with one another, their resources, their appraisal mechanisms, and their problem-solving to achieve balance and harmony within the family environment and between family members and the community within which they live.

According to Studies

What makes a difference to family well-being?

Practitioners sometimes reflect on what the impact is of a particular neurological or developmental condition, such as cerebral palsy or spina bifida, on the family. Although an important question to ask, there are also other factors that inform the well-being of families. An exhaustive review of these is beyond the scope of this chapter. However, income and ethnicity will be used to illustrate this point.

In the UK, a majority of children at risk of intellectual impairment spend their early years in very disadvantaged socio-economic circumstances (i.e. 63% live in income poverty at age 3 years). Therefore, children whose development is already compromised are growing up in conditions that will further limit their family's well-being and their own (Emerson et al 2008). When compared with other families, families of children with intellectual impairment experience greater instability and financial hardship, especially single mothers and partners in a cohabitating relationship (Parish et al 2008). When they were 36 years old, mothers of children with impairments were less likely to have job spells lasting more than 5 years and had lower earnings than mothers of children without impairments. Further, as their children grew older there was a trend for them to be less likely to have full-time jobs (Parish et al 2004). Most studies control for socio-economic indicators in an effort to remove them from explaining various outcomes, including family well-being. Yet, lower levels of income are linked to higher levels of family need for support (Almasri et al 2011). To carry this further, the extent to which parents feel supported informs their parenting behaviours and influences their child's well-being (McConnell et al 2010). The ripple effect is substantial. Although indicators of socio-economic disadvantage are sometimes referred to as 'distal factors', the process of removing their explanatory value by 'controlling for socio-economic status' not only connotes that little can be done to improve the financial circumstances of families of children with neurological and developmental conditions, it also relegates the consideration of poverty to the sidelines. Income support programmes such as federal tax incentives and matched registered disability savings programmes can make a difference to the well-being of families and should not be so readily discounted. Their impact, as well as the impact of poverty on family well-being, deserves further study.

Another factor that is often described but not accounted for in studies of children with impairments is that of ethnicity. This is unfortunate as there is some evidence that families from different ethnic backgrounds experience the impact of their child's disability in different ways; furthermore, factors that inform their experience also vary by ethnocultural background (Neely-Barnes and Marcenko 2004). As clinically obvious as this may seem, few studies have systematically examined this question. For example, the way in which children with cerebral palsy are integrated into family life in the Taiwanese culture (Kuo and Lach 2012) may be very different from how they are integrated in families living in the wealthy neighbourhoods of San Francisco. One cannot assume that family values related to integration are similar across cultures, or that they are homogeneous within any particular culture. What this means is that more studies need to be done to address these questions, making ethnicity a front- and centre-stage phenomenon, rather than a backstage one. In the meantime, practitioners can best adopt a stance of cultural naivety. Through a process of questioning, families from various cultures can 'teach' practitioners about their values related to issues such as integration and their ways of operating as a family [for illustration read Fadiman's (1998) book]. This approach is consistent with a family-centred perspective, which is considered best practice for all families.

What difference does family make to parent and child well-being?
From a family systems perspective, the family environment is one of the contexts within which parents and children grow and interact. The quality of that environment will therefore have an impact on the well-being of both. Families of children with cerebral palsy who had higher levels of unmet needs related to information and financial support were also families most likely to have parents with high levels of distress (Glenn et al 2008). The family's ability to adapt to external stimuli and changes is essential and has been shown to predict change in maternal depression over time (Baker et al 2011a) as well as parent stress (Glenn et al 2008). Similarly, it predicts change in child behaviour problems (Baker et al 2011b). The directionality of the

relationship between family environment and child behaviour is not unequivocally causal and linear, as child behaviour and functional limitations also inform the degree of burden and stress experienced by the family (Majnemer et al 2012).

This 'chicken and egg' dilemma has really *not* been resolved in the literature. The relationships are probably bidirectional and transactional, and operate in a circular feedback loop over time. The issue is further complicated by the fact that the central nervous system is implicated in the regulation of child behaviour (see also Chapter 7). In a prospective study conducted by Austin et al (2001), newly diagnosed children with epilepsy were administered measures evaluating the extent of behavioural dysregulation at that time. Even before the family had an opportunity to 'react' to the diagnosis and develop entrenched problematic patterns of interaction, levels of behavioural dysregulation were already inordinately high. The authors strongly suggested that this could be related to an intrinsic brain abnormality. This study was significant in its impact as it cast doubt on the strength of the assumption that family environment was responsible for behaviour problems among children with epilepsy.

Parents matter
It is well known that parents of children with various types of neurological and developmental conditions are at higher risk for symptoms of depression, anxiety, and stress (Singer 2006, Bailey et al 2007, Gray et al 2011). They are also at higher risk for physical health problems such as migraines, back pain, and arthritis (Lach et al 2009). Questions are sometimes raised about whether parents of children with diagnosis 'A' are better or worse off than parents of children with diagnosis 'B' – and some literature supports this proposition. For example, Abbeduto et al (2004) found that mothers of adolescents and young adults with autism reported higher levels of pessimism and higher levels of depressive symptoms than did the mothers of adolescents and young adults with Down syndrome. Others argue that comparing how well mothers of one diagnostic group are doing with another is not helpful as it masks the variability within any particular diagnosis and minimizes characteristics shared across these diagnoses (Stein and Jessop 1982). (These non-categorical issues are also discussed in Chapter 2.) In other words, there are mothers who are doing better and mothers doing less well in each of those groups, and their well-being may be more of a function of the child's behaviour than the diagnosis per se. In Abbeduto et al's (2004) study, for example, adolescents and young adults diagnosed with autism had significantly higher levels of behavioural issues than those with Down syndrome. Therefore, the difference in caregiver pessimism and depressive symptoms may be a function of the diagnosis or of the behaviour.

These observations suggest that caregiver outcomes should be investigated across neurological and developmental conditions, rather than by diagnosis, and that characteristics of the child's function such as ability to walk, reason, communicate, or regulate their behaviour might be as informative as the diagnosis per se. When caregivers of children with neurological and developmental conditions are grouped in this 'non-categorical' manner and compared with caregivers whose children do not have neurological and developmental conditions, they are worse off in terms of their physical, psychological, and health outcomes, and behavioural dysregulation issues have an additive effect (Lach et al 2009). In another non-categorical study of caregivers of children with various diagnoses associated with intellectual impairment, caregivers whose children had higher levels of social adjustment problems and mental health issues had higher rates of mental health problems than caregivers whose children did not display these difficulties (Gray et al 2011). These findings provide an example of how it is not just the child's diagnosis that has an impact on parents' well-being, but that comorbid symptoms related to other types of functional impairment play a significant role.

Factors associated with indicators of parental well-being include the presence of intellectual impairment in the child with cerebral palsy (Glenn et al 2008) and the number of children with impairments in the family (Abbeduto et al 2004, Orsmond et al 2007). Among mothers and fathers of children with fragile X syndrome, the child's level of adaptive skills predicted paternal stress while the strongest predictor of maternal stress was marital satisfaction (McCarthy et al 2006). Among mothers of adolescents and young adults with autism, anxiety was higher when social support networks were smaller and when more stressful life events were experienced (Barker et al 2011). In another non-categorical study of parents of children with intellectual impairment, both behaviour problems and low levels of hope were significant predictors of depression and anxiety among mothers, but only low levels of hope were significant for the fathers. The authors wondered whether the caregiver role, rather than gender, may account for the differences between mothers and fathers (Lloyd and Hastings 2009). The issue of directionality in relation to parental well-being and child difficulties is similar to that of family well-being and child difficulties. As researchers begin to examine the strength of both relationships (child difficulties predicting parent stress and vice versa) within the same study and over time, causal findings implicating child difficulties as stronger causal factors of parent stress than the reverse begin to form the evidence base for this relationship (McConnell et al 2010).

Parenting matters
The consideration of family matters would not be complete without a discussion about parenting. Although scholars have attempted to conceptualize and measure parenting through dimensions such as parenting practices, parenting styles, parenting behaviours, and parenting cognitions, it is almost impossible to compare studies, as what is referred to by one scholar as a parenting practice is called something entirely different by another. For example, in an effort to distinguish between parenting 'practices' and parenting 'styles', Darling and Steinberg (1993) operationalized parenting practices as parental strategies that have a direct effect on the development of specific child behaviours. Parenting practices were distinguished from parenting styles as the latter were defined as 'a constellation of attitudes towards the child that are communicated to the child and create an emotional climate in which the parents' behaviours are expressed' (Darling and Steinberg 1993: 493). Others distinguish parenting 'practices' from 'styles' by referring to the former as what parents do (e.g. spank, hug), and the latter as to how they do it (e.g. with warmth or hostility) (Locke and Prinz 2002). What Darling and Steinberg (1993) refer to as parenting style (e.g. attitudes) is referred to by Bugental and Johnston (2000) as parenting cognitions (e.g. thoughts, attributions, and beliefs held by parents with respect to their children and to their own parenting practices and behaviours). As a result, there is absolutely no conceptual consensus or consistency to guide what is meant by 'parenting'.

In an effort to create internal consistency, a typology of parenting has been created in order to group studies together for a systematic review of observational studies of parenting of children with neurological and developmental conditions (Lach et al 2010): parenting as experienced, parenting as enacted, and disability-related parenting.

PARENTING AS EXPERIENCED

Parenting as experienced is defined conceptually as the thoughts and beliefs that parents have about themselves as parents or about parenting their child. This includes parents' experience of themselves in their parenting role (i.e. how efficacious they feel, how worried they are), their beliefs and attitudes about their parenting (i.e. how parents should be towards their child), and schemata and attributions they make about their child in the parenting relationship (child's responsiveness to them).

A population-based Canadian study compared how effective parents perceived their parenting to be. Parents of children with neurological and developmental conditions were compared with parents whose children had externalizing behaviour impairments, parents whose children had both neurological and developmental conditions and externalizing behaviour impairments, and parents whose children had neither. After controlling for sociodemographic characteristics, ineffective parenting scores of caregivers of children in the 'neither' group remained significantly lower than those in the other groups, with caregivers of children in the 'both' group reporting the highest ineffective parenting scores (Garner et al 2011). These findings suggest that there is a relationship between parents' experience of how effective they are in their parenting and the complexity of their child's condition. They do not, however, confirm that having a child with both a neurological and developmental condition and externalizing behaviour impairments *leads to* ineffective parenting or vice versa. This can only be tested longitudinally, and, even then, any conclusion arrived at would be tentative as it is impossible to evaluate parents' sense of effectiveness prior to learning about their child's diagnosis.

There are some fairly robust findings connecting different aspects of the family environment to parenting as experienced. Higher levels of social support were associated with lower levels of ineffective parenting (McConnell et al 2010). Parents with higher than average levels of marital satisfaction experienced lower levels of parenting burden (Hartley et al 2011). In the latter study, mothers reported having a closer relationship than fathers with their son/ daughter with autism spectrum disorder (Hartley et al 2011). However, fathers with above-average marital satisfaction perceived themselves to have a closer parent–child relationship than fathers with below-average marital satisfaction (Hartley et al 2011). Among parents of children with severe intellectual impairment, lower levels of family distress, as indicated by level of family cohesion and conflict, were associated with lower levels of parenting distress, an indicator of a more positive parenting experience (Blacher et al 1997). Therefore, in studies that differentiated the family environment from parenting, different aspects of the family environment informed parenting as experienced. These findings also suggest that interventions could directly target how parents experience their effectiveness or how burdened they feel, or try to increase parents' perception of social support or marital satisfaction, with the expectation that parents will experience their parenting in a more positive way.

PARENTING AS ENACTED

Parenting as enacted is a term developed to capture the behavioural aspects of parenting – that is, what parents and others think they do when they parent their child. This refers to observable aspects of parenting such as how supportive, directive, critical, or autonomy-promoting a parent's behaviour is towards his or her child. The behaviour may have a positive, negative, or neutral valence, and may refer to a strategy or style that a parent uses when interacting with the child (e.g. authoritative). For example, mothers of children with Down syndrome use more teacher- and helper-like behaviours, particularly at mealtime, and fewer positive verbalizations than mothers of typically developing children (Pino 2000). In comparison with a nationally representative sample of mothers of children without impairments, mothers of adolescent and adult children with autism spectrum disorder spent significantly more time providing childcare and doing chores and less time in leisure activities. Argumentative exchanges were also more common among mothers of individuals with autism spectrum disorder. However, mothers of individuals with autism spectrum disorder reported similar levels of positive interactions as the comparison group (Smith et al 2009).

Consistency is a quality of parenting as enacted as it is observable and parents and others can generate an evaluation of the degree to which they are consistent in their 'behaviour' towards their child. In the Garner et al (2011) study noted above, caregivers of children in the 'both' and externalizing behaviour impairments groups were significantly less consistent in their parenting than were caregivers of children in the neurological and developmental condition and 'neither' groups.

In Smith et al's (2008) investigation of positive maternal behaviours maternal warmth, praise, and relationship quality were related to subsequent reductions in internalizing and externalizing behaviour problems and an abatement of autism symptoms (i.e. repetitive behaviours and social reciprocity) among adolescents and young adults with autism spectrum disorder. These findings contrast with previous work by the same research team that focused on more negative maternal behaviours, in which high levels of maternal expressed emotion (e.g. criticism and negativity) were associated with increases in maladaptive behaviours and symptoms in adolescent and adult children with autism (Greenberg et al 2006). In a follow-up study, changes in maternal criticism predicted levels of behavioural problems 7 years later (Baker et al 2011b).

Child characteristics such as less severe maladaptive behaviours, better health, and reduced social impairment, as well as characteristics of the mother (lower levels of pessimism), were predictive of more positive mother–child relationships as evaluated by measures of demonstration of warmth, criticism, and positive affect among mothers of adolescents and young adults with autism (Orsmond et al 2006). In a much more dated study using a younger sample, the degree of emotional support provided by mothers of school-aged children with epilepsy was associated with the child's confidence, flexibility, positive affect, and social acceptance (Lothman et al 1990).

DISABILITY-SPECIFIC ASPECTS OF PARENTING

Parenting a child with a neurological or developmental condition demands something more from parents than parenting a typically developing child. Parents have to find different ways of accommodating and responding to the child's behaviour and signals, both verbal and non-verbal. Although it takes time, they eventually adjust their worldviews and expectations of themselves, their family, and their child (King et al 2005). Some have shown that, through a process of reappraisal (Paster et al 2009), parents begin to appreciate the positive contribution their child makes and the reconstructed possibilities that lie ahead. Furthermore, there are things that parents do, such as bathing, dressing, and feeding, that go on indefinitely over their child's life-course. Therefore, disability-related parenting refers to those things that parents do such as attend appointments, advocate, case-manage, administer medications, communicate with their child's school, etc. that are unique to parenting a child with a neurological or developmental condition. Similarly, these parents experience worry about their child's future and courtesy stigma and they generate representations of themselves that are specific to parenting a child with a neurological or developmental condition (see also Chapter 12 on stigma). Much of this aspect of parenting is beginning to be documented through qualitative studies, as measures to capture these unique dimensions of parenting are not yet well developed (e.g. Ray 2002). These will hopefully be developed in the future, as they will help to capture the complexity of parenting children with neurological and developmental conditions.

Conclusion

The review of literature in this chapter has highlighted the important roles that parents and parenting play in the lives of families of children with neurological and developmental conditions. The logical conclusion is that interventions should focus on providing parents with adequate support to parent their child in a manner that optimizes everyone's development. The most recent meta-analysis of different types of parenting interventions provided to parents of children with neurological and developmental conditions suggests that they are more effective than no treatment (Singer et al 2007). However, there is a potential for a paradoxical message in this finding. The more empowering message is that parents and families can make a difference. The other message is that, if parents can make a difference and fail to do so, the risk is that they will feel blamed. This is a nuanced conclusion that must be addressed by practitioners who encourage and/or deliver such programmes, insofar as parenting interventions work better for some than for others, and their success is highly contingent on numerous factors, only one of which has to do with parents' adherence to the intervention and to implementing optimal parenting practices.

The role that families play in the lives of children is irrefutable: children are part of families and families are essential and important partners in the provision of care. From both an ethical and an empirical standpoint adherence to a family-centred approach to practice is not negotiable. In spite of this, implementation remains a challenge (Darrah et al 2010) and we still hear practitioners blaming families for their child's challenging behaviours, sometimes referring to them in ways that are disrespectful and disempowering of the tacit knowledge families have about their child. Notwithstanding how difficult it is to engage meaningfully with all families at all times, we recommend that practitioners remain vigilant in their efforts to adhere to family-centred principles of practice (Rosenbaum et al 1998). [A full discussion of family-centred services is beyond the scope of this chapter. Interested readers are directed to a series of reports about family-centred services on the *CanChild* website (www.canchild.ca).]

Given that some parents and families experience high levels of distress, more attention needs to be paid to their well-being during our encounters with them in practice. It is also important to remember that families of children with neurological and developmental conditions also experience positive aspects in their relationships with one another and with their child (Charles and Berman 2009). *Although the child is almost always the point of entry into the health and social service system, asking parents about their well-being as well as the well-being of their family members remains best practice* (Head and Abbeduto 2007). Enquiry about well-being should be not only about symptoms of anxiety, depression, and stress, but also about ways in which the family is managing distress, meeting each others' needs, and growing. An invitation into a conversation that balances the challenges with the hopes and successes will be a strong signal about the fact that the family matters!

REFERENCES

Key references

*Abbeduto L, Seltzer MM, Shattuck P, Krauss MW, Orsmond G, Murphy MM (2004) Psychological well-being and coping in mothers of youths with autism, Down syndrome, or fragile X syndrome. *Am J Ment Retard* 109: 237–254. http://dx.doi.org/10.1352/0895-8017(2004)109<237:PWACIM>2.0.CO;2

Almasri N, Palisano RJ, Dunst LA, Chiarello A, O'Neil ME, Polansky M (2012) Profiles of family needs of children and youth with cerebral palsy. *Child Care Health Dev* 38: 798–806. http://dx.doi.org/10.1111/j.1365-2214.2011.01331.x

Austin JK, Harezlak J, Dunn DW, Huster GA, Rose DF, Ambrosius WT (2001) Behavior problems in children before first recognized seizure. *Pediatrics* 107: 115–122. http://dx.doi.org/10.1542/peds.107.1.115

Bailey DB, Golden RN, Roberts J, Ford A (2007) Maternal depression and developmental disability: research critique. *Ment Retard Dev Disabil Res Rev* 13: 321–329. http://dx.doi.org/10.1002/mrdd.20172

Baker JK, Seltzer MM, Greenberg JS (2011a) Longitudinal effects of adaptability on behaviour problems and maternal depression in families of adolescents with autism. *J Fam Psychol* 25: 601–609. http://dx.doi.org/10.1037/a0024409

*Baker JK, Smith LE, Greenberg JS, Seltzer MM, Taylor JL (2011b) Change in maternal criticism and behaviour problems in adolescents and adults with autism across a 7-year period. *J Abnorm Psychol* 120: 465–475. http://dx.doi.org/10.1037/a0021900

Barker ET, Hartley SL, Seltzer MM, Floyd FJ, Greenberg JS, Orsmond GI (2011) Trajectories of emotional well-being in mothers of adolescents and adults with autism. *Dev Psychol* 47: 551–561. http://dx.doi.org/10.1037/a0021268

Blacher J, Shapiro J, Lopez S, Diaz L, Fusco J (1997) Depression in Latina mothers of children with mental retardation: a neglected concern. *Am J Ment Retard* 101: 483–496.

Boss PG, Doherty WJ, LaRossa R, Schumm WR, Steinmetz SK (1993) *Sourcebook of Family Theories and Methods: A Contextual Approach*. New York: Plenum Press. http://dx.doi.org/10.1007/978-0-387-85764-0

Brehaut JC, Kohen DE, Garner RE, et al (2009) Health among caregivers of children with health problems: findings from a Canadian population-based study. *Am J Public Health* 99: 1254–1262. http://dx.doi.org/10.2105/AJPH.2007.129817

Brehaut JC, Garner RE, Miller AR, et al (2011) Changes over time in the health of caregivers of children with health problems: growth curve findings from a 10-year Canadian population-based study. *Am J Public Health* 101: 2308–2316. http://dx.doi.org/10.2105/AJPH.2011.300298

Bugental DB, Johnston C (2000) Parental and child cognitions in the context of the family. *Annu Rev Psychol* 51: 315–344. http://dx.doi.org/10.1146/annurev.psych.51.1.315

CanChild (2012) Family-centred services sheets. Available at: http://www.canchild.ca/en/childrenfamilies/fcs_sheet.asp (accessed 26 June 2012).

*Charles NC, Berman RC (2009) Making space for positive constructions of the mother–child relationship: the voices of mothers of children with autism spectrum disorder. *J Assoc Res Mothering* 11: 180–198.

Cox MJ, Paley B (1997) Families as systems. *Annu Rev Psychol* 48: 243–267. http://dx.doi.org/10.1146/annurev.psych.48.1.243

Crosbie-Burnett M, Klein DM (2010) The fascinating story of family theories. In: Bray JH, Stanton M, editors. *The Wiley-Blackwell Handbook of Family Psychology*. Oxford: Blackwell Publishing, pp. 37–52.

Darling N, Steinberg L (1993) Parenting style as context: an integrative model. *Psychol Bull* 113: 487–496. http://dx.doi.org/10.1037/0033-2909.113.3.487

Darrah J, Wiart L, Magill-Evans J, Ray L, Andersen L (2010) Are family-centred principles, functional goal setting and transition planning evident in therapy services for children with cerebral palsy? *Child Care Health Dev* 38: 41–47. http://dx.doi.org/10.1111/j.1365-2214.2010.01160.x

Davis E, Shelly A, Waters E, Boyd R, Cook K, Davern M (2009) The impact of caring for a child with cerebral palsy: quality of life for mothers and fathers. *Child Care Health Dev* 36: 63–73. http://dx.doi.org/10.1111/j.1365-2214.2009.00989.x

Dykens EM (2005) Happiness, well-being, and character strengths: outcomes for families and siblings of persons with mental retardation. *Ment Retard* 43: 360–364.

Emerson E, Graham H, McCulloch A, Blacher J, Hatton C, Llewellyn G (2008) The social context of parenting 3-year old children with developmental delay in the UK. *Child Care Health Dev* 35: 63–70. http://dx.doi.org/10.1111/j.1365-2214.2008.00909.x

Fadiman A (1998) *The Spirit Catches You and You Fall Down: A Hmong Child, Her American Doctors, and the Collision of Two Cultures.* New York: Farrar, Strauss and Giroux.

Findler L, Vardi A (2009) Psychological growth among siblings of children with and without intellectual disabilities. *Intellect Dev Disabil* 47: 1–12. http://dx.doi.org/10.1352/2009.47:1-12

Fredrickson BL, Losada MF (2005) Positive affect and the complex dynamics of human flourishing. *Am Psychol* 60: 678–686. http://dx.doi.org/10.1037/0003-066X.60.7.678

Garmezy N (1996) Reflections and commentary on risk, resilience, and development. In: Haggerty RJ, Sherrod LR, Garmezy N, Rutter M, editors. *Stress, Risk, and Resilience in Children and Adolescents: Processes, Mechanisms, and Interventions*. Cambridge: Cambridge University Press, pp. 1–18.

*Garner RE, Arim RG, Kohen DE, et al (2011) Parenting children with neurodevelopmental disorders and/or behaviour problems. *Child Care Health Dev* (epub ahead of print, 9 November). http://dx.doi.org/10.1111/j.1365-2214.2011.01347.x

Glenn S, Cunningham C, Poole H, Reeves D, Weindling M (2008) Maternal parenting stress and its correlates in families with a young child with cerebral palsy. *Child Care Health Dev* 35: 71–78. http://dx.doi.org/10.1111/j.1365-2214.2008.00891.x

Gray KM, Piccinin AM, Hofer SM, et al (2011) The longitudinal relationship between behaviour and emotional disturbance in young people with intellectual disability and maternal mental health. *Res Dev Disabil* 32: 1194–1204. http://dx.doi.org/10.1016/j.ridd.2010.12.044

*Greenberg JS, Seltzer MM, Hong J, Orsmond GI (2006) Bidirectional effects of expressed emotion and behaviour problems and symptoms in adolescents and adults with autism. *Am J Ment Retard* 111: 229–249. http://dx.doi.org/10.1352/0895-8017(2006)111[229:BEOEEA]2.0.CO;2

Hartley SL, Barker ET, Seltzer MM, Greenberg JS, Floyd FJ (2011) Marital satisfaction and parenting experiences of mothers and fathers of adolescents and adults with autism. *Am J Intellect Dev Disabil* 116: 81–95. http://dx.doi.org/10.1352/1944-7558-116.1.81

Head LS, Abbeduto L (2007) Recognizing the role of parents in developmental outcomes: a systems approach to evaluating the child with developmental disabilities. *Ment Retard Dev Disabil Res Rev* 13: 293–301. http://dx.doi.org/10.1002/mrdd.20169

*Heimen T, Berger O (2008) Parents of children with Asperger syndrome or with learning disabilities: family environment and social support. *Res Dev Disabil* 29: 289–300. http://dx.doi.org/10.1016/j.ridd.2007.05.005

Hill R (1949) *Families Under Stress: Adjustment to the Crises of War Separation and Reunion*. New York: Harper.

King GA, Zwaigenbaum L, King S, Baxter D, Rosenbaum P, Bates A (2006) A qualitative investigation of changes in the belief systems of families of children with autism or Down syndrome. *Child Care Health Dev* 32: 353–369. http://dx.doi.org/10.1111/j.1365-2214.2006.00571.x

Kuo YC, Lach LM (2012) Life decisions of Taiwanese women who care for a sibling with cerebral palsy. *Health Care Women Int* 33: 646–665.

*Lach LM, Kohen DE, Garner RE, et al (2009) The health and psychosocial functioning of caregivers of children with neurodevelopmental disorders. *Disabil Rehabil* 31: 607–618. http://dx.doi.org/10.1080/09638280802242163

Lach LM, Saini M, Bailey S, et al (2010) Systematic review methods for observational studies: challenges and solutions. *Cochrane Colloquium Abstracts Journal*, October 18–22, 2010. Available at: www.imbi.uni-freiburg.de/OJS/cca/index.php?journal=cca&page=article&op=view&path[]=9635 (accessed 20 April 2012).

Lazarus R (1999) *Stress and Emotion: A New Synthesis*. New York: Springer Publishing.

Lloyd TJ, Hastings R (2009) Hope as a psychological resilience factor in mothers and fathers of children with intellectual disabilities. *J Intellect Disabil Res* 53: 957–968. http://dx.doi.org/10.1111/j.1365-2788.2009.01206.x

Locke LM, Prinz RJ (2002) Measurement of parental discipline and nurturance. *Clin Psychol Rev* 22: 895–929. http://dx.doi.org/10.1016/S0272-7358(02)00133-2

Lothman DJ, Pianta RC, Clarson SM (1990) Mother–child interaction in children with epilepsy: relations with child competence. *J Epilepsy* 3: 157–163. http://dx.doi.org/10.1016/0896-6974(90)90102-5

McCarthy A, Cuskelly M, van Kraayenoord CE, Cohen J (2006) Predictors of stress in mothers and fathers of children with fragile X syndrome. *Res Dev Disabil* 27: 688–704. http://dx.doi.org/10.1016/j.ridd.2005.10.002

McConnell D, Breitkreuz R, Savage A (2010) From financial hardship to child difficulties: main and moderating effects of perceived social support. *Child Care Health Dev* 37: 679–691. http://dx.doi.org/10.1111/j.1365-2214.2010.01185.x.

McCubbin HI, Patterson JM (1983) The family stress process – the Double ABCX model of adjustment of adaptation. *Marriage Fam Rev* 6: 7–37. http://dx.doi.org/10.1300/J002v06n01_02

McCubbin MA, McCubbin HI (1987) Family stress theory and assessment: the T-Double ABCX model of family adjustment and adaptation. In: McCubbin HI, Thompson A, editors. *Family Assessment for Research and Practice*. Madison, WI: University of Wisconsin-Madison, pp. 3–32.

McCubbin MA, McCubbin HI (1996) Resiliency in families: a conceptual model of family adjustment and adaptation in response to stress. In: McCubbin HI, Thompson AI, McCubbin MA, editors. *Family Assessment: Resiliency, Coping and Adaptation – Inventories for Research and Practice*. Madison, WI: University of Wisconsin-Madison, pp. 1–64.

McMillan E (2005) A parent's perspective. *Ment Retard* 43: 351–353.

*Majnemer A, Shevell J, Law M, Poulin C, Rosenbaum P (2012) Indicators of distress in families of children with cerebral palsy. *Disabil Rehabil* 34: 1202–1207.

Minuchin S, Nichols MP, Lee WY (2007) *Assessing Families and Couples: From Symptom to System*. Boston: Pearson/Allyn and Bacon.

*Miodrag N, Hodapp RM (2011) Chronic stress and its implications on health among families of children with intellectual and developmental disabilities (I/DD). *Int Rev Res Dev Disabil* 41: 127–161. http://dx.doi.org/10.1016/B978-0-12-386495-6.00004-7

Neely-Barnes S, Marcenko M (2004) Predicting impact of childhood disability on families: results from the 1995 National Health Interview Survey Disability Supplement. *Ment Retard* 42: 284–293. http://dx.doi.org/10.1352/0047-6765(2004)42<284:PIOCDO>2.0.CO;2

Olson DH (2000) Circumplex model of marital and family systems. *J Marital Fam Ther* 22: 144–167.

Orsmond GI, Seltzer MM, Greehberg JS, Kraus MW (2006) Mother–child relationship quality among adolescents and aduilts with autism. *Am J Ment Retard* 111: 121–137. http://dx.doi.org/10.1352/0895-8017(2006)111[121:MRQAAA]2.0.CO;2

Orsmond GI, Lin LY, Seltzer MM (2007) Mothers of adolescents and adults with autism: parenting multiple children with disabilities. *Intellect Dev Disabil* 45: 257–270. http://dx.doi.org/10.1352/1934-9556(2007)45[257:MOAAAW]2.0.CO;2

*Parish SL, Seltzer MM, Greenberg JS, Floyd F (2004) Economic implications of caregiving at midlife: comparing parents with and without children who have developmental disabilities. *Ment Retard* 42: 413–426. http://dx.doi.org/10.1352/0047-6765(2004)42<413:EIOCAM>2.0.CO;2

Parish SL, Rose RA, Grinstein-Weiss M, Richman EL, Andrews ME (2008) Material hardship in U.S. families raising children with disabilities. *Exceptional Children* 75: 71–92.

Paster A, Brandwein D, Walsh J (2009) A comparison of coping strategies used by parents of children with disabilities and parents of children without disabilities. *Res Dev Disabil* 30: 1337–1342. http://dx.doi.org/10.1016/j.ridd.2009.05.010

Patterson JM (1988) Families experiencing stress: the family adjustment and adaptation response model. *Fam Syst Med* 5: 202–237. http://dx.doi.org/10.1037/h0089739

Patterson JM (2002) Integrating family resilience and stress theory. *J Marriage Fam* 64: 349–360. http://dx.doi.org/10.1111/j.1741-3737.2002.00349.x

Pino O (2000) The effect of context on mother's interaction style with Down's syndrome and typically developing children. *Res Dev Disabil* 111: 155–169.

Raina P, O'Donnell M, Rosenbaum P, et al (2005) The health and wellbeing of caregivers of children with cerebral palsy. *Pediatrics* 115: e626–e636. http://dx.doi.org/10.1542/peds.2004-1689

Ray L (2002) Parenting and childhood chronicity: making visible the invisible work. *J Ped Nurs* 17: 424–438. http://dx.doi.org/10.1053/jpdn.2002.127172

Rodenburg R (2006) Family predictors of psychopathology in children with epilepsy. *Epilepsia* 47: 601–614. http://dx.doi.org/10.1111/j.1528-1167.2006.00475.x

Rosenbaum P, King S, Law M, King G, Evans J (1998) Family-centred services: a conceptual framework and research review. *Phys Occup Ther Pediatr* 18: 1–20. http://dx.doi.org/10.1080/J006v18n01_01

Rutter M (2006) Implications of resilience concepts for scientific understanding. *Ann N Y Acad Sci* 1094: 1–12. http://dx.doi.org/10.1196/annals.1376.002

Singer GHS, Ethridge BL, Aldana SI (2007) Primary and secondary effects of parenting and stress management interventions for parents of children with developmental disabilities: a meta-analysis. *Ment Retard Dev Disabil Res Rev* 13: 357–369. http://dx.doi.org/10.1002/mrdd.20175

Smith LE, Greenberg JS, Seltzer MM, Hong J (2008) Symptoms and behaviour problems of adolescents and adults with autism: effects of mother–child relationship quality, warmth, and praise. *Am J Ment Retard* 113: 387–402. http://dx.doi.org/10.1352/2008.113:387-402

*Smith LE, Hong J, Seltzer MM, Greenberg JS, Almeida DM, Bishop SL (2010) Daily experiences among mothers of adolescents and adults with autism spectrum disorder. *J Autism Dev Disord* 40: 167–178. http://dx.doi.org/10.1007/s10803-009-0844-y

Stein REK, Jessop DJ (1982) A noncategorical approach to chronic childhood illness. *Public Health Rep* 97: 354–362.

Trute B, Hiebert-Murphy D (2002) Family adjustment to childhood developmental disability: a measure of parent appraisal of family impacts. *J Ped Psychol* 27: 271–280. http://dx.doi.org/10.1093/jpepsy/27.3.271

Trute B, Hiebert-Murphy D, Levine K (2007) Parental appraisal of the family impact of childhood developmental disability: times of sadness and times of joy. *J Intellect Dev Disability* 32: 1–9. http://dx.doi.org/10.1080/13668250601146753

*Trute B, Benzies KM, Worthington C, Reddon JR, Moore M (2010) Accentuate the positive to mitigate the negative: mother psychological coping resources and family adjustment in childhood disability. *J Intellect Dev Disabil* 35: 36–43. http://dx.doi.org/10.3109/13668250903496328

12
STIGMA: A PERVASIVE CONTEXTUAL BARRIER

Ann Jacoby and Joan K. Austin

Overview

Illness stigma has long been a key concept in the sociology and psychology of health and illness (Weiss et al 2006). The role of stigma in the lived experience of illness, particularly chronic illness, has been the focus of a considerable body of research. Illness stigma has been identified as a significant public health issue, because it can act as a health stressor additional to the index health problem, and as a barrier to optimal health care for the primary condition of ill health. Much of the work on illness stigma has explored its meaning and significance for chronically ill adults. This chapter focuses on the issue of the nature and impact of such stigma for children and young people, with a particular focus on 'invisible' and 'intermittently visible' disabilities (and in particular epilepsy). In doing so, it draws on the wider literature on illness stigma but focuses on stigma concepts first, with particular relevance to the age groups in question. It concludes with a consideration of factors that may help children, young people, and their families address the challenges, both visible and invisible, of this important potential barrier to coping with living with a chronic neurodevelopmental condition. Throughout, the chapter draws heavily on the literature relating to the condition of epilepsy, which has been the area of our own research interests and which, we believe, stands as an excellent 'tracer' condition for the arguments presented here, as much of what the epilepsy literature offers can be generalized to the other neurodevelopmental conditions addressed in this book.

Why is ill health stigmatizing?

Any discussion of the nature of illness stigma inevitably starts with the pioneering work of Irving Goffman (1963), in whose classic text, *Stigma*, it is delineated as relating to three major categories, one of which is the stigma arising from 'abominations of the body' (Goffman 1963). Many writers on this subject have explored why and to what extent such physical incapacity and ill health should be a focus of stigma. Jones et al (1984) see illness stigma as a psychological response of the anxious 'well' when reminded of the future possibility of pain, tragedy, and death in their own lives. In a similar vein, illness stigma has been attributed to the idea of illness as posing a psychological threat, by representing some kind of danger to the taken-for-granted moral universe (Das 2001). Ablon (2002) highlights that, to appreciate why particular conditions of ill health are stigmatized over others, consideration needs to be given to the nature of the stigmatized illness, its historical connotations, and its attributed characteristics. Thus, she argues, mental illness is stigmatizing because it represents unpredictability, and leprosy because it is associated with gross disfigurements disturbing to those seeing them. Writing in relation to epilepsy, a common neurological condition of childhood, Bagley (1972) argues that stigmatizing concepts of epilepsy are based in a kind of 'anomic terror', as people with epilepsy are seen as doing what others fear doing themselves, namely losing control and reverting to 'the primitive'.

Other authors have argued for a more biologically driven basis for illness stigma, which in their analysis rests on the perceived inability of the ill to contribute effectively to society. Parsons (1951) characterized ill health as a state of deviance in relation to societal expectations and the obligations of its members, and hence as subject to social stigma. Following Parsons, Reidpath et al (2005) suggest that those experiencing chronic ill health are stigmatized because they are unable to contribute to the same extent as others in their social group. Their reduced social value to the group leads to stigma and social exclusion. Such arguments may be more clearly applicable to adult ill health than to conditions of childhood, as the social imperative to contribute to society is relevant for adults in a way that is not the case for children. Nonetheless, children with chronic illnesses may be marked out as representing not just a present but also a future drain on societal resources and as those that are likely to break the social rules of 'reciprocal exchange'.

Anthropological studies have been important in highlighting how culturally specific beliefs about the causes and prognosis of conditions of ill health determine their definition as socially relevant and the link to negative stereotypes, and hence how they are managed both individually and collectively (for some epilepsy-specific examples see Fadiman 1998, Ismail et al 2005, Allotey and Reidpath 2007, Winkler et al 2010). Such studies highlight the fact that the social course of a condition is 'organized as much by what is at stake for participants in [*their*] local world as it is by the biology of the condition' (Kleinman et al 1995). In the case of childhood illness, the participants are other family members as well as the affected child, and what is at stake for them will also be highly relevant to the process of illness adjustment, the management of potential stigma, and any associated expressions of discrimination.

What are the mechanisms for illness stigma?

Link and Phelan (2001) have proposed that stigma exists only when a series of interrelated conditions converge. In the first instance, human differences must be defined as socially relevant; next, these differences must be linked to negative stereotypes; then, such stereotypes must lead to social separation; this, in turn, creates status loss and discrimination. Crocker et al (1998) highlight the pervasiveness of many social stigmas, which are often absorbed at an early age, reinforced through the media and public consciousness, and so often accessed automatically, both by those who do not even consciously agree with them and by those who are their targets. This accessing of negative stereotypes leads to tension and anxiety and, in extremis, to rejection in the interactions between stigmatized and non-stigmatized individuals. Mulhbauer (2002) points out that such anxiety and rejection are played out not just at an individual level but also at interpersonal and institutional levels, where they are enshrined in laws and statutes aimed at control of the stigmatized group.

In the context of the present volume, then, it is important to recognize that parents of children with neurodevelopmental conditions do not operate within a family vacuum. Their attitudes and beliefs are informed by those of the wider society in which they live, as well as by their own experience of the illness in question (Marteau and Johnson 1986). Where such attitudes are negative, parents may well absorb and integrate them into their understanding of the meaning and social consequences implied by a diagnosis of a particular chronic condition in their child. This in turn may present enormous psychological challenges to them. Parents may manage such challenges by rejection or denial of societal attitudes or, conversely, by projection of their own negative attitudes onto their affected child.

Are neurodevelopmental conditions stigmatizing and, if so, why?

Ablon (2002) notes that there are particular diseases that are commonly treated 'with special fear, dread or repulsion'. She quotes Sontag (1978), who writes that, 'Any important disease whose causality is murky and for which treatment is ineffectual tends to be awash with significance' for stigma. This can certainly be said to be the case, at least historically, for a number of neurodevelopmental conditions. As an example, epilepsy has consistently been defined across time and place as an 'undesired differentness' (Goffman 1963), a condition attributable to malignant or magical causes. Even in the present day, despite scientific advances that have allowed theories of causality to be clarified and effective treatment strategies to be defined, epilepsy remains shrouded in misinformation and misbeliefs that contribute significantly to the major negative life impacts associated with this condition for young people as much as for adults (Jacoby and Austin 2007). For example, in a recent US survey of 19 000 teenagers (Austin et al 2002), only 31% said they would consider dating someone with epilepsy and 75% agreed that teenagers with epilepsy were more likely to be bullied or picked on by their peers. In a UK study (Robson 2006) college students reported that they would avoid mixing socially with a fellow student with epilepsy. Although in this study the rationale for avoidance was based on fears about managing a seizure should one occur, rather than more negative stereotypes, such expressions of rejection among peers are likely to engender internalized stigma in those at whom they are projected.

Stigma of neurodevelopmental conditions in the context of family

Role of Family Attitudes

Family members, particularly parents but also siblings and grandparents, are key actors in a stigma drama in which a child with a neurodevelopmental condition takes centre stage, and, as for any chronic childhood illness, the argument has been made that, if parents hold negative attitudes, they will be prevented from adjusting to the diagnosis of that disease in their child – and their own lack of adjustment will in turn translate into poor adjustment in their child

(Hansen and Hill 1964, Voeller and Rothenberg 1973). Where family members' reactions are negative, the child will probably learn to think negatively about his or her condition; where family members seek to hide or deny the condition, the child will learn a script of silence. Todd and Shearn (1997) investigated how parents were engaged in shaping the identities of their offspring with intellectual impairments. These authors note the centrality of parents in the interpretation of messages about the disabled child. They comment that, 'Parents are likely to be significant actors in providing their offspring with a sense of self that incorporates the social and moral meanings associated with LD' (intellectual impairments) – meanings that are almost universally stigmatizing. Likewise, Rodenburg et al (2006) showed in the context of epilepsy that parental rejection, which was rooted in negative attitudes, was a key predictor of psychopathology in the affected child.

The issue of stigma and its role in parental adjustment to the diagnosis of chronic childhood illness has also been examined by Austin et al (1984), who studied 50 parents of children aged 6 to 14 years with a definite diagnosis of epilepsy but no other medical problems. Parental attitudes were assessed using a measure that addressed five major areas, including social stigma from epilepsy, effect on the family, and activity restriction. The authors found a strong positive relationship between mothers' (though not fathers') attitudes and the level of their adjustment to their child's condition, which they suggest may reflect mothers' generally higher level of involvement in the care of their child. Maternal attitude and perception of seizure control together accounted for 60% of the variance in maternal adjustment scores. However, in contrast to previous studies that assumed negative attitudes to epilepsy on the part of parents, this study found them to hold both negative and positive attitudes in parallel, suggesting that 'parental attitudes are more complex than previously described'.

A further complexity touched on by Todd and Shearn (1997) in the context of intellectual impairment, but highly relevant for neurodevelopmental conditions generally, is that for many of those affected their impairment is recognized at birth or very early on in their life and often at a point at which they themselves will have no awareness of the significance of the label assigned to them. It has been argued that, in such circumstances, children do not have to go through the process of the biographical disruption and reconstruction required in adults developing chronic illness or impairment (Bury 1982), having been socialized to their roles from birth. However, the counterargument has been proffered that it takes time for children to become aware that they are different from their peers and that the length of the time lag may be a significant one. Parents, aware of the potential for stigma of their child's condition, may actively seek to extend the time lag, constructing a 'protective capsule' within which 'self-belittling definitions of [*the child*] are prevented from entering the charmed circle' (Goffman 1963). However, as the child ages, the parents' ability to maintain this protection and ward off stigma diminishes, and the child gradually comes to recognize his or her difference from peers and the limitations accompanying such difference. The 'final facing of facts' (Glidden and Zetlin 1992) can then be a highly fraught process for child and parent alike.

COURTESY STIGMA AND COACHING FOR STIGMA

Two concepts emerging from the illness stigma literature as key for the lived experience of children with a chronic, potentially stigmatizing illness are those of 'courtesy stigma' and 'stigma coaching'. The former embodies the idea that stigma can extend beyond the person directly labelled to include connected others, in particular other close family members. This has been shown to be the case in conditions as diverse as acquired immune deficiency syndrome or infection with the human immunodeficiency virus (Alonzo and Reynolds 1995) and Alzheimer's disease (MacRae 1999). Kleinman and colleagues (1995) explored the concept of courtesy stigma in their study of epilepsy in China. Kleinman described how in the Chinese culture epilepsy was and still is seen as representing 'loss of face', not just to the affected person but also to his or her whole family, threatening other family members' life aspirations and life chances. In the Western context, West (1979) found that parents of children with epilepsy often experienced a deep sense of shame, their child being seen as conferring shame and stigma on the whole family by virtue of being 'odd'. This idea of courtesy stigma may help to explain the levels of stress (Austin et al 1992) and even rejection of the affected child (Levin et al 1988, Suurmeijer 1995) that have been documented as sometimes present in families of children with epilepsy – and which probably extends to families of children with other neurodevelopmental conditions.

One outcome of courtesy stigma, coupled with parental acceptance of negative social stereotypes, is that parents may come to act as 'stigma coaches' to their child with a neurodevelopmental condition, teaching them that it represents an 'undesired differentness' (Goffman 1963) and a moral weight to bear. Such parents may also practise what Schneider and Conrad (1983) refer to as 'disabling talk', during which they focus on the restrictions such conditions impose and coach their affected child to conceal their condition from others. In their study parents emerged as acting forcibly as the moral arbiters of the meaning of 'having epilepsy', some treating it as a normal medical condition and others quick to inculcate a sense of shame in their affected child.

Stigma of a neurodevelopment condition in the wider social context

While family members, particularly parents, emerge as key figures in the process by which children and young people with a condition of ill health come to acknowledge its potential for stigma, there are other potential actors in this drama. It has been pointed out that school is a critical social environment for children, and teachers are key significant others, who may well endorse the negative attitudes of those closer to home (Prpic et al 2003). Ablon (2002) notes that for a child whose stigma is either visible or known, starting school 'typically constitutes the first major confrontation with societal institutions, norms and systematic public scrutiny' and signals trauma that may be 'temporary or may continue for the rest of his or her life.' Of particular relevance for children with a neurodevelopmental condition is the finding that teachers tend to hold the same negative attitudes as recorded in studies of the wider public. Studies across the world report this to be the case. Taking the example of epilepsy, studies report teachers objecting to having pupils so affected in their class, assuming such children to be less capable of high academic achievement, limiting their engagement in school activities, and perceiving them to be more aggressive and disruptive in class than other pupils (Dantas et al 2001, Bishop and Slevin 2004, Bishop and Boag 2006). Work by Katzenstein et al (2007) examined how the label 'epilepsy' affected teachers' ratings of children's academic achievement when compared with their actual academic performance. When teachers were aware that a child had epilepsy, they rated their achievement lower than when they were unaware of the diagnosis – and this was despite the fact that the children labelled as having epilepsy performed no worse than their unlabelled peers on objective tests. The authors commented that, when teachers perceive children as performing poorly solely on the basis of being labelled as having a condition to which stigma attaches, such children will be disadvantaged for receiving optimal educational support. They express concern about the potential for a 'self-fulfilling prophecy' of failure and reduced self-concept.

What is the quality of life impact of such stigma?

There is a large body of literature that documents reductions in quality of life for both children and adults with chronic ill health. Considering children and adolescents with neurodevelopmental conditions specifically, studies indicate that quality of life impairments are seen in the context of their family and social relationships (see, for example, Koller et al 1988, Todd et al 1990, Olsson and Campenhausen 1993, Jalava et al 1997, Kerr et al 2011), their educational performance and outcomes and subsequent employment status (see Evans et al 1994, Austin et al 1996, Jalava et al 1997, Chin et al 2011), and their psychological well-being (see Austin et al 1992, Lee et al 2008, Hamiwka et al 2011, Stevanovic et al 2011, Vega et al 2011). Here we briefly highlight some relevant studies.

A study by Emerson et al (2009) examined the well-being of adolescents and young adults with long-term health conditions, impairments, or disabilities, including, though not confined to, neurodevelopmental conditions. The authors reported that, when compared with their non-impaired peers, this group were significantly more likely to be living under conditions known to put their sense of well-being at risk. Thus, they were more socially isolated, had fewer educational qualifications, and were more likely to be excluded from the labour force and hence to experience poverty and hardship. Although the reductions recorded in their well-being cannot be solely attributed to the effects of stigma and discrimination, the authors nonetheless suggest that they reflect a failure of governmental policies, framed around the principles of rights and participation, to address these issues, which may represent a form of implicit stigma. In a study in the USA, Maslow et al (2011a,b) compared educational, vocational, and social status in young adults who had grown up with a chronic illness and those who had not. They found that those with a childhood chronic condition were as likely as those without to have had romantic relationships, got married, and had children, but were less likely to have graduated from college or be employed. The authors propose that further investigation is warranted of the role of mediators for poor outcomes, such as school absenteeism, cognitive impairment, and parental stress (which may itself reflect perceived stigma). They further raise the issue that some conditions of childhood ill health, including some neurodevelopmental ones, may fall outside the definition of disability that would ensure they receive the supports known to be effective in improving educational and vocational outcomes. Although not suggested by the authors, an argument can be made that stigma and discrimination are also potential mediators, of which failures in the provision of support services are an indicator.

Several authors allude to the idea that stigma – indirectly and/or in ways difficult to measure – affects quality of life outcomes for children with neurodevelopmental conditions. For example, Räty et al (2003) compared the quality of life of adolescents and young adults with epilepsy with that of their typically developing peers and found that self-ratings of level of competency in relation to activities, social relations, and school achievement were much poorer among children with epilepsy than among their typically developing peers. Although the authors recognize the possible contribution of neurological deficits to these differences, they also suggest that stigma probably played a large part in determining quality of life. Likewise, the long-term negative effects on quality of life in adulthood of a diagnosis of epilepsy in childhood have been documented by Sillanpää and colleagues (Jalava et al 1997), who note the persistence of such effects, even when epilepsy goes into remission in the childhood years. The authors also raise the spectre of stigma in explaining this apparent inconsistency in their findings. Finally, social stigma is proposed as a possible explanation for the reductions in quality of life reported by Austin et al (1996), and as potentially interfering with the ability of the adolescents with epilepsy '… to accomplish psychosocial developmental tasks successfully'. The authors also note that even when their condition was inactive (i.e. they were no longer experiencing seizures), adolescents with epilepsy fared badly, signalling the possibility of a 'double whammy' for neurodevelopmental conditions, wherein the negative effects of neurological dysfunction (which in the case of epilepsy probably persists after seizures remit) are compounded by adjustment problems that are rooted in stigma.

Austin et al's (1996) conclusions are reinforced by the findings of other authors (Ronen et al 1999, Kerr et al 2011) who explored factors contributing to the perceived impact of epilepsy on quality of life. Stigma that was feared, perceived, or experienced was identified as occupying an important role, with children and adolescents reporting feeling that they were seen by their peers as 'weird' and that they were bullied, teased, or laughed at as a result. They were also well aware of being treated differently from their siblings and peers by their parents, teachers, and peers, with negative impacts for the quality of their lives. Interestingly, Oostrom et al (2000) have reported that both children with epilepsy and typically developing children attach greater shame to having epilepsy than to having other chronic illnesses or impairments.

Coping with a neurodevelopmental condition and the role of stigma

Writing in the context of intellectual impairment, Edgerton (1967) comments that 'to find oneself as a mental retardate is to be burdened by a shattering stigma … the ultimate horror.' This then begs the question as to how people with an impairment or health condition that is so socially stigmatizing can retain a positive sense of self and how others can facilitate them doing so. Edgerton examined stigma as experienced by former inpatients with mild intellectual impairment now discharged to the community. He notes that the lives of those involved were directed towards the twin aims of denying that they were 'mentally incompetent' (Edgerton 1967: 145) and passing as 'normal', and thus to enabling themselves to preserve some sense of self-esteem. As admission of the reality of their being was totally unacceptable to them, these individuals often found complex ways to explain both their previous confinement and their present incompetencies. In their attempts to cope with the threat of stigma, they also enlisted the help of others 'in the know' who, in turn, engaged in what Edgerton refers to as a 'benevolent conspiracy' (Edgerton 1967: 217) to help them pass as 'normal' to others unaware of their condition.

In the study by Todd and Shearn (1997), parents co-resident with their now adult children with intellectual impairment were asked about their own carer careers, how they managed courtesy stigma, their perceptions of the social status of their offspring, and their offspring's self-awareness of their own social identities. The authors found that stigma was a prevalent feature of parents' lives, posing an identity problem for all family members, and they dealt with it, in a similar way to Edgerton's former inpatients, through strategies of 'non-disclosure and fictional identity-building' for their affected child, strategies which, however, had the effect of continuing to legitimate stigma.

The question of the extent to which stigma acts as a barrier to coping for disabled children with a neurodevelopmental impairment is difficult to disentangle, not only because of coping strategies such as those described by Todd and Shearn (1997) but also because it represents only one set of factors in a multifactor puzzle. Based on their work in relation to epilepsy, Austin et al (1994) propose that the issue of coping with a chronic neurodevelopmental condition, and the role of stigma in determining coping and adjustment, needs to be considered in relation to competing neurological factors. An interesting study in the UK by Chin et al (2011) involved comparison of health and socio-economic outcomes in adulthood of a population-based birth cohort of children with epilepsy and their fellow cohort members unaffected by the condition. A key factor that emerged in the analysis as significant for adult outcomes was the level of anxiety (as rated by their teachers, at the time the children were aged 11 years) that the children with epilepsy experienced about being socially accepted by both their peers and adults with whom they interacted. This factor was found to be a significant predictor of poor psychosocial outcomes in adulthood, suggesting that '… there is something intrinsic about having epilepsy that results in isolation in later life, which could be linked to societal attitudes towards epilepsy.' The authors question why children, even at the age of 11, would already experience difficulties in being socially accepted, and they go on to highlight the implications of their finding for management. They conclude that managing seizures pharmacologically, while critical, is only one element in promoting effective coping. Management also needs to be directed at behavioural/cognitive and emotional problems supported by the implementation of educational policies aimed at inclusivity.

Ablon (2002) identifies a constellation of biographical and ideological factors within the families of children with chronic health conditions and impairments that are critical for successfully coping with stigma. These include unconditional family support, clear intra-familial communication and a willingness to discuss practical and emotional issues, and seeking out the best-quality medical care and strongly supportive family members to help make decisions about available treatment options. Although written in the context of another, non-neurodevelopmental childhood condition, Atkin and Ahmad (2000) argue that families' contact with health services is another important contributing factor in their coping abilities, although one which, depending on its nature, can both help and hinder. The importance of providing counselling services and peer support programmes directly to children with chronic illnesses themselves is suggested as a means of addressing issues of negative attitudes to their illness and perceived and experienced stigma (Chesson et al 2004, Galletti and Sturniolo 2004, Funderburk et al 2007). There is evidence of the success of such interventions (Snead et al 2004). It is also worth drawing attention here to the findings from work by Admi and Shaham (2007) that support a more optimistic view than is typically proposed of coping in individuals with a chronic, potentially stigmatizing condition. These authors provide evidence from their studies of adolescents successfully working their condition into their everyday lives and drawing upon personal strengths to do so.

What needs to be done to reduce the stigma barrier?

In conclusion, then, reducing the invisible barrier of the stigma of neurodevelopmental conditions is not an easy task. It involves acting upon the social meaning of these conditions and educating both the general public and specific key subgroups about the realities of causes, treatments, and prognosis. It involves challenging negative coping strategies and fostering positive responses and resilience in the face of stigma, in both those affected and their family members and carers. It also involves seeking protection and support through appropriate health and social care structures and legislation to ensure that such protection and support is offered in an appropriate and timely fashion. Finally, it involves campaigning to make the invisible visible and to challenge the implications of stigma for those against whom it is targeted.

REFERENCES

Key references

*Ablon J (2002) The nature of stigma and medical conditions. *Epilepsy Behav* 3: S2–S9. http://dx.doi.org/10.1016/S1525-5050(02)00543-7

*Admi H, Shaham B (2007) Living with epilepsy: ordinary people coping with extraordinary situations. *Qualitative Health Res* 17: 1178–1187. http://dx.doi.org/10.1177/1049732307307548

Allotey J, Reidpath D (2007) Epilepsy, culture, identity and well-being: a study of the social, cultural and environmental context of epilepsy in Cameroon. *J Health Psychol* 12: 431–443. http://dx.doi.org/10.1177/1359105307076231

Alonzo A, Reynolds N (1995) Stigma, HIV and AIDS; an exploration and celebration of a stigma strategy. *Soc Sci Med* 41: 303–315. http://dx.doi.org/10.1016/0277-9536(94)00384-6

Atkin K, Ahmad WIU (2000) Family care-giving and chronic illness: how parents cope with a child with a sickle cell disorder or thalassaemia. *Health Soc Care Commun* 8: 57–69. http://dx.doi.org/10.1046/j.1365-2524.2000.00211.x

*Austin JK, McBride AB, Davis HW (1984) Parental attitude and adjustment to childhood epilepsy. *Nurs Res* 33: 92–96. http://dx.doi.org/10.1097/00006199-198403000-00012

Austin JK, Risinger MW, Beckett LA (1992) Correlates of behaviour problems in children with epilepsy. *Epilepsia* 33: 1115–1122. http://dx.doi.org/10.1111/j.1528-1157.1992.tb01768.x

Austin JK, Smith MS, Risinger MW, McNelis AM (1994) Childhood epilepsy and asthma: comparison of quality of life. *Epilepsia* 35: 608–615. http://dx.doi.org/10.1111/j.1528-1157.1994.tb02481.x

*Austin JK, Huster GA, Dunn DW, Risinger MW (1996) Adolescents with active or inactive epilepsy or asthma: a comparison of quality of life. *Epilepsia* 37: 1228–1238. http://dx.doi.org/10.1111/j.1528-1157.1996.tb00558.x

*Austin JK, Shafer PO, Deering JB (2002) Epilepsy familiarity, knowledge and perceptions of stigma: report from a survey of adolescents in the general population. *Epilepsy Behav* 3: 368–375. http://dx.doi.org/10.1016/S1525-5050(02)00042-2

Bagley C (1972) Social prejudice and the adjustment of people with epilepsy. *Epilepsia* 13: 33–45. http://dx.doi.org/10.1111/j.1528-1157.1972.tb04547.x

Bishop M, Slevin B (2004) Teachers' attitudes towards students with epilepsy: results of a survey of elementary and middle school teachers. *Epilepsy Behav* 5: 308–315. http://dx.doi.org/10.1016/j.yebeh.2004.01.011

Bishop M, Boag EM (2006) Teachers' knowledge about epilepsy and attitudes towards students with epilepsy: results from a national survey. *Epilepsy Behav* 8: 397–405. http://dx.doi.org/10.1016/j.yebeh.2005.11.008

Bury M (1982) Chronic illness as biographical disruption. *Soc Health Illness* 4: 167–182. http://dx.doi.org/10.1111/1467-9566.ep11339939

Chesson RA, Chisholm D, Zaw W (2004) Counseling children with chronic physical illness. *Patient Educ Counsel* 55: 331–338. http://dx.doi.org/10.1016/j.pec.2003.04.002

*Chin RFM, Cumberland PM, Pujar SS, Peckham C, Ross EM, Scott RC (2011) Outcomes of childhood epilepsy at age 33 years: a population-based birth-cohort study. *Epilepsia* 52: 1513–1521. http://dx.doi.org/10.1111/j.1528-1167.2011.03170.x

*Crocker J, Major B, Steele C (1998) Social stigma. In: Fiske S, Gilbert D, Lindzey G, editors. *Handbook of Social Psychology*. Boston, MA: McGraw-Hill, pp. 504–553.

Dantas FG, Cariri GA, Cariri GA (2001) Knowledge and attitudes toward epilepsy among primary, secondary and tertiary level teachers. *Arq Neuropsiquiatr* 59: 712–716. http://dx.doi.org/10.1590/S0004-282X2001000500011

Das V (2001) Stigma, contagion, defect: issues in the anthropology of public health. Paper presented at the US NIH conference on Stigma and Global Health: Developing a Research Agenda, 5–7 September 2001, Bethesda MD, 2001. Available at: www.stigmaconference.nih.gov (accessed 27 November 2012).

Edgerton RB (1967) *The Cloak of Competence: Stigma in the Lives of the Mentally Retarded*. Berkeley, CA: University of California Press.

*Emerson E, Honey A, Madden R, Llewellyn G (2009) The well-being of Australian adolescents and young adults with self-reported long-term health conditions, impairments or disabilities: 2001 and 2006. *Aust J Soc Issues* 44: 37–51.

Evans G, Todd S, Beyer S, Felce D, Perry J (1994) Assessing the impact of the all-Wales strategy. *J Intellect Disabil Res* 38: 109–133. http://dx.doi.org/10.1111/j.1365–2788.1994.tb00368.x

*Fadiman A (1998) *The Spirit Catches You and You Fall Down: A Hmong Child, Her American Doctors, and the Collision of Two Cultures*. New York: Farrar Straus & Giroux.

Funderburk JA, McCormick BP, Austin JK (2007) Does attitude toward epilepsy mediate the relationship between perceived stigma in children and mental health outcomes with epilepsy? *Epilepsy Behav* 11: 71–76. http://dx.doi.org/10.1016/j.yebeh.2007.04.006

Galletti F, Sturniolo MG (2004) Counselling children and parents about epilepsy. *Patient Educ Counsel* 55: 422–425. http://dx.doi.org/10.1016/j.pec.2003.06.004

Glidden LM, Zetlin AG (1992) Adolescence and community development. In: Rowitz L, editor. *Mental Retardation in the Year 2000*. New York: Springer-Verlag, pp. 1–147. http://dx.doi.org/10.1007/978-1-4613-9115-9_7

*Goffman E (1963) *Stigma: Notes on the Management of Spoiled Identity*. Englewood Cliffs, NJ: Prentice Hall.

Hamiwka LD, Hamiwka LA, Sherman EMS, Wirrell E (2011) Social skills in children with epilepsy: how do they compare to healthy and chronic disease controls? *Epilepsy Behav* 21: 238–241. http://dx.doi.org/10.1016/j.yebeh.2011.03.033

Hansen DA, Hill R (1964) Families under stress. In: Christensen H, editor. *Handbook of Marriage and the Family*. Chicago, IL: Rand McNally & Co.

Ismail H, Wright J, Rhodes P, Small N, Jacoby A (2005) South Asians and epilepsy: exploring health experiences, needs and beliefs of communities in the north of England. *Seizure* 14: 497–503. http://dx.doi.org/10.1016/j.seizure.2005.08.006

*Jacoby A, Austin JK (2007) Social stigma for adults and children with epilepsy. *Epilepsia* 48(Suppl. 9): 6–9. http://dx.doi.org/10.1111/j.1528-1167.2007.01391.x

Jalava M, Sillanpaa M, Camfield C, Camfield P (1997) Social adjustment and competence 35 years after onset of childhood epilepsy: a prospective controlled study. *Epilepsia* 38: 708–715. http://dx.doi.org/10.1111/j.1528-1157.1997.tb01241.x

Jones E, Farina A, Hastorf A, Markus H, Miller D, Scott R (1984) *Social Stigma: The Psychology of Marked Relationships*. New York: Freeman.

*Katzenstein JM, Fastenau PS, Dunn DW, Austin JK (2007) Teachers' ratings of the academic performance of children with epilepsy. *Epilepsy Behav* 10: 426–431. http://dx.doi.org/10.1016/j.yebeh.2007.01.006

Kerr C, Nixon A, Angalakuditi M (2011) The impact of epilepsy on children and adult patients' lives: development of a conceptual model from qualitative literature. *Seizure* 20: 764–774. http://dx.doi.org/10.1016/j.seizure.2011.07.007

Kleinman A, Wang W, Li S, et al (1995) The social course of epilepsy: chronic illness as social experience in interior China. *Soc Sci Med* 40: 1319–1330. http://dx.doi.org/10.1016/0277-9536(94)00254-Q

Koller H, Richardson SA, Katz M (1988) Marriage in a young mental retardation population. *J Ment Deficiency Res* 32: 93–102.

Lee A, Hamiwka LD, Sheman EMS, Wirrell EC (2008) Self-concept in adolescents with epilepsy: biological and social correlates. *Pediatr Neurol* 38: 335–339. http://dx.doi.org/10.1016/j.pediatrneurol.2008.01.011

Levin R, Banks S, Berg B (1988) Psychosocial dimensions of epilepsy: a review of the literature. *Epilepsia* 29: 805–816. http://dx.doi.org/10.1111/j.1528-1157.1988.tb04238.x

Link G, Phelan J (2001) Conceptualizing stigma. *Am Rev Sociol* 27: 363–385. http://dx.doi.org/10.1146/annurev.soc.27.1.363

MacRae H (1999) Managing courtesy stigma: the case of Alzheimer's disease. *Soc Health Illness* 21: 54–70. http://dx.doi.org/10.1111/1467-9566.00142

Marteau TM, Johnston M (1986) Determinants of beliefs about illness: a study of parents of children with diabetes, asthma, epilepsy and no chronic illness. *J Psychosomatic Res* 30: 673–683. http://dx.doi.org/10.1016/0022-3999(86)90101-7

*Maslow GR, Haydon AA, Ford CA, Halpern CT (2011a) Young adult outcomes of children growing up with chronic illness. *Arch Pediatr Adolesc Med* 165: 256–261. http://dx.doi.org/10.1001/archpediatrics.2010.287

Maslow GR, Haydon AA, Ford CA, Halpern CT (2011b) Growing up with a chronic illness: social success, educational/vocational distress. *J Adolesc Health* 49: 206–212. http://dx.doi.org/10.1016/j.jadohealth.2010.12.001

Muhlbauer S (2002) Experience of stigma by families with mentally ill members. *J Am Psychiatric Nurs Assoc* 8: 76–83. http://dx.doi.org/10.1067/mpn.2002.125222

Olsson I, Campenhausen G (1993) Social adjustment in young adults with absence seizures. *Epilepsia* 34: 846–851. http://dx.doi.org/10.1111/j.1528-1157.1993.tb02101.x

Oostrom KJ, Schouten A, Olthof T, et al (2000) Negative emotions in children with newly diagnosed epilepsy. *Epilepsia* 41: 326–331. http://dx.doi.org/10.1111/j.1528-1157.2000.tb00163.x

Parsons T (1951) *The Social System*. New York: Free Press of Glencoe.

*Prpic I, Korotaj Z, Vlašin-Cicvaric I, Paucic-Kirincic E, Valerjev A, Tomac V (2003) Teachers' opinions about capabilities and behaviour of children with epilepsy. *Epilepsy Behav* 4: 142–145. http://dx.doi.org/10.1016/S1525-5050(03)00025-8

Räty LK, Wilde Larsson BM, Söderfeldt BA (2003) Health-related quality of life in youth: a comparison between adolescents and young adults with uncomplicated epilepsy and healthy controls. *J Adolesc Health* 33: 252–258.

Reidpath D, Chen K, Gifford S, Allotey P (2005) He hath the French pox: stigma, social value and social exclusion. *Soc Health Illness* 27: 468–489. http://dx.doi.org/10.1111/j.1467-9566.2005.00452.x

Robson C (2006) Examining the social stigma of epilepsy: a qualitative analysis of attitudes, perceptions and understanding towards epilepsy and people with epilepsy among young adults in the undergraduate population. MSc thesis, University of York, UK.

*Rodenburg R, Meijer AM, Deković M, Aldenkamp AP (2006) Family predictors of psychopathology in children with epilepsy. *Epilepsia* 47: 601–614. http://dx.doi.org/10.1111/j.1528-1167.2006.00475.x

Ronen GM, Rosenbaum P, Law M, Streiner DL (1999) Health-related quality of life in childhood epilepsy: the results of children's participation in identifying the components. *Dev Psychol Child Neurol* 41: 554–559. http://dx.doi.org/10.1017/S0012162299001176

*Schneider JW, Conrad P (1983) *Having Epilepsy: The Experience and Control of Illness*. Philadelphia, PA: Temple University Press.

*Snead K, Ackerson J, Bailey K, Schmitt MM, Madan-Swain A, Martin RC (2004) Taking charge of epilepsy: the development of a structured psychoeducational group intervention for adolescents with epilepsy and their parents. *Epilepsy Behav* 5: 547–556. http://dx.doi.org/10.1016/j.yebeh.2004.04.012

Sontag S (1978) *Illness as Metaphor*. New York: Farrar, Straus & Giroux.

Stevanovic D, Jancic J, Lakic A (2011) The impact of depression and anxiety disorder symptoms on health-related quality of life of children and adolescents with epilepsy. *Epilepsia* 52: 75–78. http://dx.doi.org/10.1111/j.1528-1167.2011.03133.x

Suurmeijer TPBM (1995) The impact of epilepsy on social integration and quality of life: family, peers and education. In: Aldenkamp AP, Dreifuss FE, Renier WO, Suurmeijer TPBM, editors. *Epilepsy in Children and Adolescents*. Boca Raton, FL: CRC Press, Inc.

*Todd S, Shearn J (1997) Family dilemmas and secrets: parents' disclosure of information to their adult offspring with learning disabilities. *Disabil Soc* 12: 341–366. http://dx.doi.org/10.1080/09687599727218

Todd S, Evans G, Beyer S (1990) More recognised than known: the social visibility and attachment of people with developmental disability. *Aust NZ J Development Disabil* 16: 207–218.

Vega C, Guo J, Killory B, et al (2011) Symptoms of anxiety and depression in childhood absence epilepsy. *Epilepsia* 52: 70–74. http://dx.doi.org/10.1111/j.1528-1167.2011.03119.x

Voeller KK, Rothenberg MB (1973) Psychosocial aspects of the management of seizures in children. *Pediatrics* 51: 1072–1082.

*West P (1979) Investigation into the social construction and consequences of the label 'epilepsy'. PhD thesis, University of Bristol, UK.

Weiss MG, Ramakrishna J, Somma D (2006) Health-related stigma: rethinking concepts and interventions. *Psychol Health Med* 11: 277–287. http://dx.doi.org/10.1080/13548500600595053

Winkler AS, Mayer M, Schnaitmann S, et al (2010) Belief systems of epilepsy and attitudes toward people living with epilepsy in a rural community of northern Tanzania. *Epilepsy Behav* 19: 596–601. http://dx.doi.org/10.1016/j.yebeh.2010.09.023

13
ADVANCING THE RIGHTS OF CHILDREN WITH NEURODEVELOPMENTAL CONDITIONS

Sheila Jennings

Overview

This chapter presents a sampling of landmark litigation concerning the rights of children with impairments and disabilities. Case law is reviewed from the areas of health law, criminal law, administrative law, and child welfare law. The premise of this chapter is that decisions and their aftermath – whether they be from a civil court, human rights tribunal, or criminal court or from the court of public opinion – tell us a great deal about the areas in society in which there continues to be a withholding of full rights to children with impairments.

Introduction

It has been observed that the intersection between childhood and disability has been under-researched and undertheorized. Moreover, it has been noted that 'research on contemporary childhoods has marginalized the experience of disability while social model research on disability has marginalized the experience of childhood' (Priestley 1998). The law provides a crucial perspective for our understanding of what is taking place at this intersection.

Important civil and criminal lawsuits have been brought to court in the USA and Canada on behalf of disabled children with developmental impairments. The impact of such cases has been felt beyond the findings of courts and tribunals. There have not been many civil cases involving children with special needs because, as a pathway to systemic change, civil litigation is typically complex, drawn out, and extremely costly (Rosenberg and Yohalem 1986). It goes almost without saying that parents of children with complex care needs cannot afford the time, the energy, or the money to sue governments. Moreover, and as has been described more generally with respect to disability litigation, translation of court successes into policy-level changes has not always taken place (Rosenberg and Yohalem 1986). In Canada this is best illustrated in the case of *Eldridge* v. *British Columbia (Attorney General)* (1997), an important disability rights case, although not one concerning children with developmental disabilities.

In the Eldridge case the plaintiffs, who were deaf, sought declaratory relief, stating that the failure of the government to provide sign language interpreters was discrimination on the basis of impairment, taking the position that government practices infringed the parties' equality rights under the Canadian Charter of Rights and Freedoms. The Supreme Court of Canada held that, once a government undertakes to provide a benefit to the general population, it must ensure that those listed under the equality clause can make use of it. The problem is that although the court held as it did, that interpretive services had to be provided, it is commonly understood in Canada that such services are not necessarily made available to patients in hospitals today. The Eldridge case therefore demonstrates another limitation of equality rights litigation. Nevertheless, bringing this case to court made clear that the right exists, and the case has served to place disability rights in the public domain, which is one place where consciousness raising takes place.

In criminal law matters, where harms have been perpetrated against children with neurological or developmental conditions, it is apparent that the rights of the child have presented as being questionable or doubtful in the domain of public opinion. In some cases, such as that of 6-year-old Charles Blais, who was autistic, and Katie Lyn Baker, who had Rett syndrome, the 'disability community' was alarmed at what appeared to be a reluctance to prosecute their murders. Together, such cases signal to the 'disability community' that the rights of the child with developmental impairments in Canada are less protected than are the rights of typically developing children. Case law therefore presents an opportunity to review how children with developmental conditions fare overall in civil and criminal courts in the USA and Canada and, beyond that, in media and in the court of public opinion.

Green (2007), observing the practice of withholding full citizenship in the setting of policy, has commented that:

> Western capitalistic societies construct the concept of childhood as a period of dependency which is of limited duration and which involves predictable progress toward an independent, economically productive, adulthood. Children with disabilities who do not conform to these expectations are viewed as a 'social problem.' [emphasis added]
>
> (Green 2007: 511)

Goodley and Runswick-Cole (2011) likewise assert that '... children are seen as instrumental to solving the ills of society as they achieve "economic well-being" and "make a positive contribution".'

One must consider these statements in the context of the current ideological and economic environments. Indeed, the observation has been made that recent policies with 'neo-liberal models of citizenship and normative narratives of child development exclude disabled children' (Goodley and Runswick-Cole 2011). One may surmise that this reality may be impacting the (children with impairments) language used by advocates for children with neurological or developmental conditions such as autism in order to promote their interests. It has been suggested that by choosing names social actors generate 'an imaginary of the boundaries of inclusion and exclusion' and moreover that the use of the word 'child' in politics by various groups has permitted this word to serve '… as a unifying symbol, both consolidating a community of interest and identifying a set of politically meaningful claims' (Dobrowolsky and Jenson 2004). These theorists' positions support the view that in contemporary society a childhood with impairment is perceived as being, as noted above, a social problem that remains to be solved. It is sobering to recall that in the past 'solutions' to the perceived 'problem' have included state-sponsored mass murder of children with impairments, as was witnessed during World War II in Nazi Germany (Ronen et al 2009).

Some organizations offering services to children with developmental conditions have actually adopted the language of the productive adult-to-be child, perhaps attempting to leverage their case. For example, a Canadian Television (CTV) headline dated 24 November 2011 read 'New Autism Centre Aims to Help Self-Sufficiency' followed by 'Centre opened with a talk given by Her Royal Highness, the Countess of Wessex …'. The Countess stated in her talk that 'The Kae Martin Campus will be the first of its kind in Canada, and will help put autistic children on a path towards self-sufficiency.' One needs to ask whether in fact this is helpful. One also needs to recognize that advancing the rights of children with developmental impairments is a great deal more complex than it seems, and issues pertaining to child rights change with time, making disabled child rights a moving target.

Less than certain rights

Canadian civil courts and tribunals have heard challenges to the exclusion and denial of services and supports to children with developmental conditions on diverse issues such as the right to inclusive education (*Eaton* v. *Brant County Board of Education* [1997] 1 SCR 241); funding and support (*A.L.* v. *Ontario (Ministry of Community and Social Services)* [2006] OJ No. 4637 (CA), leave to appeal refused [2007] SCCA No. 36); specialized foster care and disability supports [*Assembly of First Nations and First Nation Child and Family Caring Society* v. *Canada* (2007)]; and access to autism educational treatments [*Auton* v. *British Columbia* (2004), *Sagharian* v. *Ontario* (2008), and *Wynberg* v. *Ontario* (2006) and others]. Bell and Petrick (2010) comment that in the Canadian context:

> A prominent theme running through autism case law in Canada – from Charter litigation to tax law – is the courts' reluctance to impose obligations on government in relation to funding for or provision of autism treatment. There are tools available to the courts to order such funding; however, the courts seem bound by the principle of judicial deference to the power of legislatures to choose their methods of dealing with social issues. Under this principle, deference is owed to the legislature when making difficult policy choices regarding the claims of competing groups or the distribution of public resources. Canadian courts have sent a message that autism advocacy is not best dealt with in the courtroom; but rather that the battle needs to be taken to the Provincial and Federal legislatures.
>
> (Bell and Petrick 2010: 1)

Across the European Union (Autism Europe 2006), at least where the right to education and related services is concerned, court decisions appear to be more favourable to children with autism. These cases arguably serve to challenge the devaluation of children with neuro-logical or developmental conditions and to expose commonly held views within the dominant culture whereby their exclusion has been a common practice.

The 'outing' of ableist positions being advanced in social institutions that run counter to the rights of the child with impairments at issue in such proceedings brings attention to the con-cerns of the 'disability community'. This community necessarily includes parents of children with neurological and developmental conditions. Some parents, as part of their advocacy, have been publishing books about their experiences in raising children with neurodevelopmental conditions. For example, *Globe and Mail* journalist Ian Brown published his award-winning book about the experiences he and his wife encountered caring for their son, Walker, who has a condition called cardiofacialcutaneous syndrome, an 'orphan' syndrome, which includes intellectual impairment. Donna Thomson, married to the High Commissioner for Canada in the UK, has written a book (with a foreword by John Ralston Saul) about her experiences parent-ing her son Nicholas, who has cerebral palsy, and, like Brown, she also speaks publicly about her experience. Miriam Edelson is a trades union activist who has also published accounts of her experiences raising her (now deceased) son, Jake, who had lissencephaly. These particular parents have had the opportunity to be heard and have used that in advocating the advancement of the rights of children with neurological or developmental conditions.

Disability rights litigation not only challenges law and policy but may also be seen to reveal mainstream or other discourses regarding childhoods with neurological or develop-mental impairment. Once out in the open, views that run counter to the rights of the child can be explored in public, allowing for confrontation of rights-infringing discourses. Outside of courts and tribunals, opportunities to address problematic approaches respecting the rights of these children also arise. Indeed some such approaches have not come before a judge, but should have, and that is an issue in itself. A well-known and much debated example of this is a case still being witnessed in the American paediatric literature: the matter of Ashley X, a case to which this discussion returns below.

In spite of the above-noted difficulties with advancing the rights of children with impair-ments through litigation, what is promising about such cases is that they place the matter of the status of these children squarely in front of the courts, the media, and the public. They increase the visibility of children with neurological or developmental conditions and force society to consider and talk about issues raised in such proceedings. Moreover, public discourses can then be read about, discussed, and heard. A prominent Canadian example was the Latimer case (*R. v. Latimer* [2001] 1 SCR 3) which was discussed extensively on Canadian radio at the time of the death of Tracy and is still being discussed to the present day. An example of the way in which discourses are revealed can be seen in the March 2012 airing of a Global Television documentary entitled 'Taking Mercy'. In this programme a reporter interviews two parents of children with developmental impairments. One of the parents interviewed is Robert Latimer (whose case is discussed further below). Latimer achieved notoriety when he killed his neurodevelopmentally disabled daughter in 1993. The other person interviewed is a mother who explains that she wishes the state to do the same thing to her now middle-aged children who have Sanfilippo syndrome. This mother, Annette Corriveau, asserts that she has the legal right to withdraw gastric feeding, but states that she cannot exercise that option as it is unacceptable to her as being 'inhumane'. The reporter states at different points in the programme that '... never before has Canadian law and morality been so conflicted' and that in the '... battle between law and morality, law won'. Such statements provide a litmus test as to where such rights 'are at' at a given point in time in some sectors of the population. In this case, the view being put forward appears to be that current Canadian criminal law offends the rights of the parents of children with severe developmental impairments. In response to that position, in an open letter to Global National Television and the Canadian Broadcast Standards Council the President of the Canadian Association for Community Living (2012) asserted that, 'There are deeply concerning shifts taking place in society whereby a "perfect storm" is making it a dangerous time to be a person with a disability.'

In the aftermath of the filicide of 12-year-old Tracy Latimer, the manner in which the media dealt with the prosecution of her father, Robert Latimer, and with the fact of Tracy's neurodevelopmental impairment shone a light on perceptions about the lives of children with impairments in the culture. It became apparent over time that community perceptions differed from those of the state. The Crown's position as stated at the trial (CBC 2010a) was that '[t]here is no dispute that through her life, Tracy at times suffered considerable pain. As well, the quality of her life was limited by her severe disability. But the pain she suffered was not unremitting, and her life had value and quality.' As this case wound its way up to the Supreme Court of Canada, Tracy's questionable status as an objectified child (Janz 1998) became evident through the many expressions of sympathy for her father. The dubious nature of Tracy's status as a child clearly resulted from her impairment, yet this reality was denied even in academic literature. For example, Sneiderman's (1997) article published in *Health Law Journal*, entitled 'The Latimer mercy killing case: a rumination on crime and punishment', stated:

> ... Latimer did not kill his daughter because he disvalued her life as a disabled person. It is true that if she had not been afflicted with cerebral palsy, he would not have killed her. Still, what explains the killing was not her disability as such. If he had killed his daughter out of contempt for her life as a disabled person, then the law would be right to hand down a denunciatory sentence. But that is not why he killed her; he killed her out of compassion and heartbreak for the pain and suffering that flowed from her disability. This is not to excuse his act, but it is enough to preclude the imposition of a denunciatory sentence.
>
> (Sneiderman 1997: paragraph 17)

The 10-year mandatory minimum sentence for second-degree murder Tracy's father served was seen by many to be harsh. Robert Latimer was recently interviewed by the Canadian Broadcasting Corporation (CBC 2011), and he proclaimed once again that he did the right thing. One must ask why he has been allowed to defend his position and why Canadians are willing to listen to him do it. One reason may be found in the normalization of this particular discourse in current culture. For example, there are open online discussions that challenge the most fundamental rights of children with developmental disabilities. Yahoo Answers carries a series of discussions with the headings 'Do you think it is cruel to keep severely disabled children alive?' and 'Why are children with severe disorders allowed to live?' Similar questions are being asked about preterm infants with severe impairments and whether or not parents and physicians ought to be permitted to withhold nourishment or treatment at birth. Writing in the UK, Freeman (2011) states that this circumstance has been described as being an area that 'has tested both ethicists and courts'. This situation for infants with severe impairments has been described as a 'complex intersection of parental rights, the best interest of the child, professional integrity, and the appropriate use of powerful medical technology' (Children's National Medical Center 2000).

Disabled child rights, and not merely best interests, are, however, in the middle of this intersection. It is an intersection that was explored through litigation in the USA in the mid-1980s in a trio of cases referred to colloquially as the Baby Doe, the Baby Jane Doe, and the Baby K cases (Children's National Medical Center 2000). These cases together addressed contested issues pertaining to, among other things, discrimination against severely impaired newborn infants and the role of the state in the treatment decisions in the early lives of children born with severe impairments. Baby Doe from Indiana had Down syndrome and an oesophogeal obstruction, Baby Jane Doe was diagnosed with an exposed spinal cord (myelomeningocoele) and hydrocephaly and microcephaly, while Baby K had been diagnosed with anencephaly.

In the US Supreme Court case *Bowen* v. *American Hospital* (1986) a decision was rendered regarding whether the federal government could regulate treatment to severely impaired newborn infants as it was attempting to do under the so-called 'Baby Doe Amendment', the amendment to the Child Abuse Prevention and Treatment Act, 1984 (CAPTA) (Moss 1987). CAPTA authorizes the US federal government to provide funding to the states respecting matters pertaining to child protection. The court in *Bowen* v. *American Hospital* struck down these federally imposed requirements for the administration of nourishment and treatment to severely ill and impaired newborn infants as having encroached upon the autonomy of individual states. In an article entitled 'Baby Doe: a tentative first step on a profound issue' Malcolm (1986) stated that this decision was 'only one step in the long and painful development of policies to govern society in the face of rapidly advancing medical capabilities'. Academic literature regarding these cases reveals differences of opinion not only on the appropriateness of state intervention but also with respect to the proper role of the US federal government in these matters. The latter point is illustrated by articles such as 'Baby Jane Doe, Congress and the States: Challenging the Federal treatment standard for impaired infants' (Newman 1989) and 'The case of Baby Doe: child abuse or unlawful Federal intervention?'(Annas 1984).

As noted elsewhere in this chapter, in Canada federal versus provincial authority over children with developmental and other impairments is likewise a contested and litigated issue, for example for First Nation Status Indian Children. Although the specifics of that dispute in Canada are obviously completely different from the specifics of the trio of cases from the USA, it is nonetheless interesting to observe some important parallels – one being that the Baby Doe dispute, like that of the First Nations Child and Family Caring Society and the Assembly of First Nations dispute with Canada, challenged the role of the federal government in meeting the perceived needs of children with impairments through child welfare provisions. A major departure in these cases is that in Canada the federal government is accused of reneging on its obligations to this particular group of children, whereas in the Baby Doe case the federal government was accused of overstepping its authority. One lesson to be learned from this is that the presence of this unique group of children poses likewise unique challenges to federal systems of government, and this in turn suggests that the reasons underpinning the challenge require greater attention be paid to it in both policy and law. Reasons include the rights of children, but another reason would be governmental interests in reducing interjurisdictional disputes as to whose obligation it is to support children with developmental and other impairments. As well, monies spent by governments defending lawsuits brought on behalf of children with impairments could and should be spent more usefully.

The life versus death disputes regarding the role of federal government in the lives of these children in the USA has been experienced in Canada too. For example, Quebec parents Marie-Eve Laurendeau and Stephane Mantha filed a lawsuit against the Montreal Children's Hospital in 2009 (CTV 2009), claiming that the hospital violated the law in its decision to disregard the parents' wishes to withdraw life support and to withhold nourishment from their infant daughter, Phébé, at her birth. According to a CTV report entitled 'Couple sues hospital for keeping sick baby alive' (2009) when young Phébé, who lives with cerebral palsy and intellectual impairment, was two and a half months old her parents were instructed by the hospital to come and collect her – apparently threatening to place Phébé into state care if they did not comply. This case raised additional important (but not new) policy concerns – for example, the critical issue of lack of support for parents in Quebec who find themselves as caregivers for children with significant additional healthcare needs. This same CTV news report noted that this child's mother had had to give up her career in order to care for Phébé full time, something that will undoubtedly carry significant economic as well as other ramifications for the family. It is unclear what happened in this case, but it appears that it may have been settled. There was a similar case in the Alberta courts in 2010 respecting infant Isaiah May. Isaiah was reported to have experienced severe brain injury at his birth, and as a result of the degree of impairments he experienced his physicians sought to remove him from his ventilator. Dick Sobsey, who is the director of the John Dossetor Health Ethics Centre at the University of Alberta, asserted in his comments to the press regarding the Isaiah May case that, 'This will be hard on the doctors and parents,' and further stated that, 'But it's not about them or who wins or loses, it's really about this baby and what's best for this baby' (Priest 2010). The May court case ended after Isaiah's parents decided to remove him from life support. He had been re-evaluated by a Canadian and an American neonatologist and they informed the parents that there was no sign of brain stem function (CBC 2010b).

These kinds of cases are not only medical and legal concerns, they are social and economic ones as well and, with all due respect to Professor Sobsey, they are not matters concerning only the baby with the impairments. Very sick and severely impaired infants do not grow up in a vacuum and the reality is that children with impairments are cared for primarily by their mothers (Yantzi and Rosenberg 2008). What was and still is evident from these kinds of cases is that different discourses exist regarding the rights of children with severe impairments at all stages of childhood. These cases suggest that the rights of children who are impaired at birth remain both socially and legally obscure not only in Canada but in other common law jurisdictions as well. One thing that would go a long way towards narrowing gaps in understanding would be for more fruitful dialogue across disciplines and the application of a gender lens to any discussion about the needs of this group of children. Of great import, and often ignored in discussions about the rights of severely impaired infants, are the practical difficulties brought up by caregiving mothers from within what McKeever (1991) referred to 20 years ago now, in the setting of severe impairments in childhood, as the discourse of feminine caregiving. For example, difficulties were expressed by the caring and caregiving mother of Phébé Mantha. It is suggested here that ignoring what a cross-section of mothers of infants with severe impairments report as their experiences and needs flies directly in the face of efforts to advance the rights of the child with developmental and other conditions.

As noted earlier, situations also arise involving children with developmental conditions that ought to have been brought to court but were not. When these cases come to the attention of professionals, the public, and disability rights advocates, they offer an opportunity for a disability rights dialogue to take place. The Ashley X matter referred to earlier is a case in point. Ashley X's controversial 'treatment plan' continues to be discussed internationally and widely in the paediatric literature (Shannon and Savage 2006, Butler and Beadle 2007) and within disability rights circles as well (Koll 2010, Kittay 2011) years after it took place. Kittay (2011) offers the unique and interesting perspective of a disability rights advocate, philosophy professor, and mother of a daughter with severe impairments. One of Kittay's main points in 'Forever small: the strange case of Ashley X' is that '… because it is hard for many to recognize and acknowledge people whose lives are significantly different, we need to reiterate the unqualified humanity of people with serious cognitive disabilities.' Her comment gets to the heart of the issue, which is that difference per se has always been problematic across and within cultures.

Turning to the facts of the Ashley X case itself, Ashley is an American girl with developmental impairments who entered puberty at the age of 6 years. Her maturation caused concern to her parents. They believed that a child with a neurodevelopmental impairment who had a woman's body would be at increased risk of sexual abuse and that her adult body would make it eventually impossible for them to look after her. In consultation with Ashley's physicians her parents decided that she should have a hysterectomy, an appendectomy, and breast bud removal and be given large doses of the hormone oestrogen so that her body would remain small and light and therefore portable. Ashley's parents have a blog (pillowangel.org), which apparently had received some 2 million hits by 2007. This blog openly discusses Ashley's surgery and the hormone therapy. Right away we can see that Ashley lacks the same rights to privacy about her medical care and her life as the rest of us, and one could also argue that, like Tracy Latimer, she has been objectified.

The ethics committee at the children's hospital where Ashley was being seen reviewed the proposed 'treatment' for Ashley at the request of her physicians and the committee approved the interventions. Later, the committee agreed that, with respect to the hysterectomy, the matter ought to have been heard by a judge prior to the surgery. Gunther and Diekema (2006), who carried out what has become known as 'the Ashley treatment', presented these interventions in their article as providing 'a new approach to an old dilemma' and one that offered 'a therapeutic option available to [profoundly disabled] children should their parents request it' (Ouelette 2008). Not everyone agreed with them, however, and a bioethical debate ensued, as revealed in the title of Brosco's (2006) article 'Growth attenuation: a diminutive solution to a daunting problem'. Brosco concluded his paper with this comment:

> Although we believe that attempts to attenuate growth are ill advised, we applaud Gunther and Diekema for publishing this case report. By focusing on a critical issue and beginning the debate, they help to advance our ethical dialogue as we struggle to define our core values in words, laws, and deeds. If high-dose estrogen treatment is on the right track, the collective community response will bestow general approval on growth attenuation; if not, the criticism may suffice to proscribe this mode of treatment. Only with further research and public discussion will we learn whether attempts to attenuate growth run with or against our fundamental values in caring for children with profound developmental disabilities.
>
> (Brosco 2006: final paragraph, no page)

In her article 'Growth attenuation, parental choice and the rights of disabled children: lessons from the Ashley case' Ouellette (2008) referenced a letter to the editor of the *Archives of Pediatrics and Adolescent Medicine* on the topic of the Ashley treatment as follows:

> This is the denial of the child's basic right as a human being to be free from the unwarranted and unnecessary manipulation of [her] basic biological functions merely to satisfy the needs of a third party … Children with severe developmental disabilities are, first and foremost, human beings. The manipulation of a child's physical development relegates those receiving such treatment to a less than human category.
>
> (Ouellette 2008: 218)

This letter forms part of the public dialogue on the rights of the child with developmental impairments that Brosco (2006) suggested would come from the community and which is mentioned above in relation to disputes about treatment of all kinds where children with developmental conditions are concerned. The upshot of Ouelette's (2008) discussion is that the law failed Ashley X as a child with a developmental impairment. As Ouellette notes, a court order was required by law for the physicians to perform Ashley's hysterectomy; however, it was not obtained.

First Nation aboriginal children with developmental impairments
Historically important and legally interesting cases involving young people with developmental impairments are currently before the courts in Canada and are being followed closely by the media and the international human rights community. Lavallee (2005) drew medical attention to the dire situation of on-reserve children in *Paediatrics and Child Health* in 2005 (Nathanson 2011). The case was further brought to the attention of the medical community by paediatrician Noni MacDonald and lawyer Amir Attaran in their *Canadian Medical Association Journal* editorial. They stated that:

… those who defend the status quo say that Canada's geography makes health care delivery for complex chronic illness difficult and costly. The same critics usually omit to mention that Canada's geography – its petroleum, timber, minerals and waterways, much of it within First Nations traditional territory – also makes it wealthy. Geography is no excuse for the pusillanimous, inequitable distribution of wealth, such that advanced care exists only in the South and First Nations children and communities endure psychological and cultural stress to access it. The point isn't what portion of the cost the federal, territorial and provincial governments each pay but rather, that the wrangling stops so that the right care, at the right place, at the right time can be provided for people on First Nations reserves.

(MacDonald and Attaran 2007: 321)

Four boys are currently named in the news media or in litigation and are being held up as representative of other on-reserve First Nation young people with impairments who need care in relation to their conditions and who are unable to access it: Jordan River Anderson, Jeremy Meawasige, Dewey Sumner, and Noah Buffalo Jackson.

Jordan River Anderson (now deceased) was a very young boy from the small community of Norway House in Manitoba. Jordan was born with Carey–Fineman–Ziter syndrome, a rare neuromuscular condition. As a child from an isolated reserve, Jordan required specialized foster care in order to be discharged to live in the community and, because that was not being made available to him, he lived on a hospital ward. The federal government of Canada and the provincial Manitoba government could not agree who would pay for his medical and developmental supports. On-reserve Status Indian children are funded off reserve only when hospitalized. In Jordan's case, there were disputes between a variety of government offices for over 2 years, and Jordan passed away before he could leave the hospital to go and live in the community. In the aftermath of this situation, a complaint was brought in the Canadian Human Rights Tribunal (CHRT) in 2007 by the First Nations Child and Family Caring Society and the Assembly of First Nations. The allegation is that Canada provides less funding for child welfare services to First Nation children on reserves than is provided to children off reserve. The issue of inequitable funding was brought as a claim of discrimination pursuant to the Canadian Human Rights Act. Canada, as may be seen in its Statement of Particulars, denied the allegations. This case is of international import and interest; Amnesty International is an intervener in the case. Their memorandum of fact and law sets out obligations on Canada to meet the needs to First Nation on-reserve children in international law. In 2011 Canada brought a motion to have the case dismissed and it was. The Ruling of the CHRT has been appealed, and further hearings will commence in February 2013.

Jeremy Meawasige is a Micmac youth from the Pictou Landing First Nation in Nova Scotia. Jeremy has a number of neurodevelopmental conditions including autism, cerebral palsy, and hydrocephalus (Peters 2011). His mother and their Band council brought an Application in the Federal Court in 2011 and at the time of writing the litigation is ongoing. The facts of this case are that after Jeremy's mother, Maurina Beadle, had a stroke and became impaired herself she was no longer able to provide the required level of care for her son. The solution that the Province of Nova Scotia proposed was that Jeremy be institutionalized, possibly out of the province. In response to this plan, Jeremy's mother is aptly quoted in the press as saying, 'When reporters ask me what I'll do if Jeremy is moved to an institution, I tell them, "Over my dead body. He won't get no love in an institution"' (Peters 2011). In the Application claims are made in part for an order quashing the decision of the manager of social programmes at Aboriginal Affairs and Northern Development Canada for denying funding for home care and in-home supports, and a declaration that the government of Canada violated the equality section of the Charter of Rights and Freedoms by denying Jeremy Meawasige and Maurina Beadle the equal benefit of the Social Assistance Act. As it is estimated that there are some 50 such disputes involving young people in this kind of situation annually (MacDonald 2012) one can expect to see more such applications being brought to court on behalf of children with developmental impairments in the future; indeed, this seems to be happening as new cases are being brought forward.

Dewey Sumner is a 9-year-old male with developmental and other impairments living on Pinaymootang First Nation reserve in Manitoba. Dewey has hydrocephalus, along with a congenital condition described as causing other conditions such as autism, seizures, and glaucoma (Sanders 2012). His mother Harriet Sumner-Pruden (Assembly of First Nations Health Forum 2011) has recently filed a complaint with both the provincial and the federal human rights tribunals with respect to the cap on Aboriginal Affairs and Northern Development Canada funding for school assistance that is negatively impacting her son. She is seeking services (Sanders 2011) over the 2.5 hours of special education he currently receives per day.

Institutional living and children with developmental disabilities

For those who believe the institutionalization of children with impairments is a thing of the past, cases such as Jeremy's serve to demonstrate that this is not the case. Not only are young people placed in institutional settings as a result of the lack of services and supports, such offers of placement are often accompanied by a request that the parent relinquish custody.

In Ontario this result has been achieved through child protection applications being brought to court showing that the parent has legally abandoned his or her child so that, through a legal fiction, placements may be found for children with developmental impairments using child welfare funding frameworks. The Ontario Ombudsman launched an investigation into this situation, conducted by his own legal counsel, and in 2005 released its report *Between a Rock and Hard Place: Special Investigation: Parents Forced to Place their Children with Severe Disabilities in the Custody of Children's Aid Societies to Obtain Necessary Care.* The Ombudsman has updated his investigation since then. The 2008–2009 follow-up report revealed that the practice continued. In the 2010–2011 report it is stated that:

> … complaints to the Ombudsman about services and treatment for children with severe special needs have continued to increase over the past few years. In 2010–2011, there were 44 such complaints – up from 39 in 2009–2010 and 24 the previous year. Although not all of these cases involved parents who had reached the point of turning their children over to Children's Aid Society care, most raised real concerns about the availability of services for these children.
>
> (Ontario Ombudsman 2010–2011)

Of importance here, it does not appear that children with developmental impairments are typically represented by legal counsel through these proceedings, regardless of whether children are or are not from reserves. As we saw in the case of Ashley X, a different standard of rights is at times applied where children with developmental impairments are concerned. One is challenged by this reality to ask why developmental impairment status goes hand in hand with requests for parental legal abandonment of a child. One is also challenged to ask further what this says about the status of these children and their parents. After all, in child welfare court the state is ordinarily and rightly expected to make its case when requesting a reduction of parental rights. Yet, this is not the case where children with developmental impairments are in need of placements; indeed, in some cases, (as illustrated above) parents are expected to acquiesce to their own loss.

A fourth aboriginal young person whose story has been reported is Noah Buffalo Jackson, who has cerebral palsy and who is not able to walk or talk. Noah lives with his mother Chief Carolyn Buffalo of Alberta's Montana First Nation Reservation (Gentleman 2008). Chief Buffalo has stated that, if she hopes to acquire services for her son, she must legally abandon him in exchange for services off reserve. In 2012 in a *Canadian Medical Association Journal* editorial paediatrician Noni MacDonald (2012) again drew attention to the situation of First Nation on-reserve children with additional needs.

Aboriginal identity, childhood, Status Indian legal status, impoverishment, and racism intersect with disability status, such that children with developmental impairments who are Status Indians are so marginalized that they cannot access even basic services or support in their own federally funded communities, nor do they qualify for them in provincially funded jurisdictions. The policy mechanism called Jordan's Principle that was put in place to address the policy gap is being disregarded by involved parties (as illustrated by cases such as those of Jeremy and Noah). The social care 'system' has no other funding mechanism for these children and young people with developmental impairments to access services. Under these circumstances health outcomes can only be suboptimal, especially if one considers the intensive care needs of these children. Indeed, Nathanson (2011) states that children are dying for want of appropriate services – in wealthy Canada. If ever there were an example of how identity plays a role in power dynamics affecting the health outcomes of children, the barriers to care experienced by children such as Jordan River Anderson, Jeremy Meawasige, Dewey Sumner, and Noah Buffalo Jackson demonstrate how it plays out in Canada.

The dynamics of power also become apparent where children with developmental impairments have single mothers; it is suggested this confers an additional marginalized status on a child with a developmental condition, and this has been alluded to elsewhere (Petrenchik 2008). It is no accident that it is often single mothers who are bringing these cases to court. In Ontario, single mother Anne Larcade brought a class action for certification proceedings against the Ontario government's Ministry of Community and Social Services on behalf of her son Alexandre Larcade and other children and young people who, like Alexandre, live with developmental impairments and lack needed services. This litigation took place at a time when purse strings were being tightened in the province of Ontario.

To summarize the pleadings in this case, single mother Anne Larcade sought to bring an action for class certification that, in 2000, the Children's Aid Society advised her that she would have to agree to a court order for wardship to obtain services for Alexandre. She had learned of a provision of the Child and Family Service Act (CFSA), called special needs agreements and, in 2001, entered an arrangement for a special needs agreement with the Ministry. She alleged that Ontario had breached its duty by failing to establish criteria and procedures for entering special needs agreements. She also alleged that the requirements of families with special needs children were not fairly assessed, and that agreements were entered on an ad hoc basis resulting in uneven and inequitable access to services. Her pleadings further set out that in 1997 the Ministry underwent a restructuring and, although the special needs agreement portion of the CFSA was never repealed, the Ministry ended access to these agreements. She claimed that the decision to end the use of special needs agreements by government was reckless or was made in bad faith as Ontario knew or ought to have known that, given the dependency of special needs children and the lack of available resources, termination of special needs agreements would cause 'immediate and terrible pain, hardship, and suffering'. She further claimed that Ontario owed a duty of care to provide special needs agreements to those eligible under the special needs agreements of the CFSA and had breached that duty by ceasing to issue and/or terminating these agreements without ensuring that adequate alternative services were available to the respondents and other members of the proposed class [pleadings are set out in full in the Court of Appeal decision in *A.L.* v. *Ontario* (2006)].

This case is interesting on many levels. For one thing, it exposed contradictory perspectives among individual judges hearing the matter at different stages of the litigation. For example, in a step in the litigation prior to the rendering of the final disposition at the Court of Appeal, Madam Justice McFarland in chambers stated [in her reported endorsement in *Larcade* v. *(Ontario) Ministry of Community and Social Services* (2005)] that she would not endorse an order for the stay that the Crown sought during the litigation, stating strongly:

> As for the balance of convenience, in my view it favours the respondents. This action concerns the interests of children who are profoundly disabled – among the most vulnerable members of our society. Complex litigation such as this action takes years to resolve. This action was started in February 2002 and it is just at the certification stage. The application for leave to appeal, if all goes according to schedule, will be resolved likely by the end of September unless an oral hearing is ordered. Thereafter if leave is granted the appeal must be perfected and a date set for a hearing. Optimistically that is unlikely to happen until the spring of 2006 at the earliest. All the while the children who are members of this class are getting older. In my view, particularly where children are involved we must do everything in our power to move matters forward.
>
> (Decision dated 15 July 2005: paragraph 12)

On the other hand, at the Court of Appeal, where the case was dismissed, Justice Sharpe, for the Court of Appeal's unanimous finding (Jaffey 2006) that the case could not go forward, stated that '... government priorities ought to be founded on general public interest rather than on individual interests' (Jaffey 2006). Yet, as someone seeking class certification for this group of children with impairments, Anne Larcade was by definition not in court to advance her 'individual' interests. Moreover, and with all due respect to His Honour, the care needs of children who are severely impaired are of public interest, especially so in a society claiming to care about its most vulnerable citizens.

Other jurisdictions

Canada boasts universal access to health care pursuant to the Canada Health Act, something that the USA does not have. It is intriguing in this differential context to contemplate the respective situations for children with developmental impairments in these two very different policy settings. One might deduce from this fundamental difference that children with developmental conditions would necessarily be worse off in the USA than they are in Canada. As a blanket assumption, however, this is not supportable based at least on a very general review of policy provisions and case law.

Looking strictly at medical care offerings one might argue that all Canadian children, regardless of impairment status, receive the same level of medical care and therefore are better off than their American counterparts. However, even that assertion is subject to debate. Moreover, for the group of children under discussion here there are disparities in care across the country, with large tertiary teaching centres having more to offer than small local hospitals. In any event, this population of children requires a great deal more care of all kinds than is made available to them under the provisions of the Canada Health Act. For example 'there is no legal obligation' for provinces or territories to cover costs for home care, which renders 'families vulnerable to limited public support' (Peter et al 2007). It is precisely here, in a domain *outside* of what is offered by the Canada Health Act, that it is most interesting to look at what has been taking place in law and policy in the USA.

As the Canadian and American federally organized systems of government are so very different from one another, completely different systems of support have resulted, and it is not feasible to compare them along key policy axes. However, one can deduce from American legislation and case law, as well as media reports and the large academic literature, that the US federal government conducts itself as if it perceives there to be an obligation on the part of the state to support children with impairments and to do so in a family setting. This is not to say that the American system of supports manages to meet all of the needs of children with severe impairments. It does not, and there is an ample literature describing where policy gaps and shortcomings lie. For example, there is literature demonstrating that American parents are also at times forced to relinquish custody of their children with impairments in exchange for government support and services (Simmons 2008) in a similar manner to what has been taking place in Canada.

In an article entitled 'Medicaid managed care for children with special health care needs: examining legislative and judicial constraints on privatization' Reed and Meyer (2004) refer to the 'conservation of public responsibilities to children with special health care needs through legislative mandates and judicial decisions...'. There does not appear to be any doubt that there is a public responsibility (as there was voiced in the words of Mr Justice Sharpe in the Larcade case in Ontario, for example). They state that:

> ... it should be evident that our concern about children with special health care needs is not about democratic accountability and lost opportunities for citizen participation. What is actually at stake for these children and their families is the potential loss of ongoing institutional protection and support. For this reason, congressional response in the form of the Balanced Budget Act of 1997 is significant. It reflects a conservation of previous public commitments.
>
> (Reed and Meyer 2004: 236)

The obligation of the US state is also made apparent from the overt willingness on the part of the federal government to respond publicly to lobbying and to wade into public policy issues concerning children with impairments in the media. For example, it did so with respect to the situation of Katie Beckett (Shapiro 201, see below) and it did so with respect to outside interest groups' attempts to influence standards of care for sick and impaired newborn infants. With respect to the era of the Reagan administration in particular, it is interesting that within it the Surgeon General, a paediatric surgeon by the name of C. Everett Koop, actively and very publicly advocated for newborn infants, children, and young people with impairments (National Library of Medicine, undated). I suggest that this perceived obligation and level at which it is experienced and plays out in US politics is not at all the same in Canada. Of course this can be explained in part by the nature of the division of powers in Canadian federalism. At the same time there is more to it, as seen in the comments made by President Reagan over 30 years ago (Shapiro 2010) with regard to the predicament of then 3-year-old Katie Beckett who had severe impairments. Reagan stated:

> By what sense do we have a regulation in government that says we'll pay $6000 a month to keep someone in a hospital that we believe would be better off home, but the family cannot afford one-sixth of that amount to keep them at home?
>
> (Shapiro 2010)

The issue that Julie Beckett (Katie's mother) confronted and was assisted with in 1981 is the same issue that confronted the parents of Jordan River Anderson and the mother of Jeremy Meawasige in Canada in the current era. They all wanted government funding for non-institutional care.

In 1978 as an infant Katie acquired encephalitis, which ultimately rendered her partially paralysed and requiring a respirator to breathe. Her parents wished to care for her at home but, under the regulations prior to the changes wrought by President Reagan on her behalf, in returning home her parents' income would have made her ineligible for Supplemental Security Income (SSI), a Medicaid programme provided by the Social Security Administration (Hevesi 2012). According to Hevesi (2012), President Reagan heard about Katie Beckett from Vice President Bush who had himself been told of her predicament by an Iowa Republican Congressman. As a result of President Reagan's interest and intervention the Tax Equity and Fiscal Responsibility Act (TEFRA) Medicaid Eligibility Option, also referred to as the Katie Beckett waiver (Semansky and Koyanagi 2004), came into force in 1982. This waiver permitted Katie and other children to live at home 'without the loss of federal support'. In addition, a

Review Board was put in place to deal with other cases like this one (Hevesi 2012). Semanski and Koyanagi (2004) in 'The TEFRA Medicaid Eligibility Option for children with severe disabilities: a national study' offer a discussion of policy where care for poor, near-poor, and middle-income American children with developmental impairments are concerned. One important thing noted about the Katie Beckett matter is that it brought to national attention the right of the child with significant impairments to live at home. In Canada the highest profile situations that correspond with that of Katie Beckett's situation and that manage to make the press do not seem to attract prime ministerial comment. Children in Canada who are medically fragile and technology dependant routinely live at home in Canada now; the problem is that the funding and services that are made available to their parents are such that some parents are placing their children in state care.

That Republicans in the USA have over the years taken up the cause of the support of children with impairments of all kinds serves as a reminder that one needs to be careful about criticizing the political right in the setting of childhood impairment policy formation. Republican Congressman Pete Sessions, for example, has worked hard to advance the rights of children with impairments, having advocated for and introduced the Dylan Lee James Family Opportunity Act in 2005 (www.petesessions.com/downsyndrome.htm). This was a bill to amend the Social Security Act to permit families to buy coverage under Medicaid for their children with impairments. This Act is stated to have been 'designed to help families of children with [impairments] stay together and stay employed, without losing their access to appropriate health care for special needs' (www.petesessions.com/downsyndrome.htm). Unfortunately the status of this bill appears to be noted as having 'died' (www.govtrack.us). One might speculate that the presence of politicized 'American family values' and perhaps more robust family policy overall have played a major role alongside a strong federal government in putting children with developmental impairments in the political limelight. At the same time, one might also want to interrogate overall the importance of personal experience of being the parent of a child with a developmental impairment in political consciousness raising. Congressman Sessions is the parent of a child with Down syndrome, President Reagan lost an infant at birth, and Julie Beckett wanted her daughter to live with her. The work of these and the many other childhood disability advocates in Canada, the USA, and elsewhere underlines the point that when it comes to parenting children with severe impairments the personal and the private are also by necessity profoundly political.

American law for children qualifies children with special healthcare needs as a distinct category in their legislative provisions. Kruger (2001) informs that offerings for children with special healthcare needs 'work within the policy context of state Title V programs'. Her article sets out in detail Title V Program development over the course of a 20-year period (a review of which is beyond the scope of this discussion) and refers also to other legislation that has been instrumental to the evolution of programming for children. She notes that 'the enactment of Medicaid (Title XIX) in 1965 had a large impact on Title V programs because it broadened the funding base for the economic burden of payment of direct care services for low-income families and children' (2001). She further references the Developmental Disabilities Act, which she notes was initially enacted in the 1970s and which is now referred to as the Developmental Disabilities Assistance and Bill of Rights Act, 2000, as well as the

Social Security Amendments of 1972. Importantly, and of relevance to this discussion, the latter brought in the SSI Program 'to assist families by providing monthly cash payments to low income children with disabilities'. She advises that in 1976 funds from SSI/Disabled Children's Program were used to connect poorer children with impairments to community services (Kruger 2001) through a referral system and to a Title V agency that 'provided care and service coordination' (Kruger 2001).

The point of bringing up selected individual pieces of legislation is simply to demonstrate that policy for children with developmental impairments in the USA has been front and centre for some time and present in a robust manner, unlike the situation in Canada. One can look to the field of education law to see yet additional evidence of this. Moreover, an extensive body of disability-in-childhood research exists in the USA, erecting a platform from which state policies can be launched in an informed manner. Research too is an area of deficit in Canada. In addressing the policy situation for children with complex care needs in Canada, Carnevale et al (2008) state that 'we know that these children commonly receive sub-optimal care because they "fall between the cracks" due to ambiguous categories, exclusionary criteria or service gaps.' Petrenchik (2008) comments in a publication that same year that 'it is challenging, if not impossible to develop population based strategies and measure their effectiveness in the absence of meaningful descriptions of the target populations', adding 'in the absence of reliable surveillance and monitoring activities'. While it is true that there is vastly more research on the needs of children with impairments in the USA than in Canada, this is not to say that a great deal is known about the experiences of children with more severe impairments overall. Scambler (2005) a medical sociologist in England stated, for example, that:

> There is a need to take account of people with different types of disabilities [impairments] and particularly the experiences of people with profound multiple disabilities and degenerative disabilities. These groups are barely represented in the literature, if at all, and yet their experiences are often very different to those of people with less severe or static disabilities.
>
> (Scrambler 2005: 158)

It has been observed that shifting ideological frameworks, shifting legal standards, and ever-changing policy make advancing disability rights a challenge (Rioux 2003). This very phenomenon was witnessed in the area of disabled child rights in the United States *in the aftermath* of the landmark Supreme Court decision *Sullivan* v. *Zebley* (1990). Doolittle (1998) explains that young Brian Zebley was a child living with multiple impairments who was nevertheless denied SSI child disability benefits. Brian Zebley, who was born in 1978, lived with congenital brain abnormality, visual and intellectual impairments, developmental delays, and partial paralysis (Erkulwater 2006). The *Sullivan* v. *Zebley* (1990) matter was brought as a class action lawsuit on behalf of children whose claims for SSI benefits had been denied (Doolittle 1998). According to Erkulwater (2006) over 300 000 children were represented by the class. As in the (smaller) Canadian case of *Larcade* v. *(Ontario) Ministry of Community and Social Services* (2005), a lower court at one stage in the litigation dismissed the class complaint in the Zebley matter (United States Social Security Administration Office of Disability Adjudication and Review 2012). The difficulty of then proceeding as a class in these cases on both sides of the border demonstrates that a reliance upon litigation as a tool to advance the rights of children with disabilities can be precarious. Erkulwater (2006) in her book *Disability Rights and the American Social Safety Net* comments that the Zebley case 'was one of the few social security cases to have ever reached the Supreme Court'. She states that '… latecomers to disability litigation, the Supreme Court did not hear a social security case until 1968 and when it did it always sided with [the Social Security Administration].' There was clearly something compelling to the US Supreme Court about the plight of lower-income disabled children who were left out of the scheme of benefits.

Doolittle (1998) explains regarding Brian Zebley that 'the reason he was denied was because his conditions did not match [the Social Security Administration's] listed adult or childhood impairments.' Upon a review the court held that, in determining eligibility for benefits, the Social Security Administration had to allow for an individual functional assessment and the court required additional disabling conditions be added to the list such as Down syndrome, fetal alcohol syndrome, and other serious hereditary, congenital, or acquired conditions (Doolittle 1998).

On a political note, Erkulwater (2006) advances the position that Brian Zebley had become 'a casualty of the Reagan administration's purge of the disability rolls at the age of 5'. This is an interesting observation in light of the progressive steps President Reagan took in the Katie Beckett case, and forces one to confront the relationship between social assistance and disability overall. The title of Doolittle's (1998) article 'Welfare reform: loss of supplemental security income (SSI) for children with disabilities' drives this connection home. In pointing this out, Erkulwater (2006) draws attention to an important pathway that exists between disability in childhood and poverty in childhood. Both Litt (2004) and Doolittle (1998) explain that further changes came about in disabled children's SSI benefits in 1996 through the Personal Responsibility and Work Opportunity Reconciliation Act, which is described as being 'a retrenchment' (Doolittle 1998) from advances made to the right to support children with impairments in the Zebley (1990) case. Doolitte (1998) and Litt (2004) draw attention to a most economically vulnerable sector of the disabled child population in the USA, namely those who are cared for by a single mother. These authors also flesh out the connections between poverty and childhood disability, supporting a position that disabled child rights cannot be advanced in the face of poverty. They likewise both look at the economic and political context for such negative changes to the support of children with impairments in the USA in the mid-1990s, with Litt (2004) asserting that children below the low-income cut-off in the USA are twice as likely to report a limitation or impairment as those who are economically above the poverty line.

In 'Profiling health and health related service for children with special health care needs with and without disabilities [impairments]' (Houtrow et al 2011) hypothesize 'that CSHCN [children with special health care needs] with disabilities have more severe and less stable health conditions than other CSHCN and have more extensive health service needs, but have higher rates of unmet needs and less commonly receive care within a medical home than other CSHCN.' They further hypothesized that 'after controlling for health condition severity and sociodemographic characteristics often associated with health care inequities, CSHCN with disabilities have increased odds of unmet service need'; indeed, their study found that both health and social challenges faced by children with special healthcare needs with impairments were more pronounced (Houtrow et al 2011), pointing to another highly vulnerable population in need in that jurisdiction. What their findings indicate overall is that in the USA, as elsewhere, more attention must be paid to the policy needs of children with the most severe conditions.

Although it is beyond the scope of this chapter to provide a more thorough comparative analysis of the matter of advancing the rights of children with developmental conditions outside North America, there is space to touch upon a couple of other places in which the rights of such children are being considered in policy and in law. Bulgaria and Latin America by way of example are both places with less wealth and fewer resources than the USA or Canada. As examples, they highlight the fact that disabled child rights are not simply tied to the ability of a nation state to pay to support these children but rather are tied to multifarious other things such as ideology and the political desire for change. Rechel (2008) in 'Access to care and the right to life of disabled children in Bulgaria' explains that:

> Children with disabilities may experience premature death not simply because of their medical conditions, but because they do not receive optimal physical care and emotional stimulation, they are neglected or have accidents, are not brought in time to hospital when ill, or because nobody has the expertise to treat their conditions. The underlying cause of all these pathways is lack of political guarantees of their right to life and health care, and failure to implement child protection policies for children without parental support and children with disabilities. In a culture where children are highly valued, it is difficult to understand why there has been little societal engagement with the rights of disabled children. Possible clues may be sought on the one hand in the Communist tradition of presenting a society free of evil and disease, and on the other hand in the still-prevailing stigma attached to disability and the discriminatory low value accorded to a life with disability.
>
> (Rechel 2008: 220)

Disabled children in Bulgaria are described by Rechel (2008) as having at one time been hidden away in barns, attics, and basements and as having been significantly harmed as a result of such practices. A human rights lawyer representing a non-governmental organization (cited by Rechel 2008) has stated that in Bulgaria there is a continuing belief that emanates from the medical model of disability whereby the presence of impairment in childhood continues to be seen as a situation requiring long-term care in an institutional setting. Rechel (2008) also reports that physicians in Bulgaria continue to suggest that children with impairments be placed in state care. Analyses such as this one by Rechel (2008) are important. They reveal that, although children remain in institutions in many places across the world, there is a growing awareness of and knowledge about the conditions of their care and the need for social change regarding their care. Comparative analyses serve to show that the difficulties that disabled children experience as rights bearers are global. For example, Amnesty International, as discussed above, is involved with and observing the situation for First Nations on-reserve children in Canada who have developmental conditions, in a similar way to the human rights lawyer quoted in Rechel (2008) observing what has been taking place in Bulgaria.

Childhood with a developmental condition in Canada is an oppressed status, as it is in Bulgaria and elsewhere. This is true although disability policy milieus for children differ greatly in Canada and Bulgaria. Moreover, it would be a mistake to assume that, because Canada is a wealthy nation with universal access to medical treatment, children with developmental conditions have greater legal rights in Canada. Canadian courts have demonstrated at times a reluctance to deal directly with issues (submitted here) that rest at the heart of state obligations to children with impairments. In not doing so, courts have made establishing the right to support of children with developmental conditions judicially elusive. Even with the various published reports of an outspoken provincial Ombudsman, as in the case of Ontario (Ontario Ombudsman 2005, 2008–2009, 2010–2011), making the case for the state's obligation to children with developmental impairments has proved challenging. The weak response of the Canadian state to the findings of the Ontario Ombudsman is both curious and concerning. Ombudsman's Offices elsewhere, such as in the case of Colombia, have had greater influence in promoting disabled child rights in courtroom settings it would seem. For example:

> As a consequence of a 1995 complaint filed by the Ombudsman (T-020/95) on behalf of 229 children with a broad spectrum of disabilities (Down's Syndrome, cerebral palsy, hydrocephaly, amongst others) the court required the social security agency to recommence treatment and the provision of medication for children on the basis that it would improve their quality of life.
>
> (Courtis 2008: 197)

Moreover, in his chapter 'The right to life and the right to health of children with disabilities before the courts: some Latin American examples' Courtis (2008) explains that in Latin America 'Constitutional, legislative and judicial evolution in this field has been dramatic.' He further states that:

> ... the field of children's rights and that of children with disability have been groundbreaking areas ... The acknowledgement of the positive duties stemming from civil rights has been an important entry point for the growing recognition of enforceable rights to access social services.
>
> (Courtis 2008: 197)

One can hope that in our ever-shrinking world, court decisions elsewhere in favour of the rights of the child with developmental (and other) impairments will be felt in Canada. Some legal theorists argue that international human rights norms may, in part at least, be diffused in just this manner. Toope and Rehaag (2004), for example, in 'Globalization and instrument of choice: the role of international law', reference Jinks's (2002) article 'Respondent: the legalization of world politics and the future of U.S. human rights policy' as stating that '... an increasingly precise body of universally-applicable human rights standards developed through various global associational processes will increasingly constrain policy options of nation states. Democratic polities will be governed, in part by exogenously-defined legal norms' (see Toope and Rehag 2004: 432, footnote 4). If this is indeed the case, then Canada may have to take notice of rights advances made by such children elsewhere and may not be able to continue on its current path where children with developmental conditions are concerned.

Conclusion

The above discussion has set out some ways in which the relatively recent legal and academic medical literature together have been grappling with the matter of the rights of children with developmental conditions. The discussion has also demonstrated that advancing the rights of children with impairments is a complex undertaking. For example, as seen in the Latimer case, it was the Crown (the state) that argued in favour of the rights of the child with a developmental condition, and it was public opinion that was not in overall support of those same rights. In other situations, for example in Ontario, the Ombudsman, lawyer André Marin, criticized the Ontario government in 2009 regarding the loss of custody of disabled children to the state in exchange for services by saying that the situation '… is one of the most morally repugnant things that government has done …' (Page 2009). In this case it is the state that is presented as reneging on its obligations to children with developmental impairments.

It is clear that where situations have been contested for lack of equality, the results for children with developmental impairments have been uneven. Rioux (2003) commented on the unevenness in equality rights advocacy, observing that 'Shifting legal and philosophical standards of equality … further complicate the impact of the various formulations of disability.' As discouraging as this has been, there is no question that the status quo is not tenable and that over time it will need to accord with the rights of the disabled child, both in the domestic and the international frame.

REFERENCES

Key references

Amnesty International Canada. Memorandum of Fact and Law (provided by Mr Craig Benjamin, campaigner for the Human Rights of Indigenous Peoples, Amnesty International Canada). Memorandum retrieved from: www.amnesty.ca/resource_centre/AIC_Memorandum_ChildServices.pdf

Annas GJ (1984) The case of baby Jane Doe: Child abuse or unlawful Federal intervention? *Am J Publ Health* 74: 727–729.

Answers.Yahoo.Com (2011) Do you think it is cruel to keep severely disabled children alive? Retrieved 19 April 2011 from: http://answers.yahoo.com/question/index?qid=20111025144024AA3UFQf

Assembly of First Nations Health Forum. Ottawa, 7–9 November 2011. Retrieved 23 March 2012 from: www.afn.ca/uploads/files/events/afn_health_forum_booklet.pdf

Attorney-General of Canada. Statement of Particulars in the matter of *Assembly of First Nations and First Nations Child and Family Caring Society* v. *Indian and Northern Affairs Canada* (2007), provided to the author by Dr Cindy Blackstock, Executive Director, First Nations Child and Family Caring Society of Canada.

Autism Europe (2006). Autism and Case Law. Protecting the Right to Education for Children with Autistic Spectrum Disorders. Retrieved 21 March 2012 from: www.autismeurope.org/files/files/caselaw-uk.pdf

Bell D, Petrick T (2010) Autism and the law. Published by Guild Yule LLP. Retrieved 22 March 2012 from: http://guildyule.com/cms/images/M_images/pdf/autism%20and%20the%20law%20-%20themes%20in%20recent%20litigation.pdf

Brosco JP (2006) Growth attenuation: a diminutive solution to a daunting problem. *Arch Pediatr Adolesc Med* 160: 1077–1078.

Brown I (2009) *The Boy in the Moon. A Father's Search for His Disabled Son*. London, UK: Random House.

Burke PJ (2004) Media representation in the case of Tracy Latimer. Retrieved 16 March 2012 from: http://patburke.info/media_representation_and_tracy_latimer-burke.pdf

Butler GE, Beadle EA (2007) Manipulating growth and puberty in those with severe disability: when is it justified? *Arch Dis Child* 92: 567–568. http://dx.doi.org/10.1136/adc.2007.116327

Canadian Association of Community Living (CACL) Website. Posting of correspondence by Laurie Larson, President of CACL, dated 30 March 2012. Open letter and formal complaint to Global TV for biased, damaging media coverage. Retrieved 19 April 2012 from: www.cacl.ca/news-stories/blog/open-letter-and-formal-complaint-global-tv-biased-damaging-media-coverage

Carnevale FA, Rehms RS, Kirk S, McKeever P (2008). What we know (and do not know) about raising children with complex continuing care needs. *J Child Health Care* 12 [editorial].

CBC (2010a) Compassionate homicide: the law and Robert Latimer, 6 December. Retrieved 21 March 2012 from: www.cbc.ca/news/canada/story/2010/12/06/f-robert-latimer-compassionate-homicide.html

CBC News Edmonton (2010b) Baby Isaiah dies in Edmonton hospital, 11 March. Retrieved 7 July 2012 from: www.cbc.ca/news/canada/edmonton/story/2010/03/11/edmonton-baby-isaiah-court-appearance-cancelled.html

CBC News Montreal (2011) Interview Podcast. Latimer still defends killing daughter, 17 February. Retrieved 21 March 2012 from: www.cbc.ca/news/canada/montreal/story/2011/02/17/robert-latimer-defends-decision-to-kill-disabled-daughter.html

Children's National Medical Centre (2000) Baby Doe and Baby Jane Doe Regulations. Paediatric Ethicscope Vol 11, No. 1. Retrieved 24 November 2012 from: www.sris.org/prog/samples/cnmc/doctors/Ethic00.pdf

Courtis C. (2008) The right to life and the right to health of children with disabilities before courts: some Latin American examples. In: Clements L, Read J, editors. *Disabled People and the Right to Life, The Protection and Violation of Disabled People's Most Basic Human Rights*. New York: Routledge, pp. 195–207.

CTV News Staff (2009) Couple sues hospital for keeping sick baby alive, 13 March. Retrieved 4 July 2012 from: www.ctvnews.ca/couple-sues-hospital-for-keeping-sick-baby-alive-1.379178

CTV News (2012). New autism centre aims to help with self sufficiency, 24 November. Retrieved 20 March 2012 from: http://toronto.ctv.ca/servlet/an/local/CTVNews/20111124/toronto-autism-training-centre-111124/20111124?hub=TorontoNewHome

Dobrowolsky AZ, Jenson J (2004) Shifting representations of citizenship: Canadian politics of women and children. *Social Politics Int Stud Gender State Soc* 11: 154–180. http://dx.doi.org/10.1093/sp/jxh031

Doolittle DK (1998). Welfare reform: loss of supplemental security income (SSI) for children with disabilities. *J Soc Pediatr Nurs* 3: 33–44. http://dx.doi.org/10.1111/j.1744–6155.1998.tb00207.x

Edelson M (2000) *My Journey with Jake: A Memoir of Parenting and Disability*. Toronto, ON: Between the Lines.

Edelson M (2005) Battle cries: Justice for kids with special needs. Toronto: Sumach Press.

Erkulwater JL (2006) *Disability Rights and the American Social Safety Net*. Ithaca, NY: Cornell University Press.

Federal Court of Canada Website – National List – Ottawa Sittings. Retrieved 27 March 2012 from: http://cas-ncr-nter03.cas-satj.gc.ca/portal/page/portal/fc_cf_en/National_List

Freeman M (2011) Children at the edge of life: parents, doctors, and children's rights. In: Rioux MH, Basser LA, Jones M, editors. *Critical Perspectives on Human Rights and Disability Law*. Boston, MA: Martinus Nijhoff, pp. 117–136. http://dx.doi.org/10.1163/ej.9789004189508.i-552.37

Gentleman K (2008) Aboriginal kids suffer while governments bicker. CapitalNewsOnline. Retrieved 19 March 2012 from: http://www4.carleton.ca/jmc/cnews/03042009/n2.shtml

Global Television (2012) 16X9 Program, Taking Mercy, aired 16 March 2012. Global Television Taking Mercy Live Blog. Retrieved 5 April 2012 from: www.globalnews.ca/live+blog+taking+mercy/6442601396/story.html

Goodley D, Runswick-Cole K (2011) Problematizing policy conceptions of 'child' 'disabled' and 'parents' in social policy in England. *Int J Incl Educ* 15: 71–85.

GovTrack.US. Retrieved 7 July 2012 from: www.govtrack.us/congress/bills/109/s183

Green SE (2007) We're tired, not sad: benefits and burdens of mothering a child with a disability. *Soc Sci Med* 64: 150–163. http://dx.doi.org/10.1016/j.socscimed.2006.08.025

Gunther DF, Diekema DS (2006) Attenuating growth in children with profound developmental disability: a new approach to an old dilemma. *Arch Pediatr Adolesc Med* 160: 1013–1017. http://dx.doi.org/10.1001/archpedi.160.10.1013

Hevesi D (2012) Katie Beckett, who inspired health reform, dies at 34, 22 May. NewYorkYimes.com. Retrieved 5 July 2012 from: www.nytimes.com/2012/05/23/us/katie-beckett-who-inspired-health-reform-dies-at-34.html

Houtrow AJ, Okumura MJ, Hilton JF, Rehm RS (2011). Profiling health and health related services for children with special health care needs with and without disabilities. *Academic Pediatr* 11: 508–515. http://dx.doi.org/10.1016/j.acap.2011.08.004

Jaffey J (2006) Appeal court overturns class action authorization on care for disabled children. *The Lawyers Weekly* 26 (30).

Janz HL (1998) Disabling images and the dangers of public perception: a commentary on the media's 'coverage' of the Latimer case. *Constitut Forum* 9: 66–70.

Jinks D (2002) Legalization of world politics and the future of US human rights policy. *St Louis Law J* 46: 357–376.

Kittay EF (2011) Forever small: the strange case of Ashley X. *Hypatia* 26: 610–631. http://dx.doi.org/10.1111/j.1527–2001.2011.01205.x

Koll M (2010) Growth, interrupted: nontherapeutic growth attenuation, parental medical decision making, and the profoundly developmentally disabled child's right to bodily integrity. *Univ Illinois Law Rev* 1: 225–264.

Kruger BJ (2001) Title V-CSHCN: a closer look at the shaping of the national agenda for children with special health care needs. *Policy Politics Nurs Pract* 2: 321–330. http://dx.doi.org/10.1177/152715440100200411

Lavallee TL (2005) Honouring Jordan: putting First Nation children first and funding fights second. *Paediatr Child Health* 10: 527–529.

Litt J (2004) Women's carework in low-income households: the special case of children with attention deficit hyperactivity disorder. *Gender Society* 18: 625–644. http://dx.doi.org/10.1177/0891243204267399

MacDonald N (2012) Aboriginal children suffer while governments ignore Jordan's Principle. *Can Med Assoc J* 184: 853. Retrieved 20 March 20 2012 from: www.cmaj.ca/content/early/2012/03/05/cmaj.120193.full.pdf

*MacDonald N, Attaran A (2007) Jordan's principle, government's paralysis. *Can Med Assoc J* 177: 321. Retrieved from: www.cmaj.ca/cgi/content/full/177/4/321

McKeever PT (1991) Mothering chronically ill. Technology-dependant children: an analysis using critical theory. PhD dissertation, Faculty of Sociology, York University, York, UK.

Malcolm AH 1986). Baby Doe Decision: a tentative first step in a profound issue. *The New York Times*, 11 June 1986. Retrieved 25 November 2012 from: www.nytimes.com/1986/06/11/us/baby-doe-decision-a-tentative-first-step-on-a-profound-issue.html

Moss K (1987) The 'Baby Doe' legislation: its rise and fall. *Policy Studies J* 15: 629–651. http://dx.doi.org/10.1111/j.1541–0072.1987.tb00751.x

Nathanson A (2011) Legislating Jordan's Principle: an indirect success. *Manitoba Law J* 35: 215–232.

National Library of Medicine. Profiles in Science. The C. Everett Koop Papers. Retrieved 6 July 2012 from: http://profiles.nlm.nih.gov/ps/retrieve/Narrative/QQ/p-nid/86

Newman SA (1989) Baby Doe, Congress and the states: challenging the federal treatment standard for impaired infants. *Am J Law Med* 15: 1–60.

Ontario Ombudsman (2005) Between a rock and hard place. Special Investigation: Parents forced to place their children with severe disabilities in the custody of Children's Aid Societies to obtain necessary care. Retrieved 20 March 2012 from: www.ombudsman.on.ca/Ombudsman/files/8d/8d42b2f4–3cd1–4a30–8c63–0f8f849338bc.pdf

Ontario Ombudsman (2008–2009) Case update – Annual Report of 2005 SORT Report entitled Between a rock and hard place. Special Investigation: Parents forced to place their children with severe disabilities in the custody of Children's Aid Societies to obtain necessary care. Retrieved 20 March 2012 from: www.ombudsman.on.ca/Files/sitemedia/Documents/Investigations/SORT%20Investigations/special-needs-children_0809.pdf

Ontario Ombudsman (2010–2011) Case update – Annual Report of 2005 SORT Report entitled Between a rock and hard place. Special Investigation: Parents forced to place their children with severe disabilities in the custody of Children's Aid Societies to obtain necessary care. Retrieved 20 March 2012 from: www.ombudsman.on.ca/Investigations/SORT-Investigations/Completed/Children-with-special-needs---em-Between-a-Rock-an/Case-update---Annual-Report-2010–2011.aspx

*Ouelette AR (2008) Growth attenuation: parental choice and the rights of disabled children. Lessons from the Ashley X case. *Houston J Health Law Policy* 8: 207–244.

Page S (2009) Ombudsman probes custody-for-care claims; Ottawa parents among 12 cases Marin says emit a 'certain stench'. *The Ottawa Citizen*, 7 February 2009. Retrieved through the Proquest Newspaper database.

Peter E, Spalding K, Kenny N, Conrad P, McKeever P, Macfarlane A (2007). Neither seen nor heard. Children and homecare policy in Canada. *Soc Sci Med* 64: 1624–1636.

Peters M (2011) It's a matter of Jordan's Principle. *The Dominion*, 5 October. Retrieved 20 March 2012 from: www.dominionpaper.ca/articles/4180

*Petrenchik T (2008) Childhood Disability in the Context of Poverty: A Discussion Paper Prepared for the Ontario Ministry of Children and Youth Services. *CanChild* Publication. Retrieved 18 April 2012 from: www.canchild.ca/en/ourresearch/resources/ChildhoodDisabilityintheContextofPoverty_CanChild.pdf

Pillowangel.org. Retrieved 20 March 2012 from: http://pillowangel.org/

Priest L (2010) The two faces of a life or death dilemma. The Globe and Mail.com, 27 January. Retrieved 6 July 2012 from: www.theglobeandmail.com/news/national/the-two-faces-of-a-life-or-death-dilemma/article4303882/

*Priestley M (1998) Childhood disability and disabled childhoods: agendas for research. *Childhood* 5: 207–223. http://dx.doi.org/10.1177/0907568298005002007

Rechel B (2008) Access to care and the right to life of disabled children in Bulgaria. In: Clements L, Read J, editors. *Disabled People and the Right to Life, The Protection and Violation of Disabled People's Most Basic Human Rights*. New York: Routledge, pp. 208–231.

Reed CM, Meyer, KP (2004) Medicaid managed care for children with special health care needs: examining legislative and judicial constraints on privatization. *Publ Admin Rev* 64: 234–242. http://dx.doi.org/10.1111/j.1540–6210.2004.00364.x

Rioux M (2003) On second thought: constructing knowledge, law, disability, and equality. In: Herr S, Gostin L, Koh H, editors. *The Human Rights of Persons with Intellectual Disabilities: Different But Equal*. London: Oxford University Press, pp. 287–317. Retrieved 5 April 2012 from: scholar.googleusercontent.com/scholar?q=cache:1wZwI1bik2YJ:scholar.google.com/+On+Second+Thought%3B+Constructing+Knowledge,+Law,+Disability,+and+Equality&hl=en&as_sdt=0,5&as_vis=1

Ronen GM, Meaney B, Dan B, Zimprich F, Stögmann W, Neugebauer W (2009) From eugenic euthanasia to habilitation of 'disabled' children: Andreas Rett's contribution. *J Child Neurol* 24:115–127. http://dx.doi.org/10.1177/0883073808321763

Rosenberg NS, Yohalem JB (1986) Litigation on behalf of mentally disabled children: targets of opportunity. *Mental Physical Disability Law Reporter*. Retrieved 15 March 2011 from: www.bazelon.org/LinkClick.aspx?fileticket=UOLJtBxcDCw%3D&tabid=222

Sanders C (2011) Gaps remain for special needs kids. *Winnipeg Free Press*, 2 March. Retrieved 22 March 2012 from: www.winnipegfreepress.com/local/gaps-remain-for-first-nations-special-needs-kids-115170099.html

Scambler S (2005) Exposing the limitations of disability theory: the case of juvenile Batten disease. *Soc Theory Health* 3:144–164. http://dx.doi.org/10.1057/palgrave.sth.8700045

Semansky RM, Koyanagi C (2004) The TEFRA Medicaid eligibility option for children with severe disabilities: a national study. *J Behav Health Services Res* 31: 334–342.

Shannon SE, Savage TA (2006) The Ashley treatment: two viewpoints. *Pediatr Nurs* 32: 175–178.

Shapiro J (2010) Katie Beckett: patient turned home-care advocate. Retrieved 20 October 2011 from the National Public Radio website: www.npr.org/templates/story/story.php?storyId=131145687

Simmons T (2008) Relinquishing custody in exchange for mental health services: undermining the adoption and safe families Act's promise of reasonable efforts towards family preservation and reunification. *J Law Family Studies* 10: 377.

Sneiderman B (1997) The Latimer mercy killing case: a rumination of crime and punishment. *Health Law J* 5: 1–26.

Thomson D (2010) *The Four Walls of My Freedom*. Toronto, ON: McArthur and Company.

Toope SJ, Rehaag S (2004) Globalization and the instrument of choice: the role of international law. In: Eliadis, Hill M, Howlett M, editors. *Designing Government: From Instruments to Governance*. Montréal, QB: McGill–Queens University Press, pp. 322 –341.

United States Social Security Administration Office of Disability Adjudication and Review (2012). HALLEX Hearings, Appeals and Litigation Law Manual, Vol. 1, Chapter I-5-4, Court Cases I-5-4-28. *Sullivan v. Zebley*. Issued 7 February 1992. Baltimore: United States Social Security Administration Office of Disability Adjudication and Review. Retrieved 27 November 2012 from: http://ssa.gov/OP_Home/hallex/I-05/I-5-4-28.html

Yantzi NM, Rosenberg MW (2008)The contested meanings of home for women caring for children with long-term care needs in Ontario, Canada. *Gender Place Culture* 15: 301–315.

Cases and law

A.L. v. *(Ontario) Ministry of Community and Social Services*, A.L. and A.E.L., a minor by his litigation guardian [2005] Ontario Superior Court of Justice, Divisional Court. Note: Order in the Special Needs Children Class Action proceeding retrieved from: http//fixcas.com/news/2005/larcade.htm

A.L. v. *(Ontario) Ministry of Community and Social Services* [2006] OJ No. 4637 (CA), leave to appeal refused [2007] SCCA No. 36.

A.L. v. *Her Majesty the Queen in the Right of Ontario, Ministry of Community and Social Services* [2007] SCCA No. 36. Re. Status of application for leave to appeal dismissed without costs (without reasons) 10 May 2007.

Auton (guardian ad litem *of)* v. *British Columbia (Attorney General)* [2004] 3 SCR 657.

Bowen v *American Hospital Association*, 476 US 610 (1986) (Baby Doe case).

Child and Family Service Act RSO 1990, c. C11.

Eldridge v. *British Columbia (Attorney General)* [1997] 3 SCR 624.

First Nations Child and Family Caring Society and Assembly of First Nations v. *Attorney General of Canada (Representing the Minister of Indian and Northern Development Canada)* (2007). Decision dated 14 March 2011 may be accessed at the Canadian Human Rights website in PDF format. Ruling retrieved 20 March 2012 from: http://chrt-tcdp.gc.ca/NS/pdf/Ruling%202011%20CHRT%204.pdf

Larcade v. *(Ontario) Ministry of Community and Social Services* [2005] OJ No. 3156.

Pictou Landing Band Council and Maurina Beadle v. *Attorney General of Canada* [2011]

R. v. *Latimer* [2001] 1 SCR 3. Retrieved 24 November 2012 from: www.canlii.org/en/ca/scc/doc/2001/2001scc1/2001scc1.pdf

Sagharian v. *Ontario (Minister of Education)* [2008] ONCA 411 (ON CA)

Sullivan v. *Zebley*, 493 US 521 (1990).

The US Department of Health and Human Services. Administration for Children and Families. The Developmental Disabilities Assistance and Bill of Rights Act of 2000. PUBLIC LAW 106–402–30 October 2000. 114 STAT. 1677. Retrieved 9 July 2012 from: www.acf.hhs.gov/programs/add/ddact/DDACT2.html

Wynberg v. *Ontario* (2006) 82 OR (3d) 561 (Ont. CA)

Section B Methods and Measurement

14
MEASUREMENT CONCEPTS, STANDARDS, AND PERSPECTIVES

Aileen M. Davis

Overview

Clinical researchers increasingly are using patient-reported outcome (PRO) measures in effectiveness research and in day-to-day monitoring of patients. As in disciplines where quantitative values are generated (e.g. laboratory medicine), issues of measurement are fundamental and germane in the application and interpretation of PROs. Measurement properties, typically reliability, validity, and responsiveness (when change in response to natural history or an intervention is relevant), are critical to interpreting scores on a measure. However, these measurement properties are not characteristics of the PRO itself but an interaction of the measure and the context in which it is used. This chapter provides background on fundamental concepts of health measurement. It focuses in particular on the specification of the health concept being measured, the population of interest, the purpose(s) for measuring (context), and the necessary properties of measures (content and face validity, scaling, reliability, construct validity, and responsiveness, including defining response to treatment). Additionally, the chapter presents recommended standards for measurement properties and their implications for measure application.

Setting the context

CONCEPT, PURPOSE, AND POPULATION

One of the most challenging statements clinician researchers need to specify in relation to outcome measurement is 'I need a measure of "x" concept to describe, predict or evaluate change in "y" outcome in "z" patient or patient group.' Defining the concept is critical. Clearly defining the phenomenon of interest – be it health-related quality of life, impairment, or some other concept – is fundamental to specifying the relevant items to be included in a PRO. Simply providing a label of the concept is insufficient as the same label frequently is used for different phenomena (as discussed in Chapters 3 and 15). For example, the literature includes many measures of 'function', but a review of the items shows that some of these instruments include items such as range of motion and strength, whereas others include items related to difficulty with walking, dressing, and so on. Similarly, health-related quality of life (HRQL) has been defined in numerous ways. Specifying the concept, often using a theoretical framework (e.g. the World Health Organization's International Classification of Functioning, Disability and Health from 2001, discussed in Chapter 4) or specified definition of health (Huber et al 2011; see Chapter 2), facilitates a common understanding of the phenomenon being measured.

Measures are generally used for one or more purposes: to describe, predict, or measure change in status (Kane and Kane 1981, Kirschner and Guyatt 1985). The requisite measurement properties are based on the purpose(s) for which the measure will be used and the standards of measurement differ depending on whether the measure is applied at a group or individual level. A measure used for description at a single point in time does not require test–retest reliability or evaluation of responsiveness. A measure used to predict a second concurrent or future event requires demonstration of predictive validity, while a measure of change needs to demonstrate responsiveness. As described in more detail below under reliability, measures applied in decision making at the individual level require much higher reliability to be confident that change beyond day-to-day variability has occurred. Table 14.1 provides an overview of the purposes of measures and the minimum necessary measurement properties that are described in more detail later in the chapter.

Content and face validity
The content of a PRO needs to include items that are important from the perspective of all the relevant stakeholders, and not just the clinician researcher. In the case of measures for children and adolescents, research has shown that children as young as 5 years old can participate in generating items (Ronen et al 1999). Additionally, the perspectives of parents, caregivers, and teachers may be important.

The actual items chosen also need to reflect the nature of the experience of the patient group to avoid floor and ceiling effects. For example, if only very easy mobility items are included in a group with very little difficulty in mobility, almost everyone will have

TABLE 14.1
Purpose of measurement and minimal measurement properties for the specified patient population

Purpose	Reliability	Validity	Responsiveness
Description	Internal consistency (sometimes) interrater	Content and face; construct	NA
Prediction	Internal consistency; test–retest	Content and face; construct; concurrent and/or predictive	NA
Change	Internal consistency; test–retest	Content and face; construct	Responsiveness (group level); MCID and/ or PASS (individual response)

NA, not applicable; MCID, minimally important difference; PASS, patient acceptable symptom state.

near-perfect scores and no mobility challenges will be identified. In contrast, very difficult items for a group with severe mobility restrictions would result in almost all being identified as being immobile. Hence, the breadth of item difficulty included in a measure needs to reflect the complexity of the issues in the relevant patient group.

Face validity is a judgement that the items seem to be measuring the phenomena of interest and that the item wording and the response options are clear.

From items to scores

Item responses for PROs typically use either a dichotomous 'no/yes' response or an ordinal polytotomous Likert-type response (e.g. strongly agree to strongly disagree) or rating scale (e.g. 'none' to 'extreme') over a number of ordered categories. In the context of HRQL, impairment, or symptoms, response options are often based on the amount of difficulty, limitation, frequency, or intensity. Generating scores from these response options requires consideration of how responses to individual items are aggregated and also decisions about whether to create a single summary score or to create individual domain scores (e.g. separate summary scores for each symptom and functional limitation dimension).

The classic test theory approach (see, for example, Nunnally 1978 or Kerlinger 1986) evaluates the interrelationships of items through inter-item and adjusted item–total correlations. (The item–total correlation is adjusted for the contribution of the individual item to the total score.) Generally, items that are intercorrelated and have item–total correlations in the range of 0.30 to 0.70 are considered to be associated but not so highly related as to result in redundancy of information. The chosen items are tested for internal consistency or scale homogeneity with Cronbach's alpha (α) (for multiple response items) or Kuder–Richardson 20 (for binary responses). Failure to achieve scale homogeneity may occur if the items actually consist of two or more phenomena with relatively little interrelationship. Furthermore, a high Cronbach's α does not guarantee that a scale is measuring a single attribute, as a 'satisfactory' index of homogeneity may be achieved by a group of items with two or more attributes that have some intercorrelation. Cronbach's α is also influenced by the number of items so the alpha must be interpreted with caution when the number of items is over 15, particularly if the items represent redundant concepts. For research- and group-level comparisons, an internal consistency of 0.80 (DeVellis 1996) is acceptable. Factor analysis is often used for further clarification of dimensionality.

Factor analysis refers to a group of statistical techniques that create a linear combination of variables (based on correlations or the covariance of the items) (Norman and Streiner 2008). The purpose of factor analysis is to determine groups of items that are intercorrelated, and thus are potentially measuring a single phenomenon. Exploratory factor analysis is used when there are no a priori hypotheses about which specific items will be related to a given factor. In contrast, confirmatory factor analysis (CFA) prespecifies the items that will form each specified factor (Brown 2006). The methods of factor analysis are beyond the scope of this chapter, but there are numerous statistical approaches, the most common of which is maximum likelihood estimation. Irrespective of method, a factor analytical solution, demonstrating that items 'load' on (or are associated with) a factor (or domain) that clinically and/or conceptually makes sense, is evidence from a classic test theory approach that the items can be summed to a total 'domain' score. In some cases, these domain scores are factor analysed and, based on the results, are summed to an overall summary score. For example, the Short Form-36 (SF-36) (Ware 1993, Ware et al 1994, Ware and Kosinski 2001) – has items aggregated to eight domain scores, and the domain scores have been aggregated to two component scores using a factor analytical approach.

In the last decade, item response theory (IRT) methods that have long been used in education to create standardized tests have been applied in health measurement. These models use a probabilistic approach to create a hierarchy of item difficulty and ultimately a summary score for a unidimensional construct. Item response theory creates an item characteristic curve for each item, and items are then chosen with favourable characteristics to represent the range of the attribute. Inclusion of items that are not part of the unified construct would result in poor characteristics (usually poor discrimination) (Bond and Fox 2001, Wilson 2005).

The Rasch model approach to IRT utilizes the one-parameter logistic model in which the slope of the item is 1 (Rasch 1960). In this model, the data must fit the model and scores generated for the participant are interval-level data. Proponents of this model argue that the Rasch model is the only model that produces functional form and interval-level scores that meet the requirements for measurement. These requirements are invariance where item difficulty is the same irrespective of the person score (e.g. stairs have a consistent level of difficulty and it is the people who have different abilities on the stairs as reflected by their score); invariance in that order of item difficulty is maintained irrespective of the context (i.e. item 'a' is always more difficult than item 'b'); the item-response function is the same for all items (i.e. the slope is 1); and the thresholds are the same between response options (i.e. the distance at which there is a 50% chance of choosing one option or the other is the same between response options) (Wilson 2005). Other people utilize a one-parameter IRT model where the slope is a constant (not necessarily 1) or a multiparameter model in which the data are used to determine the parameter estimates in the model. The derived model is used to calculate the scores. Proponents of the Rasch approach argue that functional form and the requirements for measurement are not met by IRT models or by CFA. It should also be noted that CFA can produce solutions that are equivalent of up to a two-parameter IRT model (Brown 2006).

Perhaps the most significant contribution of the Rasch and IRT models in the context of health measurement is the development of item banks and the implementation of computer adaptive testing (Haley et al 2006, PROMIS Network Center 2012). An item bank consists of items, representing a unidimensional construct, that have been calibrated in a hierarchy of difficulty. An item bank often includes hundreds of calibrated items such that a very precise measure can be achieved by obtaining responses to a very small number of items. Based on the responses to an initial small number of items, a computer software algorithm chooses the next item to be answered from the item bank. The process continues until the participant's score is obtained to the desired level of precision. Figure 14.1 demonstrates how this might work where there is a set of 10 items and three are asked initially. It is assumed that the respondent cannot perform the most difficult item asked, 'hiking for 2 hours', but reports no difficulty with the next most difficult item presented, 'rising from the floor'. The person's score, therefore, lies within the range of difficulty of these two items. The response to the next items posed ('climbing one flight of stairs') indicates no difficulty, but the person has an inability to 'run to catch a bus'. As there is only one item remaining between these two

		Round 1	Round 2	Round 3
Most difficult ↑	**Item**			
	Running a marathon			
	Hiking for 2 hours	×		
	Running to catch the bus		×	
	Walking 2 hours on flat ground			√
	Climbing one flight of stairs		√	
	Rising from the floor	√		
	Bending to pick a pencil from the floor			
	Rising from a chair	√		
Least difficult ↓	Walking in the house			
	Rolling over in bed			

Fig. 14.1 An example of an item bank with 10 items.

items, the respondent has a difficulty score either equivalent to climbing one flight of stairs or to the remaining item, walking 2 hours on flat ground. The respondent indicates that they are able to walk 2 hours on flat ground – the more difficult item – which then generates his or her score. In this example, although the measure or item bank included 10 items, the precise person score was achieved by responding to only six items. One can imagine the increased efficiency when multiple domains (item banks) with many items are used.

Rasch and IRT methods support unidimensional scale scoring, i.e. subscale scores. While there are some advantages to a single summary score for a PRO because of its perceived simplicity and its use in economic analyses, subscale scores may be more informative for a number of reasons. Specifically, if an intervention such as pain medication is likely to impact one construct more than another (e.g. pain intensity vs physical function) or if there is likely to be differential recovery (e.g. pain intensity may improve more rapidly than physical function as joint motion, muscle strength, and flexibility may also need to improve and can, now that pain is controlled), subscale scores may demonstrate effects of the intervention that may be diluted through a single summary score that would combine the pain and physical function items. Additionally, subscale scores may be more helpful in interpreting the outcome of clinical studies and may assist patients in understanding the expected course of their recovery over a number of outcomes.

Reliability

A measure is reliable when the same score is obtained when repeated by the same rater (intra-rater reliability or test–retest reliability in the case of self-administered measures) or different raters (interrater reliability) when there has been no change in status. Validity, described more fully later in the chapter, is supported when a body of evidence supports that a measure has relationships with another phenomenon as hypothesized (Messick 1989). For example, if you stand on a weigh scale and obtain radically different and inconsistent measurements, you would conclude that the scale was neither reliable nor valid. However, if you stood on the scale and obtained the same measurement that was consistently 5 kg less than the 'true' weight, you would conclude that the scale was reliable but not valid.

Reliability is the basic and essential quality of a scientific measurement. Scientific investigation can be performed only if the measure used in testing hypotheses is reliable. Additionally, change in a reliable measurement can more confidently be attributed to clinical change. Treatment decisions are often based on the detection of a change in a clinical state and such change must be differentiated from measurement variability/error (i.e. poor reliability) to avoid incorrect treatment decisions, either failure to treat or unnecessary treatment. Finally, reliable measures reduce the number of patients required in clinical trials by reducing the variability or 'noise' of the measurement.

In the case of PROs measurement variability can arise from the measure itself (e.g. the wording of items on a questionnaire may be poor and allow for multiple interpretations) or from rater variability in administered questionnaires. Clear, standardized instructions and interviewer training reduce such variability.

Historically, psychometricians used internal consistency, such as Cronbach's α, as a measure of reliability, arguing that repeated measures might be affected by learning effects (patients remembering their previous responses leading to falsely high reliability) or that a patient's clinical state might change between measurements (falsely lowering reliability). Each item (in a homogeneous measure) is considered to measure roughly the same phenomenon such that the questionnaire functions as if the measure were being repeatedly performed. However, test–retest reliability (where the measure is repeatedly examined on two [or more] occasions by the same rater) is now the most commonly performed test of reliability for PROs. Clinician researchers perform test–retest reliability because it more closely matches the clinical situation of measurement of a phenomenon on repeated occasions. However, Cronbach's α and the intraclass correlation coefficient (ICC), discussed below, bear mathematical equivalence and in many situations provide the same results as long as patients do not change between measurements (Bravo and Potvin 1991).

Reliability is quantified using statistics of concordance (or agreement), although there is a body of literature that has used tests of association (or trend). Tests of association such as correlation coefficients provide a minimal estimate of reliability because two measurements could correlate well but never agree (e.g. a perfect association but no agreement would occur if there were a systematic 10-point increase for all participants on the second administration compared with the first). Furthermore, correlation coefficients such as Pearson's r, Spearman's rho, or Kendall's tau do not correct for chance agreement. Poor correlation between measures indicates poor reliability, and thus reliability needs to be confirmed with an index of concordance such as the kappa statistic or ICC.

Percentage agreement and the kappa statistics are used as measures of concordance for binary or ordinal data. The per cent agreement is expressed by the number of occasions the scale provided the same answer (for each individual patient) as a percentage of the number of comparisons; however, it does not correct for chance agreement. The kappa statistic evaluates the incremental improvement in agreement of the measure, adjusting for agreement caused by chance alone. For ordinal scales, agreement may be quantified either with the unweighted kappa or the unweighted per cent agreement. These unweighted indices assume that a disagreement of one level is equivalent to a disagreement of two or more levels apart. For example, the difference between a response of 1 ('not at all') and 2 ('a little') would have the same weight as a difference between 1 ('not at all') and 3 ('a moderate amount'). Weighted per cent agreement and weighted kappa both assign weights to the disagreement, with greater discrepancies receiving a greater weight. The weights assigned to disagreement are arbitrary. However, the most common weighting scheme is to grade disagreements according to the number of separated categories. For example, a difference of one is assigned a weight of one, a difference of two is assigned a weight of two, and so on. This quadratic weighted kappa is frequently used as it is equivalent to the ICC (Fleiss and Cohen 1973).

The ICC is used to evaluate the reliability for continuous measurements as a ratio of variability between and within participant scores. The ICC is derived from an analysis of variance table and the appropriate formula depends on the need for generalizability of the results (Portney and Watkins 2000). If the results will be generalized to only a specific group of examiners evaluating the same group of patients, or the same group of respondents as in the case of self-report, a 'fixed effects' model is appropriate. In the more common situation of generalization of the results to a theoretical group of all patients and all examiners, the 'random effects' model is appropriate. 'Mixed effects' models are appropriate for either a fixed group of examiners on a sample of patients or a fixed group of patients examined by a sample of examiners (Portney and Watkins 2000).

The standards for reliability depend on whether decisions need to be made at a group or an individual level, with individual-level measurement requiring much higher reliability and less random variability. Somewhat arbitrary standards have been described for both the kappa and ICC statistics. For the kappa, 0 to 0.20 is referred to as 'poor', 0.20 to 0.40 is 'acceptable', 0.40 to 0.60 is 'fair', 0.60 to 0.80 is 'substantial', and 0.80 to 1 is 'almost perfect agreement' (Landis and Koch 1977). For the ICC, 0.80 is recommended for group-level use and 0.90 or higher is recommended for individual-level application (Nunnally 1978). It is highly recommended that 95% confidence intervals be calculated, with particular attention paid to the lower bound. At a group level, lower levels of reliability result in more variability which increases the required sample size for a desired effect with a specified power and significance level (Fleiss 1986). At an individual level, reliability is critical in determining how much change is required (boundaries of error) to ensure that any observed change is not just day-to-day variation.

For determining the boundaries of error for measuring change (which Stratford has termed 'minimal detectable change' [MDC] at 95% confidence), the formula is (Stratford 2004):

$$MDC_{95} = Z_\alpha \times SD \sqrt{(2[1-r])}$$

where r is the test–retest ICC, Z_α is the z-score for the desired level of confidence, and SD is the standard deviation at one point in time. The multiplier '2' takes into account a doubling of the chance of error by taking data from two sets: test and retest.

As an example, at a 95% confidence level for a measure with score range 0 to 100 with a standard deviation of 20, the MDC_{95} for test–retest reliability of 0.90 and 0.95 would be 17.5 and 12.4, respectively. Hence, with a reliability of 0.90 an individual would need to change more than 17.5 points to be sure that true change had occurred, and with a reliability of 0.95 a change of 12.4 points would be required. If reliability were 0.85, a change of 21.5 points would be required.

For the sake of completeness and considering the statements above regarding the use of alpha as a measure of reliability, a measure of precision (McHorney and Tarlov 1995) can also be calculated. In much of the psychology literature, this is referred to as 'reliable change' (Jacobson et al 1999). Reliable change is calculated as:

$$MDC_{95} = Z_\alpha \times SD \sqrt{(1-r)}$$

where r is Cronbach's α, Z_α is the z-score for the desired level of confidence, and SD is the standard deviation at one point in time.

Note that r in this formula is alpha and also that there is no doubling effect as alpha is based on one measure rather than repeated tests. In situations where the intent is to make a decision at the individual level, such as placing a child in a special education class based on test scores, Cronbach's α >0.90 is recommended (Nunnally 1978). If one were to solve the formula, it becomes evident that lower values of alpha reduce the precision of the score estimate.

Bland–Altman plots, which define limits of agreement, have also been described as a method of differentiating between measurement variability and true clinical change when a change in a measurement is observed between clinical observations (Bland and Altman 1986, 1995). Limits of agreement are the mean difference between two measurements ± 2 standard deviations. If a measurement difference exceeds the limits of agreement, then the difference is often presumed to represent 'true' clinical change rather than change that could be due to error (day-to-day variability in scores). The MDC_{95} is equivalent to the Bland–Altman limits of agreement when they are set around zero (no change) rather than the mean observed difference.

Sample size calculations for reliability studies are based on the number of raters, the alpha and beta error, and either the confidence interval around the estimate (Streiner and Norman 2008) or testing that the coefficient is different from some arbitrary value that is set a priori (Donner and Eliasziw 1987). Most test–retest reliability studies for PROs seeking to achieve an ICC of at least 0.80 with a lower 95% bound of 0.70 require between 30 and 40 participants.

Validity

Validity is not an all or none phenomenon; rather, it involves a building of evidence that supports the meaningfulness of results with the measure; that is, the evidence and theoretical rationales support the inferences of or actions based on test scores (Messick 1989).

There are numerous types of validity, some of which are necessary only in relation to specific purposes of a measure, as noted in Table 14.1. The literature is confusing in that multiple terms are used for the same type of validity, and terms sometimes are used in unusual ways. While the terminology will be presented it is most important to think about what the hypothesis is that one is attempting to test to support validity.

Construct validity is requisite for PROs as most of the outcomes of interest are not tangible phenomena but rather attributes or constructs such as anxiety, depression, HRQL, satisfaction, etc. Hence, a mini-theory is created through the formulation of hypotheses about the magnitude and direction of the relationships of the measure of interest and other measures. These hypotheses may include relationships that would be expected to converge (convergent construct validity), whereas divergent construct validity (sometimes referred to as discriminant validity) would be tested when one expects opposing relationships between measures. Correlational analyses are typically conducted to explore these issues.

Known group/extreme group validity (sometimes referred to as discriminant validity, as it differentiates between two or more groups) is tested through a hypothesis defining groups between/among which a difference in the construct of interest is expected. Appropriate parametric or non-parametric statistics are used to evaluate differences in the measure scores, based on the number of groups.

CFA and multitrait multimethod analyses are special analytical techniques for testing construct validity. CFA was introduced above and is an analytical process whereby an a priori model of items related to a specified construct is tested. A multitrait multimethod approach is a way of summarizing the many correlation coefficients in the matrix when one is evaluating a measure with multiple constructs in relation to at least one other measure that has multiple constructs (Campbell and Fiske 1959). Hypotheses are generated about the constructs that will be strongly related and those that are expected to have lower or divergent relationships. The average of the convergent correlations should be higher than the average of the divergent correlations and no individual correlation from the divergent relationships should be higher than the correlations of the convergent relationships. Table 14.2 provides a simple hypothetical example of multitrait multimethod validity.

Predictive validity evaluates how well a measure predicts another current (concurrent predictive validity) or future event. Various forms of regression techniques are used to test

TABLE 14.2
Multitrait multimethod construct validity based on two different measures evaluating similar constructs

| Measure B | Measure A | | | |
	Pain	Mobility	Depression	Social function
Pain	0.75			
Mobility	0.61	0.69		
Depression	0.56	0.55	0.71	
Social function	0.43	0.34	0.44	0.64

Hypothetical correlation coefficients are presented for the bivariate relationships between constructs. The convergent correlations are on the diagonal and have a mean of 0.70, and the divergent correlations have a mean of 0.49.

prediction and the form is dependent on the type of outcome date (Harrell et al 1996). The statistical methods for determining a predictive model can be complex, as the model itself needs to be validated. Large samples with large numbers of events may allow random splitting of the sample with the expectation that the results would agree in the two samples. With smaller samples, bootstrapping may be used. The analysis is run multiple times using a proportion of the sample (about 75–80% of the cases) and should provide a stable model.

Responsiveness, response to treatment, and score interpretation

RESPONSIVENESS

Responsiveness has been defined in many ways in the literature, but the definition by DeBruin et al – the ability of an instrument to accurately detect change when it has occurred (DeBruin et al 1997) – is considered the most versatile (Beaton 2000, Beaton et al 2001). The component of accurate detection of change focuses on mathematical issues of effect size while the construct of change (within participant, between participant, hybrid incorporating both within and between) is emphasized by the component of 'when change has occurred'. An instrument can never be declared to 'be responsive'. Rather, as with reliability and validity, responsiveness reflects the application of the measure in a certain context and to a certain type of change, and evidence builds over time.

Having defined the construct of change and described the expected magnitude and direction of the change, the mini-theory is tested using mathematical and statistical techniques. Responsiveness is reported using a standardized change score or effect size for unpaired or paired data (Cohen 1989). The most common approach is for paired data for PROs (as baseline or pretreatment scores are known to impact the final score) and this is commonly referred to as the standardized response mean (SRM). The SRM is calculated by dividing the mean change score by the standard deviation of the score change. Responsiveness of a measure for an intervention of interest allows predetermination of study sample size.

RESPONSE TO TREATMENT

Responsiveness provides information at a group level but it does not help the clinician or clinician scientist understand who has responded to treatment. Rather the minimal clinically important difference (MCID) or the Patient Acceptable Symptom State (PASS) defines who has responded based on achieving important change (Jaeschke et al 1989, Goldsmith et al 1993) or a defined threshold acceptable state, respectively (Tubach et al 2006). Although the MCID has been calculated based on score distributions (Wyrwich et al 1999a,b, Norman et al 2003), the Food and Drug Administration in the USA now requires that patient-based anchor methods be used to determine the MCID (US Food and Drug Administration 2012). These methods include the use of a question asking people how much better or worse they are and calculating the change score at which a specified proportion of respondents felt they had achieved important improvement (or worsening) (Jaeschke et al 1989, Juniper et al 1994). Similarly, the PASS asks people to indicate their satisfaction with their level of symptoms, function, or some other construct and calculates the PASS based on the final state score for a prespecified proportion of people who are satisfied. The 75th centile is commonly used.

Recent work indicates that using both the MCID and PASS may more accurately define who has responded to treatment (Beaton et al 2011).

The MCID and PASS are challenging in that they are affected by a number of factors. These include, but are not limited to, the effect of the baseline scores and the fact that MCID values must be larger than day-to-day variability (as described above under 'Reliability') (King 2011). Some authors suggest that the MCID should be calculated across the tertiles of the baseline score (Tubach et al 2006). The PASS is less affected by baseline score, but precision, as described above, must be considered (Tubach et al 2006).

There may also be a need to interpret the meaning of a score on a measure outside the context of an intervention, for example between groups of people with different health conditions or among those with a health condition, healthy control individuals, or the general population (so called normative data). These comparator groups usually are matched by age and sex to the patient group of interest and ideally are selected from a population of similar socio-economic status to ensure that other known factors related to health status do not confound the comparison. Healthy control individuals are people without the condition. In contrast, normative data may include some individuals with the condition or other conditions, as would be found in the general population.

Conclusions

This chapter has provided an overview of the concepts of measurement, largely reflecting the use of PROs. In presenting the methodological approaches and standards for measurement, the implications for measure application have been presented. Understanding the concepts and standards of measurement, reliability, validity, and responsiveness of a measure used for a given purpose, with specified interventions in a specified patient population, is critical to applying and interpreting data. The quality and interpretability of study results are only as good as our measures.

REFERENCES

*Key references

Beaton DE (2000) Understanding the relevance of measured change through studies of responsiveness. *Spine* 25: 3192–3199.

*Beaton DE, Bombardier C, Katz JN, Wright JG (2001) A taxonomy for responsiveness. *J Clin Epidemiol* 54: 1204–1217. http://dx.doi.org/10.1016/S0895-4356(01)00407-3

*Beaton DE, van Eerd D, Smith P, et al (2011) Minimal change is sensitive, less specific to recovery: a diagnostic testing approach to interpretability. *J Clin Epidemiol* 64: 487–496. http://dx.doi.org/10.1016/j.jclinepi.2010.07.012

Bland JM, Altman DG (1986) Statistical methods for assessing agreement between two methods of clinical measurement. *Lancet* 1: 307–310. http://dx.doi.org/10.1016/S0140-6736(86)90837-8

Bland JM, Altman DG (1995) Comparing methods of measurement: why plotting difference against standard method is misleading. *Lancet* 346: 1085–1087. http://dx.doi.org/10.1016/S0140-6736(95)91748-9

Bond TG, Fox CM (2001) *Applying the Rasch Model: Fundamental Measurement in the Human Sciences.* Mahwah, NJ: Lawrence Erlbaum Associates, Inc.

*Bravo G, Potvin L (1991) Estimating the reliability of continuous measures with Cronbach's alpha or the intraclass correlation coefficient: toward the integration of two traditions. *J Clin Epidemiol* 44: 381–390. http://dx.doi.org/10.1016/0895-4356(91)90076-L

*Brown TA (2006) *Confirmatory Factor Analysis for Applied Research*. New York: The Guildford Press.

*Campbell DT, Fiske DW (1959) Convergent and discriminant validation by the multitrait–multimethod matrix. *Psychol Bull* 56: 81–105. http://dx.doi.org/10.1037/h0046016

Cohen J (1989) *Statistical Power Analysis for the Behavioural Sciences*, 2nd edition. Hillsdale, NJ: Lawrence Erlbaum Associates.

DeBruin AF, Diederiks JPM, DeWitte PL, Stevens FCJ, Philipsen H (1997) Assessing the responsiveness of a functional status measure: the Sickness Impact Profile versus the SIP68. *J Clin Epidemiol* 50: 529–540. http://dx.doi.org/10.1016/S0895-4356(97)00047-4

DeVellis RF (1996) A consumer's guide to finding, evaluating, and reporting on measurement instruments. *Arthritis Care Res* 9: 239–245. http://dx.doi.org/10.1002/1529-0131(199606)9:3<239::AID-ANR1790090313>3.0.CO;2-O

Donner A, Eliasziw M (1987) Sample size requirements for reliability studies. *Stat Med* 6: 441–448. http://dx.doi.org/10.1002/sim.4780060404

Fleiss JL (1986) *The Design and Analysis of Clinical Experiments*. New York: John Wiley and Sons.

*Fleiss JL, Cohen J (1973) The equivalence of weighted kappa and the intraclass correlation coefficient as measures of reliability. *Educ Psychol Meas* 33: 613–619. http://dx.doi.org/10.1177/001316447303300309

Goldsmith CH, Boers M, Bombardier C, Tugwell P (1993) Criteria for clinically important changes in outcomes: development, scoring and evaluation of rheumatoid arthritis patient and trial profiles. OMERACT Committee. *J Rheumatol* 20: 561–565.

*Haley SM, Ni P, Ludlow LH, Fragala-Pinkham MA (2006) Measurement precision and efficiency of multidimensional computer adaptive testing of physical functioning using the Pediatric Evaluation of Disability Inventory. *Arch Phys Med Rehabil* 87: 1223–1229. http://dx.doi.org/10.1016/j.apmr.2006.05.018

*Harrell FE Jr, Lee KL, Mark DB (1996) Multivariable prognostic models: issues in developing models, evaluating assumptions and adequacy, and measuring and reducing errors. *Stat Med* 15: 361–387. http://dx.doi.org/10.1002/(SICI)1097-0258(19960229)15:4<361::AID-SIM168>3.0.CO;2-4

Huber M, Knottnerus JA, Green L, et al (2011) How should we define health? *BMJ* 343: 1–3.

Jacobson NS, Roberts LJ, Berns SB, McGlinchey JB (1999) Methods for defining and determining the clinical significance of treatment effects: description, application, and alternatives. *J Consult Clin Psychol* 67: 300–307. http://dx.doi.org/10.1037/0022-006X.67.3.300

Jaeschke R, Singer J, Guyatt GH (1989) Measurement of health status. Ascertaining the minimal clinically important difference. *Control Clin Trials* 10: 407–415. http://dx.doi.org/10.1016/0197-2456(89)90005-6

Juniper EF, Guyatt GH, Willan A, Griffith LE (1994) Determining a minimal important change in a disease-specific quality of life questionnaire. *J Clin Epidemiol* 47: 81–87. http://dx.doi.org/10.1016/0895-4356(94)90036-1

Kane RA, Kane RL (1981) *Assessing the Elderly: A Practical Guide for Measurement*. Toronto, ON: Lexington Books.

Kerlinger FN (1986) *Foundations of Behavioral Research*, 3rd edition. New York: Holt, Rhinehart and Winston.

*King MT (2011) A point of minimal important difference (Mid): a critique of terminology and methods. *Exp Rev Pharmacoecon Outcomes Res* 11: 171–184. http://dx.doi.org/10.1586/erp.11.9

*Kirschner B, Guyatt G (1985) A methodological framework for assessing health indices. *J Chron Dis* 38: 27–36. http://dx.doi.org/10.1016/0021-9681(85)90005-0

Landis JR, Koch GG (1977) The measurement of observer agreement for categorical data. *Biometrics* 33: 159–174. http://dx.doi.org/10.2307/2529310

*McHorney CA, Tarlov AR (1995) Individual-patient monitoring in clinical practice: are available health status surveys adequate? *Qual Life Res* 4: 293–307. http://dx.doi.org/10.1007/BF01593882

*Messick S (1989) Validity. In: Linn RL, editor. *Educational Measurement*, 3rd edition. New York: Macmillan, pp. 12–103.

Norman G, Streiner D (2008) Principal components and factor analysis. In: *Biostatistics: The Bare Essentials*, 3rd edition. Hamilton: BC Decker Inc., pp. 194–209.

Norman GR, Sloan JA, Wyrwich KW (2003) Interpretation of changes in health-related quality of life: the remarkable universality of half a standard deviation. *Med Care* 41: 582–592. http://dx.doi.org/10.1097/01. MLR.0000062554.74615.4C

Nunnally JC (1978) *Psychometric Theory*, 2nd edition. New York: Oxford University Press.

*PROMIS Network Center (2012) Patient Reported Outcomes Measurement Information System (PROMIS). Available at: http://www.nihpromis.org/ (accessed 26 January 2012).

Portney LG, Watkins MP (2000) Statistical measures of reliability. In: *Foundation of Clinical Research: Applications to Practice*, 2nd edition. Norwich, CN: Appleton and Lange, pp. 557–586.

Rasch G (1960) *Probablislistic Model for Some Intelligence and Attainment Tests*. Chicago, IL: University of Chicago Press.

Ronen GM, Rosenbaum P, Law M, Streiner DL (1999) Health-related quality of life in childhood epilepsy: the results of children's participation in identifying the components. *Dev Med Child Neurol* 41: 554–559. http://dx.doi.org/10.1017/S0012162299001176

*Stratford PW (2004) Getting more from the literature: estimating the standard error of measurement from reliability studies. *Physiother Can* 56: 27–30. http://dx.doi.org/10.2310/6640.2004.15377

Streiner DL, Norman GR (2008) Reliability. In: *Health Measurement Scales: A Practical Guide to Their Development and Use*, 4th edition. Oxford: Oxford University Press, pp. 167–210.

Tubach F, Dougados M, Falissard B, Baron G, Logeart I, Ravaud P (2006) Feeling good rather than feeling better matters more to patients. *Arthritis Rheum* 55: 526–530. http://dx.doi.org/10.1002/art.22110

*US Food and Drug Administration (2012) *US Department of Health and Human Services Food and Drug Administration, Center of Drug Evaluation and Research (CDER), Center for Biologics Evaluation and Research (CBER), Center for Devices and Radiological Health (CDRH) Guidance for Industry Patient-Reported Outcome Measures: Use in Medical Product Development to Support Labeling Claims*. Rockville, MD: US Food and Drug Administration.

Ware JE Jr (1993) *SF-36 Health Survey: Manual and Interpretation Guide*. Boston, MA: Nimrod Press.

Ware JE, Kosinski M (2001) *SF-36 Physical and Mental Health Summary Scales: A Manual for Users of Version 1*, 2nd edition. Lincoln, RI: Quality Metric Incorporated.

Ware JE, Kosinski M, Keller SK (1994) *SF-36® Physical and Mental Health Summary Scales: A User's Manual*. Boston, MA: The Health Institute.

*Wilson M (2005) *Constructing Measures: An Item Response Modeling Approach*. Mahwah, NJ: Lawrence Erlbaum Associates.

World Health Organization (2001) *International Classification of Functioning, Disability and Health*. Geneva: World Health Organization.

Wyrwich KW, Nienaber NA, Tierney WM, Wolinsky FD (1999a) Linking clinical relevance and statistical significance in evaluating intra-individual changes in health-related quality of life. *Med Care* 37: 469–478. http://dx.doi.org/10.1097/00005650-199905000-00006

Wyrwich KW, Tierney WM, Wolinsky FD (1999b) Further evidence supporting an SEM-based criterion for identifying meaningful intra-individual changes in health-related quality of life. *J Clin Epidemiol* 52: 861–873. http://dx.doi.org/10.1016/S0895-4356(99)00071-2

15

PRACTICAL CONSIDERATIONS IN CHOOSING HEALTH, HEALTH-RELATED QUALITY OF LIFE, AND QUALITY OF LIFE MEASURES FOR CHILDREN AND YOUNG PEOPLE

Nora Fayed

Overview

Selecting the appropriate instrument for one's specific clinical or research purposes can be a daunting task. The literature on general psychometric properties such as reliability, validity, and responsiveness can be jargon laden and present barriers to selecting an instrument. This chapter outlines basic issues of instrument selection for scales already developed and applied in the paradigm of classic test theory, while providing information about essential concepts that can be generally applied.

A common scenario

A community-based health service programme manager wants to know about the health-related quality of life (HRQL) of children served by the programme. She consults with colleagues and the literature and develops a short list of three instruments to consider implementing. Now the manager must decide which instrument to choose.

Introduction: why should I be interested in this topic?

The introductory chapters of this book discuss what it means for a child, adolescent, or young adult to be healthy and have a good quality of life. If these outcomes are essential to one's professional goals, they need to be assessed appropriately. Measuring broad outcomes such as health, HRQL, and quality of life (QOL), and their component elements (such as physical and emotional functioning, healthy relationships, community participation, and integration), or satisfaction with any of the above, can be achieved through the use of measurement

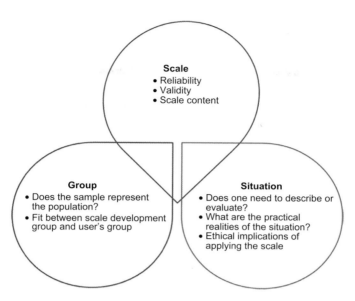

Fig. 15.1 Elements important in selecting a scale.

instruments. Because these outcomes cannot be observed with the naked eye they can be difficult to measure, and rating scales are the instruments needed to assess these topics.

Historically, guides for measurement present information about reliability as well as the 'three Cs' of instrument validity (content, construct, and criterion). These concepts have been presented in some detail in Chapter 14, and are discussed briefly here, but the emphasis is on selecting instruments according to the best fit between the *group* being assessed, the *test* itself, and the *situation* to which the test is being applied (Fig. 15.1). This approach provides instrument users with some basis to judge the most appropriate scale for their purpose. Instruments can be used for any of several purposes – to describe, discriminate, predict, or measure change. When selecting an instrument we need clear evidence that the measure can do whichever of these functions is required. In reality, appropriate scale selection usually involves a balance of weighing priorities. Shortcuts to making the best choice for one's programme, patients, or research study should be avoided.

The scale: what are the necessary basics?

Why Check Reliability and What Does It Actually Mean?
Many reviews discuss reliability but few explain why it is important. The extent to which an instrument is reliable imposes a ceiling on the extent to which it can be valid, because without good reliability one cannot have confidence in the 'truthfulness' of an observation collected with that instrument. Many people think of reliability as consistency, or the ability of an instrument to reproduce very similar scores when all other factors are held constant. This is only

part of the story of reliability. Reliable scales must be able to demonstrate consistent scores across a range of the thing being measured (e.g. HRQL/QOL). For example, an HRQL scale that consistently provides the same score for the same individual when his/her life situation remains constant is reliable only if the scale has the capacity to show the same consistency for individuals of higher or lower levels of HRQL. Thus, in order for the programme manager to choose a reliable scale, the instrument must (1) provide consistent scores (when all other factors being measured remain the same) while (2) demonstrating the ability to reproduce the range of changes that are truly present (show the difference in scores across the continuum of HRQL/QOL). Although reliability is typically thought of as an estimate of consistency, it is most importantly an index of variability (Streiner and Norman 2008). A good HRQL scale should show a stable score for any individual person when his or her life has remained constant, but the scale should also detect the range of HRQL that is truly present among a group of individuals being measured. Thus, in order for an instrument to be reliable, it must vary but in a consistent manner.

WHAT IS INTERNAL CONSISTENCY AND WHAT DOES IT INDICATE ABOUT SCALE QUALITY?

Internal consistency indicates how closely the items in a scale or subscale are related to one another. The presumption is that high internal consistency implies that a uniform concept is being measured (i.e. the instrument demonstrates 'unidimensionality'). Although internal consistency is the most often reported index of reliability for health and QOL scales in child research, there is increasing recognition that the index points to how well the content of the scale is related to a uniform construct as opposed to a scale's ability to detect variation in the sample being measured. Internal consistency as an index of reliability should be interpreted with great caution when applied to multidimensional health and HRQL/QOL scales, because by definition these instruments are composed of subscales that might not be highly related to one another – nor should they be. For example, the KIDSCREEN HRQL instrument has subscales of General Physical Health, Emotions and Mood, Social Acceptance, and Home Environment. These subscales, all relevant to HRQL, are tapping different dimensions of HRQL and thus should not be subject to one measure of internal consistency for the overall scale. The programme manager from our scenario should interpret the popular guideline – namely, that a scale should report a level of internal consistency greater than 0.7 to 0.8 overall – as irrelevant to the overall HRQL score. The manager should look for internal consistency scores at or above those values for subscales only (Streiner and Norman 2008, Mokkink et al 2010).

The most popular statistical test of internal consistency is Cronbach's alpha (α). Cronbach's α provides an indication of how closely the items in the scale are related to each other, and it can be influenced by two factors: (1) the 'real' consistency of the items on the scale; and (2) the total number of items. Knowing this, Cronbach's α can be inflated when scales have more items. One should be cautious of scales that report this statistic as its sole index of reliability, especially if there are more than 15 items in the calculation of α (Streiner and Norman 2008).

When choosing an instrument, it is useful to seek out the average *item–total correlation* as a measure of internal consistency to show how much each item correlates with the total or subscale score or the *range of inter-item correlation* (which shows how much the items correlate with each other). Unlike Cronbach's α these indices provide an estimate of consistency uninfluenced by the number of items.

Checking for test–retest reliability

Test–retest reliability is important to health, HRQL, and QOL scales because it provides information about how well an instrument can produce the same scores over time when no other factors have changed. In the context of child HRQL/QOL reports, test–retest is important because this method often demonstrates a child's ability to understand a concept by reporting the same responses across two or more time points when nothing else has changed.

Critics of HRQL/QOL self-report scales for children often question children's ability to report consistently on their lives. Test–retest scores provide evidence about the consistency of the test and also whether children can provide consistent assessments of themselves when nothing else has changed. On the other hand, 'learning effects' or the duplicating of responses when children recall their previous responses, should be addressed. It is therefore important to determine the time between test applications of an instrument and child self-report scales in order to decide whether test–retest reliability was assessed properly. Children are constantly in a state of change and their development can spurt and slow through a variety of changes over time. The test–retest administration period should be reported by the instrument developer or in the manual and should be sufficiently long that the respondent will have forgotten the responses to the scale but short enough that the respondent has not had significant changes in his or her life experience for any reason (including natural development). An interval of 3 days to 2 weeks is probably acceptable, but the time interval needs to be balanced with the child's stage of development. For example, 2 weeks is too long to obtain a reliable test–retest score on an infant scale but is acceptable for an 18-year-old.

Checking for interrater reliability

Interrater reliability (comparing two people's rating on a measure) is often not applicable to self-report scales that are used to measure health, HRQL, and QOL because the respondent is the same child and cannot be varied. However, functioning or disability scales that are clinician administered can and should be tested between raters to ensure that they work the same way regardless of which clinician is performing the evaluation. In an interrater reliability test, a developer should show that efforts were made to keep all facets of applying the test constant while only the raters varied. The separate raters should have at most minimal opportunity to influence the others' scoring (e.g. by avoiding discussions between rating sessions about how to score the test), so the developer should report how the procedure was performed.

The issue of interrater reliability (in self-report scales such as health status, HRQL, and QOL) is worthy of attention when comparing scores from both child and caregiver or proxy responders. This issue of parent versus child respondents is discussed in further detail in Chapter 17. Suffice to say, empirical work has repeatedly demonstrated that agreement between child and parent responses on these scales is not only unrealistic but is probably an inappropriate goal, particularly when the construct being measured is the subjective experience of the child, as it is in scales assessing HRQL and QOL.

Judgement is always needed to evaluate whether the reliability reported from a study will be applicable to the user such as the programme manager in the scenario. Reliability is a property not solely of the scale but also of the application of the scale to a *group* of children and a real-life *situation*. Thus the programme manager in the scenario should be looking for applicability to his or her specific needs. To make this decision, the group of children and the situation on which the reliability was reported should be related to the needs of the community-based programme to which the measure might be applied.

VALIDITY: ANOTHER COMMONLY USED TERM, BUT WHAT DOES IT REALLY MEAN?
Validity has been described as a characteristic of a scale that demonstrates that it measures what it purports to measure. However, that may mislead one into believing that validity is a trait of the scale. Measurement scientists prefer to think about an instrument's validity relative to a particular context and purpose, i.e. how valid is this scale for this group of children in a particular context (Cronbach 1955, Messick 1995, Kane 2001, Streiner and Norman 2008)? The discussion below on validity focuses on desirable scale traits that users such as the programme manager can apply to a particular group, context, and purpose. By doing so, users can be more confident about the conclusions that can be drawn from the results obtained with the scale.

Content and content validation
There is a great deal one can do to decide whether a scale is appropriate for one's purposes by reviewing its content and reports of how content was developed. The content of health status, HRQL, or QOL patient-reported scales can be found in the questions children and families are asked when filling out a questionnaire. The standards for sound content development have changed over the years. Whereas older instruments emphasized statistical techniques such as factor analysis, extracting items from existing instruments, literature review, and expert opinion, current standards also include the need for theoretical/conceptual guidance in the creation of the measure, qualitative input from children and families, and cognitive interviewing. Content validity is judged to be appropriate when the items on the scale are representative of the construct being measured. When selecting an instrument, one should consider how the candidate items were developed, how the final group of items was narrowed down, and the extent to which the content of a scale applies to one's group of children and the situation for which the instrument is being used.

What sources did developers use to generate content: theory, literature, expertise, or qualitative input?
There are many sources of information for developing candidate items for instruments, including a theory that describes and defines the construct being measured; the definition and application of that construct in empirical research; previously developed instruments that contain related items; expert opinion and expert groups that generate ideas for items; and children and parents who participate in qualitative research and report on what a construct means to them.

The use of theory to generate items is an important and often overlooked area of content development. Without conceptual definitions, the interpretation of instrument scores in a study, or relative to the literature, can be difficult. This is especially true of health status, HRQL, and QOL instruments, because the name of the scale is not always well matched to its content, and developers have varying ideas about what those concepts mean. Some tools are called HRQL but it is unclear how their content is distinct from health status-based instruments. This problem often arises because developers have differing theoretical orientations about what these concepts represent. For example, some writers define HRQL as those bio-psychosocial areas of life affected by a child's health condition, while others consider HRQL to represent a child's personal and subjective view on his or her overall health. (See Chapters 2 and 3 for more discussions of the concepts of HRQL.)

This discordance about what concept a scale is measuring can be confusing for selecting instruments. Users should therefore apply three criteria to decide on the appropriateness of conceptual content: (1) the theory or conceptual basis used to develop the instrument is declared; (2) the content of the instrument is consistent with the theory or concept; and (3) the theory is consistent with the use to which the tool will be applied (Fayed et al 2011). The programme manager who wants to measure HRQL must first determine what that construct means relative to a conceptual view, then consider whether the items in the scale correspond with that view, and finally ask whether that view of HRQL is suitable for explaining and predicting what is happening among the clinical or study group. Avoiding this step will make it difficult to interpret the meaning of scores, or changes in scores, once the scale is applied.

Many scale items are taken from literature review. One has only to type search terms such as 'child health' into MEDLINE and a breadth of topics will emerge that will alert people to what components might constitute the construct of health – ranging from reducing infectious disease to promoting language development. The disadvantage of this approach is that the available literature could be limiting one's understanding of the concept under discussion or even be out of date. For example, if a search for child health articles were performed in the 1970s, there would be a great deal of research about infectious disease, birth rates, and mortality. Today, nutrition, active lifestyle, weight maintenance, and nurturing family environments are considered essential components of child health that should not be overlooked when generating items to measure the concept.

Expert consensus was once considered the most important element of content development in rating scales. Experts such as health services researchers have detailed knowledge of specific areas of child health and HRQL, and this can be beneficial for generating items for a rating scale. However, experts are by definition people with a particular locus and focus of experience and can therefore introduce a bias into the creation or prioritization of content. Health professional experts often have a biased experience because they see the people most significantly affected by the conditions about which they have expertise. Problems often arise when experts are the only source of item development, or if expert opinions are the main method of narrowing candidate items into the final list of items. Both approaches might result in bias or items that are not the most suitable for measuring the construct of interest in a real clinical or community situation.

Finally, direct (qualitative) input from children and families themselves is an excellent source of content in health and HRQL scales. This type of information is particularly useful because one needs to know the issues that are perceived as the most important or relevant to the children and families responding to questionnaires. Children and families will use their own language for the constructs of interest and will highlight important elements thereof. For example, qualitative focus groups used in the development of the CHEQOL instrument for children with epilepsy (Ronen et al 2001) resulted in identification of areas of QOL such as normalcy and belongingness that were found to be HRQL priorities for children who have the condition. Child and parent interviews provided ideas about how to write items in everyday language and overcome the jargon that could be introduced into questionnaires by developers. Appropriate item wording can also be checked in the content reduction stage with cognitive interviewing. More discussion of qualitative methodology is found in Chapter 16.

How did the developers refine the content of their scales (factor analysis and/or cognitive interviewing)?
The items in most scales do not usually include all the items from the content-generating stage discussed above. Instead, a process of psychometric testing is needed in order to: (1) make sure that there is a short enough list to keep the burden of answering the scale low, while (2) being representative of the construct, and (3) making sure that the items included in the final version perform well when measuring the construct of interest. Sometimes there is a trade-off in meeting these objectives. Regardless, a user can look for certain elements with respect to content reduction to see if the instrument developers have engaged in 'good science' for their scale.

Many instrument developers have organized their items into subscales using exploratory factor analysis. This technique is used to reduce the number of items in a scale and organize items into subscales based on assessing common themes. A factor analysis provides evidence about how certain items are related to one another and hence which ones should be assembled in a subscale. The analysis on its own still requires a great deal of decision making and interpretation, thus a developer should either explain the steps involved or how a theory, a framework, or qualitative evidence guided the interpretation and decision making of the process. This should involve some statements about why certain items were dropped from the original list of items or how they were reworded to relate with ('load on to') certain factors if they were not fitting well.

Cognitive interviewing is a technique used by scale developers to probe how items are understood by respondents and the cognitive processes respondents use to answer questions. There has been minimal work in this area in child health research, although the technique has a great deal of potential for discovering how children interpret the phrasing and scaling of items (Geiselman and Padilla 1988). New scales often use this technique to develop well-constructed items and modify or discard other items. Cognitive interviewing is a suitable method for checking items and interpreting the results of factor analysis.

Putting it all together: selecting instruments using content overlap
Determining the overlap between the content of an instrument and the domains that require measurement need not be complex or lengthy, but it should be systematic. Use of a matrix or comparison table can be very helpful for deciding how much a scale overlaps with one's purposes. Content overlap is important for all types of scale selection. In health and QOL assessment for children, this is particularly true because the actual content and items vary

so much from scale to scale that one cannot know by the title alone what is being measured. Fortunately, the content of most of the popular health and QOL scales available for children is often posted on scale websites or available on request from the developer as long as they are being accessed for content review purposes.

Once an instrument is obtained, one can perform one's own simple content mapping or use more complex published content mappings to construct a comparison table that shows whether there is correspondence between the instrument content and one's study or clinical purpose. The International Classification of Functioning, Disability and Health (ICF), described in Chapter 4, is particularly useful for this purpose because it provides a standard language to determine content overlap in functioning, disability, and health outcomes (World Health Organization 2001). The content of many health and QOL scales is increasingly being made available using ICF terms in the peer-reviewed literature (Geyh et al 2007, Fayed and Kerr 2009, Fayed et al 2011, 2012).

The programme manager in the case scenario who seeks to assess HRQL for the children in the programme has learned from clinician feedback focus groups and review of goal-setting reports that priority areas for the programme include: overall emotional functions, behavioural issues, friends and peer relationships, acceptance by peers, school performance, and parental support. The manager can now construct a simple matrix to review whether these domains are actually measured by three frequently applied generic instruments, as illustrated in Table 15.1.

According to the manager's matrix, the Health Utilities Index (HUI) addresses very few priority areas for the programme. The PedsQL and KIDSCREEN both address the child's emotional functions, peers, and school to some extent; however, there is greater content coverage with the KIDSCREEN and the identified priorities than with the PedsQL. Finally, domains of parental support and friends are addressed only by the KIDSCREEN. The manager has therefore determined that KIDSCREEN has the best content match for the programme but decides to also consider the psychometric properties of both the PedsQL and KIDSCREEN.

Scale content summary

By assessing content of health status, HRQL and QOL self-report scales users have an opportunity to evaluate whether an instrument is appropriate for their purposes without needing to have much psychometric sophistication. Users should look for scales that were developed with more than one source of input (theory, literature, experts, or interviews); provide clear and consistent messages about the theoretical basis or definitions for the concept being measured; minimize bias and use a systematic and empirically driven process to finalize the eventual group of items; and cue children and parents to provide responses that are easily understood and interpreted. Once these criteria have been met, users should assess the extent to which there is good overlap and fit between the content of the scale and the situation in which it will be applied.

Testing construct validity: what is it and how do you know if it is there?

Construct validity concerns the extent to which the scale represents the construct its intended to measure. In a practical sense, construct validity is assessed by exploring how well a scale

TABLE 15.1
The programme manager's matrix for comparing scale content and programme needs

Priority area (with ICF categories)	Peds QL[a]	KIDSCREEN[b]	HUI-III[c]
Child's Emotional and Mental Health			
b152 Emotional Functions	+++	++++	+
Child's General Behaviour			
d250 Managing One's Own Behaviour			
Child's School Performance			
d163 Thinking			+
d175 Solving Problems			+
d820 School Education	+++	+++	
Child's Friendships and Peer Relationships			
d7 Interpersonal Interactions and Relationships and Interactions			
d750 Informal Social Relationships (friends, acquaintances, peers)	+	++++++++	
d9205 Socializing			
Child's Parental Support			
d760 Family Relationships	+	++	
e310 Immediate Family		++	
e410 Individual Attitudes of Immediate Family Members		++	
Child's Acceptance from Peers		+++	
e320 Friends		+	
e420 Attitudes of Friends			
e425 Attitudes of Acquaintances, Peers, Colleagues, Neighbours, and Community Members	++	++	

[a]Varni et al 2001. [b]Ramjil et al 2006. [c]Feeny et al 1995. The + signs reflect the relative strength of the evidence that a specific measure actually assesses in relation to the priority areas listed in the left column.

performs relative to related outcomes based on relationships that are known to exist or are expected to be observed. For example, a QOL scale (based on a subjective definition of QOL) should be highly related to other scales of life satisfaction. In order to assess the construct validity of instruments, there needs to be a solid understanding of how the concept being measured should or could relate to other concepts to which the instrument is being compared. Developers can demonstrate a scale's construct validity by showing that it is related to an analogous instrument ('convergent' validity) or that the scale demonstrates poor agreement with a concept to which it is inversely related ('divergent' validity). For example a depression scale should demonstrate a strong negative correlation with a happiness scale. The same depression scale that distinguishes children with low, medium, and high levels of negative affect demonstrates discriminant validity. In other cases, construct validity is demonstrated based on how well scale scores predict a related outcome or future event. For example, one would expect school-aged children with higher scores of life satisfaction and social support to have lower levels of health risk behaviours in early adolescence. If an instrument is used for decision making, then the scores should show that they can accurately predict the outcome that is the basis for that decision (predictive validity). This means that if HRQL scores are used to determine which children receive access to services, then the scores should be highly predictive of a child's true need for services. As construct validity is explored through the relationship of a scale to related outcomes, correlation statistics are often used. Deciding whether a measure shows construct validity means that one must assess if the relationships observed between the measure in question and other variables or outcomes are what would be reasonable and expected.

The last form of validity addressed by the three Cs, 'criterion' validity, is actually a special case of construct validity, whereby a scale is compared with a 'criterion standard' that measures the same construct. Criterion validity is rather suspect in the field of health status, HRQL, and QOL measurement because there are arguably no ideal scales in this field, only scales that are more or less popular, and those that are more or less suited to a particular concept of health, HRQL and QOL, a particular group of children, or a particular situation (such as programme evaluation).

Regardless of the methods used to support construct validity (convergent, divergent, predictive), one must always *make a case* as to whether the validity tests reported are applicable to the group and situation to which the scale will be applied. Instrument reports should therefore provide some a priori hypotheses about how the scale will perform relative to the comparison outcomes or scales (Mokkink et al 2010). Failure to report an a priori hypothesis is problematic, because a developer is easily able to adjust the interpretation of his or her scale after the results are obtained, as opposed to testing pre-stated hypotheses about whether the scale represents the construct of interest based on the way the tool was created.

The group: to whom can the scale be applied?

A group may be a collection of people who have a shared experience or trait. The trait could be a diagnosis such as epilepsy, and the experience could be stigma or discrimination. Sample refers to children or families that are drawn from a larger group that encompasses all the people who share that experience or trait. If a group is composed of everyone with the experience or trait, it is called a population. These terms are important, because an instrument user always needs to think about how well the sample used to develop or validate a scale represents the population from which it was drawn and to which it might be applied in his or her study. Thus the programme manager in the case scenario must also think about how closely the group sampled in the scale development relates to the group in the community-based programme.

In the field of health and HRQL/QOL measurement, many instruments have been developed with a focus on a particular group of children who represent a population. The PedsQL, for example, was developed with children using community paediatricians, hospital in- and out-patient services, as well as rheumatology and diabetes clinics (Varni et al 2001). However, once an instrument is validated, developers and users often apply it to groups thought to be

215

analogous or related in some way. This method cuts down on the time and resources required in creating a new instrument for every population; however, problems can arise if the items in the instruments are not re-examined relative to the new group. If an instrument was developed using a sample of children with cancer, and another researcher wishes to apply the instrument to children with epilepsy, the items should be assessed and retested with the new responders, i.e. children with epilepsy and/or their parents, using the content validation techniques discussed earlier. Failure to do so might result in measuring elements that are not relevant to the new group, or, worse, may fail to include items that are vital to measuring the construct of interest in the new group. Thus, if a scale is being applied to a new group, some re-evaluation of the construct at the item level should be performed.

When deciding whether to adopt a scale, one should also check demographics and basic descriptive statistics in the original measurement development sample. Were the range and median age of the children applicable to the user's intended application group? Even if the diagnosis of the children matches up, one must decide if there are other features, such as function or severity of impairment, that can help one decide if the scale development and validation sample match the target group.

The situation: which applications of the scale are suitable?

DESCRIPTION AND EVALUATION

In assessing the situation to which an instrument is applied it is important to ask: why is this concept important in the first place? Perhaps the manager in the case scenario wants to show a policy maker or director the special needs of the service group. If so, then an instrument should be able to distinguish between the service group and the general population. In the manual of the instrument, the manager should look for evidence of discriminative validity, demonstrating that there are meaningful differences observed between the children with a health condition and children in the general population. Given the programme manager's goal, they would also be looking at whether the developers have published any norms for the general population of children. Information about whether subscales can discriminate between groups would also be helpful for deciding on whether a scale can suitably describe a group of children. For example, a mobility scale or subscale should be able to demonstrate marked differences in average scores between groups of children with cerebral palsy who have level 1 and level 5 mobility impairment as described by the Gross Motor Function Classification System (Palisano et al 1997).

If a user wants to capture what changes occurred in a group as a result of an event such as an intervention or the loss of a service, then evidence must be provided that the scale can capture change. What will be needed is an instrument containing items that measure domains of the construct that are expected to change as a result of that event. For example, was there a significant and meaningful difference in the range of motion values of children with cerebral palsy when the measure was applied before and after botulinum toxin intervention? A statistically significant change is insufficient for demonstrating that a scale adequately captures change, because, if the sample size is large enough, changes may be statistically significant, even if they are not big enough to be clinically important. In measuring health, HRQL, and

QOL, few scales report in the original development paper their potential for capturing change – for which specific validation evidence is needed (Rosenbaum et al 1990) – so one might need to look for evidence of responsiveness in studies that have at least two time points to get a sense of whether the instrument can pick up changes.

Statistical indicators of responsiveness include effect sizes, standard error of measures, Guyatt's responsiveness index, and receiver operating characteristic (Guyatt et al 1987). All these indicators are related to how big a change score is observed. Each one has advantages and disadvantages that are beyond the scope of this chapter. One must also always consider whether the instrument is measuring a construct that is likely to change following an intervention. For example, if one defines QOL based on the World Health Organization definition: 'a [child's] perception of their position in life', is this likely to change with the introduction of an antiepileptic drug with a better side-effect profile? Constructs that are important to describe a child's life are not always the same as the constructs that are expected to change with intervention.

An instrument that can perform well for descriptive purposes as well as evaluative purposes is ideal but often difficult to find – and one needs evidence of the validity of the measure to do those tasks depending on the situation. Therefore, the manager in the scenario needs to set priorities and use them to decide which scale is the most appropriate. This a priori goal setting will be useful when the time comes to interpret scale scores between groups or across time.

PRACTICAL REALITIES/UTILITY OF SCALE APPLICATION

As every clinician and health services researcher is aware, the practical realities of the measurement situation will weigh heavily in the decision on which instruments to adopt. Factors such as time to complete an instrument, how easily the tool can be interpreted or scored, and how easily the results can be used are all important. This is especially true for self-report scales for children who might not have the attention span or patience for long research-oriented scales, despite the programme manager's need to collect good-quality information with rigorous tools. Evidence suggests that from the age of 6 or 7 children are capable of reporting validly and reliably with self-report tools, even for scales with 25 questions, under appropriate conditions (Riley 2004).

We recommend pilot testing scales that are being considered with children and their families to determine their feasibility, and varying the conditions of the testing situation. One can find out how much of the scale is completed when it is provided to patients waiting to attend their health services appointment or when they are asked to come 10 minutes early for their appointment to complete the scale. Does having a service provider check the completion of the questionnaire with families improve data quality? These are important elements to explore before deciding on the feasibility of questionnaire administration in a health services assessment situation. More details of many of these elements are discussed in Chapter 17 on self- and proxy reports.

The cost of using a scale will certainly influence whether it can be adopted and sustained. Most scales require some form of permission or a fee provided to the instrument developer. Some scales involve reporting the results back to the instrument developer to obtain reference data and interpretation. It is therefore important to be mindful of the sustainability of adopting such scales as an ongoing cost, especially if the price can increase over time. In fact the fees associated with the use of many scales are nominal and are often not related to the instrument's quality. Additionally, users in hospital, university, and not-for-profit community-based settings typically have a reduced fee.

ETHICS OF SCALE APPLICATION (SEE ALSO CHAPTER 18)
When adopting a scale, what factors make the scale selection unethical? First, it can be considered unethical if a scale was selected inappropriately for its intended purpose, in particular if the scores are used as the basis for decision making (Messick 1995). The programme manager who is attempting to decide between three generic, albeit very different, scales may be facing difficult choices about resource allocation for the children with cerebral palsy in her facility. A health economics approach to evaluation is commonly suggested in this situation, and for this reason the HUI III may be considered (owing to it econometric basis). The HUI assesses areas of health that are rated as highly important by a general 'healthy' population of adults – such as walking, hearing, vision, cognition, and emotions. Using this approach, interventions that improve these health domains will be rated by the HUI as the ones that show the most improvements. Thus, compensatory or rehabilitative interventions, such as wheelchair provision, that improve overall mobility but not walking are unlikely to demonstrate change using such an approach. This manager cannot therefore ethically apply the general population's valuation of health domains to children with cerebral palsy who prioritize different, albeit worthy, areas for health interventions. For these reasons, the application of this scale to this situation is unethical because of a mismatch between the purpose of the instrument and the consequences of applying the tool.

Second, the ethics of exposing children to many complex and personal questions contained in self-report measures should be considered (Waters et al 2009, Fayed et al 2011). This is particularly true for children who might not have considered the implications of their health condition in the ways that measures ask about them. For example, many scales ask children about whether they experience difficulties in their family or friendships as a result of their impairment or health condition (e.g. from the PedsQL: 'I cannot do things that other kids my age can do') (Varni et al 2001). Questionnaires that focus only on problems, difficulties, and challenges highlight the negative aspects of having an impairment or health condition and can cue children into a negative self-concept. Thus it is important to seek out instruments that balance negative topics (such as pain, sadness, isolation, or bullying) and negative phrasing (e.g. difficulty with…, problems with…) with neutral phrasing and positive topics (personal strengths, empathy, or positive relationships) in order to ensure a balanced approach to child assessment with rating scales.

Conclusions
Determining the fit among a measure's content and psychometric performance (reliability and validity) and its applicability to a group of children and a clinical or health-research situation involves judgement and potential trade-offs with utility and ethical considerations. In particular, selecting health status, HRQL, and QOL scales for children presents many special considerations that can influence how well any measure performs in a real-life situation.

Instrument users must therefore understand how to select measures that provide the best fit to their intended purposes and groups in order to have trustworthy and interpretable results collected from rating scales.

REFERENCES

*Key references

Cronbach LJ, Meehl PE (1955) Construct validity in psychological tests. *Psychol Bull* 52: 281–302. http://dx.doi.org/10.1037/h0040957

Fayed N, Cieza A, Bickenbach J (2009) Comparing quality of life scales in childhood epilepsy: what's in the measures? *Int J Disabil Commun Rehabil*. Available at: www.ijdcr.ca/VOL08_03/articles/fayed.shtml (accessed 24 February 2011).

*Fayed N, Schiariti V, Bostan C, Cieza A, Klassen A (2011) Health status and QOL instruments used in childhood cancer research: deciphering conceptual content using World Health Organization definitions. *Qual Life Res* 8: 1247–1258. http://dx.doi.org/10.1007/s11136-011-9851-5

Fayed N, Bickenbach JE, Cieza A (2012) Illustrating child-specific linking issues using the Child Health Questionnaire. *Am J Phys Med Rehabil* 91(Suppl. 1): S189–S198. http://dx.doi.org/10.1097/PHM.0b013e31823d53cf

Feeny D, Furlong W, Boyle M, Torrance GW (1995) Multi-attribute health status classification systems. Health Utilities Index. *PharmacoEconomics* 7: 490–502. http://dx.doi.org/10.2165/00019053-199507060-00004.

Geiselman RE, Padilla J (1988) Cognitive interviewing with child witnesses. *J Police Sci Admin* 16: 236–242.

Geyh S, Cieza A, Kollerits B, Grimby G, Stucki G (2007) Content comparison of health-related quality of life measures used in stroke based on the International Classification of Functioning, Disability and Health (ICF): a systematic review. *Qual Life Res* 16: 833–851. http://dx.doi.org/10.1007/s11136-007-9174-8

*Guyatt G, Walter S, Norman G (1987) Measuring change over time: assessing the usefulness of evaluative instruments. *J Chronic Dis* 40: 171–178. http://dx.doi.org/10.1016/0021-9681(87)90069-5

Kane MT (2001) Current concerns in validity theory. *J Educ Meas* 38: 319–342. http://dx.doi.org/10.1111/j.1745-3984.2001.tb01130.x

*Messick S (1995) Standards of validity and the validity of standards in performance assessment. *Educ Meas* 14: 5–8. http://dx.doi.org/10.1111/j.1745-3992.1995.tb00881.x

Mokkink LB, Terwee CB, Patrick DL, et al (2010) The COSMIN checklist for assessing the methodological quality of studies on measurement properties of health status measurement instruments: an international Delphi study. *Qual Life Res* 19: 539–549. http://dx.doi.org/10.1007/s11136-010-9606-8

Palisano R, Rosenbaum P, Walter S, Russell D, Wood E, Galuppi B (1997) Development and reliability of a system to classify gross motor function in children with cerebral palsy. *Dev Med Child Neurol* 39: 214–223. http://dx.doi.org/10.1111/j.1469-8749.1997.tb07414.x

Ramjil L, Alonso J, Berra S, et al; KIDSCREEN group (2006) Use of a children questionnaire of health-related quality of life (KIDSCREEN) as a measure of needs for health care services. *J Adolesc Health* 38: 511–518. http://dx.doi.org/10.1016/j.jadohealth.2005.05.022

Riley AW (2004) Evidence that school-age children can self-report on their health. *Ambulat Pediatr* 4: 371–376. http://dx.doi.org/10.1367/A03-178R.1

Ronen GM, Rosenbaum P, Law M, Streiner DL (2001) Health-related quality of life in childhood disorders: a modified focus group technique to involve children. *Qual Life Res* 10: 71–79. http://dx.doi.org/10.1023/A:1016659917227

Rosenbaum P, Cadman D, Russell D, Gowland C, Hardy S, Jarvis S. (1990) Issues in measuring change in motor function in children with cerebral palsy. A special communication. *Phys Ther* 70: 125–131.

*Streiner DL, Norman GR (2008) *Health Measurement Scales: A Practical Guide to their Development and Use*. New York: Oxford University Press.

Varni JW, Seid M, Curtin PS (2001) PedsQL (TM) 4.0: Reliability and validity of the Pediatric Quality of Life Inventory (TM) version 4.0 Generic Core Scales in healthy and patient populations. *Med Care* 39: 800–812. http://dx.doi.org/10.1097/00005650-200108000-00006

Waters E, Davis E, Ronen GM, Rosenbaum P, Livingston M, Saigal S (2009) Quality of life instruments for children and adolescents with neurodisabilities: how to choose the appropriate instrument. *Dev Med Child Neurol* 51: 660–669. http://dx.doi.org/10.1111/j.1469-8749.2009.03324.x

World Health Organization (2001) *International Classification of Functioning, Disability and Health.* Geneva: WHO Press.

16

COMPLEXITY IN THE LIVES OF CHILDREN AND YOUNG PEOPLE WITH NEUROLOGICAL AND DEVELOPMENTAL CONDITIONS: THE ROLE OF QUALITATIVE RESEARCH

Debra Stewart

Overview

This chapter describes qualitative research as applied to the lives of children and young people with neurological and developmental disabilities. Descriptions of qualitative studies with different populations of children and young people demonstrate the value of this type of research in developing an understanding of issues of health, disability, quality of life, and participation. This is accomplished through exploration of the perspectives and experiences of the people who know the most about how these concepts affect their daily lives – the children and young people themselves and their families. Many additional examples of qualitative research with these populations are described in other chapters of this book (see, for example, Chapters 17 and 22).

Introduction

This book addresses an important paradigm shift in the field of neurodevelopmental disabilities. This shift is moving health care beyond the traditional 'medical model' perspective of children and young people with disabilities and its primary focus on biological impairments and component-based physical, cognitive, and related neurodevelopmental outcomes. Today's view involves a biopsychosocial concern with broader issues of health and health-related functioning. New models and definitions of health, functioning, and disability, such as the International Classification of Functioning, Disability and Health (ICF) (World Health Organization 2001) (see Chapter 4) are propelling this paradigm. Views of health and disability are expanding to acknowledge a dynamic interaction between person and environment. The ICF (World Health Organization 2001) in particular is encouraging healthcare professionals to look beyond impairments and address the experiences, perceptions, relationships, and views of children and young people with disabilities and their families. Concepts of quality of life and participation (Chapters 3 and 5, respectively) are now recognized and valued as important and relevant outcomes for the people with whom we work in health care and rehabilitation.

It can be challenging to define, describe, and measure these evolving issues and outcomes because of their complexity and conceptual nature. Furthermore, our relative lack of knowledge of these new concepts can make them difficult to study using exclusively traditional quantitative methods. In the past few decades qualitative research methods have been used to increase our knowledge of these biopsychosocial concepts. Miller and Crabtree (2005: 609) advocate for qualitative research methods to explore the 'lived clinical experiences' of the people with whom we work. Qualitative research findings can challenge our ingrained biomedical beliefs and complement and expand our notions of 'evidence' beyond what can be learned from randomized controlled trials (Miller and Crabtree 2005). Qualitative findings provide important information about the diversity of clinical practice, dynamic interactions, complexities, and multiple perspectives, which are all relevant concepts within the new biopsychosocial paradigm.

What is qualitative research?

Qualitative research involves a large number of designs, methods, and theoretical underpinnings. One definition of qualitative research used by many experts comes from Denzin and Lincoln (2005: 3):

> Qualitative research is a situated activity that locates the observer in the world. It consists of a set of interpretive, material practices that make the world visible. These practices transform the world. They turn the world into a series of representations, fieldnotes, interviews, conversations, photographs, recordings and memos to self. At this level, qualitative research involves an interpretive, naturalistic approach to the world …

Some of the key elements of qualitative research that are common to all types of methods and traditions are:

- It aims to 'paint a picture' in a holistic way and is therefore suited to addressing complexity and dynamic processes that are part of the human experience.
- It uses distinct methodologies of data collection and analysis to create data that represent the views, experiences, and perceptions of people.
- It seeks patterns, commonalities, and differences within the textual data.
- It is conducted in the daily environments (natural settings) of the people with whom the researchers are working (Denzin and Lincoln 2005, Cresswell 2007, Richards and Morse 2007).

Qualitative research is a different form of enquiry from quantitative research. Whereas quantitative research usually uses many subjects and a relatively small number of variables, qualitative research tends to study a larger number of variables with a small number of individuals (called 'participants' or 'informants'). This enables the qualitative researcher to explore complex issues or 'phenomena' that involve a wide range of variables and their interactions. Inherent in all qualitative research is the expectation of learning about the 'meanings' of a phenomenon, as this is how we make sense of the world around us.

Researchers in the practice area of paediatrics have used qualitative research methods in the past decade to gain a better understanding of the complex issues that are emerging within health care and rehabilitation. Some of the key clinical issues or concepts that have benefited from qualitative enquiry include what is meant by 'participation', 'quality of life', and 'developmental trajectories and transitions'. Examples of qualitative studies of these issues are described below to illustrate how qualitative enquiry has contributed to our knowledge base and influenced changes in theory and practice.

THE PARTICIPATION OF CHILDREN WITH PHYSICAL IMPAIRMENTS IN LEISURE OCCUPATIONS

A longitudinal study by researchers at the *CanChild* Centre for Childhood Disability Research identified patterns and predictors of the recreational participation of children with physical impairments in Ontario, Canada (King et al 2006, Law et al 2006, 2007). Following this study, researchers were interested in learning about the meaning and perceptions of the children and young people themselves about their participation. Qualitative methods were used to gain a deeper understanding of recreational participation (Heah et al 2007, Harding et al 2009). Harding et al (2009) used a case study design with photographs and interviews to learn more about the strong interconnection between childhood activities and settings. Another qualitative study demonstrated that children with physical impairments enjoy the same activities as their peers without impairments (Heah et al 2007). The researchers also found that parents play an important role in providing opportunities for their children's participation.

Similar themes about participation were described in a qualitative study of adolescents with physical impairments (Stewart et al 2012). Interviews with 10 young people aged 17 to 19 years revealed that these young people with impairments enjoyed the same social activities as their peers. Environmental supports and barriers to participation identified by these participants were similar to those found in the qualitative studies with children: one of the key environmental supports was parents (Stewart et al 2012).

In addition to building our understanding of environmental barriers and supports for participation, these qualitative studies made us more aware of the dynamic interactions between participation and environment and the importance of providing children and young people with impairments with opportunities to participate in a variety of activities for positive development (Petrenchik and King 2011). Qualitative methods proved to be valuable in putting this knowledge into action, using interviews and focus groups to develop a measure of participation and environment (Bedell et al 2011).

THE DEVELOPMENT OF QUALITY OF LIFE MEASURES FOR CHILDREN AND ADOLESCENTS

The concept of quality of life has gained increased attention in health care over the past two decades, but until recently there was very little literature related to children and young people

(Renwick et al 2003; see also Chapter 3). Qualitative enquiry is being used by several groups of researchers in different countries to develop age-appropriate measures that fit with the views of children, young people, and parents. In Canada, Ronen et al (1999, 2001) conducted a qualitative study using focus groups with 29 children with epilepsy and, separately, with their parents, to learn about their experiences. The researchers used a modified focus group methodology that involved stratifying the focus groups into similar age groupings of the child participants, and then utilizing creative techniques of drawing environmental maps and using play-dough to ensure that the groups were child focused (Ronen et al 2001). Qualitative analysis of the transcripts from all focus groups revealed five dimensions about living with epilepsy, which the researchers used to develop a self- and proxy health-related quality of life measure for children with epilepsy (CHEQOL-25) (Ronen et al 2003).

In Australia, qualitative methods were also used to develop and evaluate a condition-specific quality of life measure (the Cerebral Palsy Quality of Life Questionnaire for Children, CP-QOL-Child) (Waters et al 2005). Researchers went further in the development of this measure by using a grounded theory approach to identify the domains that were appropriate for adolescents (Davis et al 2008). Finally, the researchers acknowledged the importance of including both child/young person and parent perceptions in a measure of quality of life by interviewing 28 children and 35 parents to explore the extent of agreement between the two groups (Parkinson et al 2011).

In the UK Morris et al (2007) used separate focus groups of children and parents to explore how children are affected by foot and ankle problems. The researchers used life-mapping techniques to consider children's activities during the day (i.e. in the morning, at school, after school, at home, and during holidays) (Morris et al 2007). Figure 16.1 illustrates a day in the life of a child with a foot and ankle problem, as recorded by one of the participants in

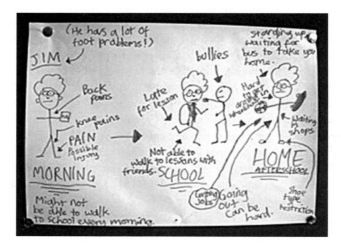

Fig. 16.1 'A day in the life of a child with foot and ankle problems', as recorded by one of the participants in a focus group of young people 12 to 15 years old. Reproduced with permission from Morris et al (2007).

a focus group of young people aged 12 to 15 years. This mapping method was used in order to depersonalize the issues being discussed and enabled the researchers to discuss potentially sensitive issues more openly without putting individual children in a vulnerable position. The findings of this enquiry helped the research team develop a questionnaire to measure how children with foot impairments are affected by foot and ankle problems from the child's own perspective (Morris et al 2009).

Qualitative methods have also been used by healthcare researchers to build an in-depth understanding of the complexity of quality of life. Renwick et al (2003) used a grounded theory approach and interviewed parents of children with developmental conditions about 'quality of life' to develop a conceptual framework for assessment and intervention. This qualitative enquiry promoted a family-centred approach to health care, as the views and experiences of parents formed the basis of the framework (Renwick et al 2003).

QUALITATIVE RESEARCH ON DEVELOPMENTAL TRAJECTORIES AND TRANSITIONS
At the beginning of the new millennium, there was a lack of knowledge of the developmental pathways or trajectories of children with developmental coordination disorder (DCD) (Missiuna et al 2006, 2007). A series of qualitative studies provided much-needed information about the impact of DCD on the lives of children and their families over time, and this information contributed to significant changes in service delivery. A phenomenological study with 13 parents of children with DCD revealed a number of themes about the challenges parents faced in trying to learn about their child's condition and to get help (Missiuna et al 2006). The theme of 'negotiating the maze' represented the many pathways followed by parents to get a diagnosis and services for their child. The results of this study highlighted the importance of early identification and intervention that included parents in the process, which led to the development of educational materials designed to empower parents on this complex journey.

In a key article about the developmental trajectories of children with DCD, Missiuna et al (2007) found that parents' concerns evolved over time from motor and play concerns in early childhood to self-care, school-based, and peer-related problems in middle childhood, and then to issues of self-esteem and emotional challenges in late childhood. This study demonstrated the troubling trajectory that children with DCD could experience without intervention and support.

A second qualitative study focused on developmental issues faced by adolescents and young adults with DCD (Missiuna et al 2008). Interviews with nine young adults about their adolescent experiences demonstrated the important role that context or environment plays in the performance of young people with mild motor delays. The participants in this study developed strategies over time to manage their coordination difficulties in different environments and also sought the best 'person–environment match' as they made the transition into adult life. These findings have promoted a greater emphasis on environmental interventions and adaptations to support young people with motor difficulties as they develop over time. These two qualitative studies contributed rich information about the developmental trajectories of children and adolescents with DCD and showed that, in the longer term, motor coordination issues are not the major focus of concern for parents, or for the young adults, and therefore perhaps should not be the primary focus of intervention. They also provided the rationale and direction for subsequent longitudinal studies that have demonstrated secondary physical health and mental health consequences of DCD that are of greater concern and that might be prevented through adaptation of tasks, increased understanding, and changes in the environment (Cairney et al 2009, 2010, Missiuna et al 2011).

In another area of practice, in the 1980s and 1990s clinicians and researchers began to explore the transition to adulthood for young people with impairments. As knowledge about this developmental process was relatively limited, qualitative research methods provided important information to guide practice, policy, and future research. Qualitative studies in the late 1990s explored the experiences of young people with different types of neurodevelopmental conditions as they finished high school and were discharged from paediatric health care and rehabilitation services (for example, Doyle et al 1994, Fraser 1994). Qualitative research was used to identify the factors that influenced the developmental journey of young people with impairments, which were personal (e.g. sex, self-determination, functional skills) and environmental (physical, social, cultural, institutional, policy) in nature (Stewart et al 2001). Many transition services began to address these many factors through programmes to assist young people to build their own capacity for self-determination for adult life (Powers 2001, Turnbull and Turnbull 2006) and to remove environmental barriers to adult transitions, such as lack of communication between paediatric and adult services (Berg 2011).

Qualitative enquiry has built knowledge and understanding about the complexities involved in the developmental transition from adolescence to adulthood. Recent research is focusing more on these complexities, recognizing the dynamic nature of any transition in terms of person–environment interactions (Stewart et al 2009, Gorter et al 2011). This is promoting the emergence of transition services that are based on biopsychosocial models and address all aspects of the young person in transition, as part of his or her natural life-course. More information about this area of practice is provided in Chapter 22.

QUALITATIVE RESEARCH WITH CHILDREN AND YOUNG PEOPLE

In the past, research on children and young people has not asked them directly about their own opinions and experiences (Vander Laenen 2009). The different types of qualitative research that are described in this chapter demonstrate how this form of enquiry can answer questions about complex issues and phenomena related to personal meanings and individual lived experiences. The studies highlighted here also provide some valuable strategies for involving children and young people in research. Qualitative methods can ensure that the voices of young people are heard and represented, but it can be difficult at times to engage children and adolescents as active participants. Some of the strategies that have worked well in the studies presented here include:

- Use art/drawing and other forms of visual media, such as photographs and videos, with children to encourage them to express feelings and experiences that may be difficult to verbalize. The use of online chat, email messages, and other forms of social media can also be relevant and motivating for children and young people.
- Use young person-friendly forms of interviewing such as focus groups, in which children and adolescents are more likely to open up and share experiences. Serving pizza and giving tokens of appreciation have always helped too!

- Conduct more than one interview with the same person. Focus the first interview on general feelings and experiences, then come back later to explore issues in greater depth, after the first interview transcript has been sent to the participants to read over. Providing the interview questions ahead of time gives young people time to think about experiences they can share.

As illustrated in this chapter there are many benefits of doing qualitative research with children and young people as active participants. Other chapters in this book use qualitative research methods to address the complexity that is inherent in the lives of children and young people with neurological and developmental conditions, and those who live and work with them.

Five traditions of qualitative research in health care and rehabilitation

There is wide array of qualitative traditions of enquiry. The choice of tradition or methodology is usually based on the fit between the research question, the type of data, and the chosen qualitative methodology (Richards and Morse 2007). The first and most important area of fit that all researchers need to examine is the fit between the research question and the methodology. Questions that ask about experiences, perceptions, and meanings fit best with qualitative enquiry, and the wording of a specific question will guide a researcher to choose a specific methodology or tradition. Table 16.1 outlines the types of questions that fit best within the qualitative traditions that are described in this chapter.

TABLE 16.1
Examples of research questions that fit within different qualitative traditions

Qualitative tradition	Examples of research questions
Ethnography: focus is on gaining understanding about the culture	What is daily life like for parents of preterm infants with neurological impairments who are in an NICU (neonatal intensive care unit)?
	(What is the culture of an NICU?)
Phenomenology: focus is on uncovering the meaning of human experience	What is the experience of children with neurodevelopmental disorders during their transition into the state school system? *or*
	What is the meaning of transition into the state school system for children with neurodevelopmental disorders?
Grounded theory: focus is on generating or modifying theory and usually considering a process	How do healthcare practitioners who work in newly formed transition clinics define and describe their practice? *or*
	What is the process that healthcare practitioners use in their practice within a newly formed transition clinic?
Case study: focus is on understanding the meaning of 'cases' within a setting or context	What factors influence a successful outcome in children with epilepsy during the process of changing their medication?
Participatory action research: focus is on social change	What changes are needed in school-based therapy services for children with developmental coordination disorder, from the perspective of different stakeholders (children, parents, therapists, school personnel, policy analysts)?

Four common qualitative traditions are often employed in health care and rehabilitation research: ethnography, phenomenology, grounded theory, and case study. Each tradition represents different disciplines of study and each explores different aspects of a phenomenon. A fifth approach to qualitative enquiry, known as participatory action research, or PAR, (Kemmis and McTaggart 2005) is also included, as it is being used by healthcare researchers to examine social change and macro-level community issues (Cresswell 2007). The descriptions below illustrate the distinct focus of each tradition, with examples of studies in health care and rehabilitation for each.

ETHNOGRAPHY

The focus of ethnographic enquiry is the culture of a group. The term culture is viewed broadly to include the shared beliefs, values, language, and patterns of behaviours of a group of people (Cresswell 2007, Richards and Morse 2007). A cultural group can be large, such as the population of children with neurodevelopmental conditions, or it can be small, such as staff at one children's rehabilitation programme.

Ethnography works well when we want to learn more about the daily lives of a cultural group – e.g. its shared patterns of behaviour, what it values. The researcher needs to become immersed in the daily lives of the members of the group being studied. This is often referred to as entering the field or 'fieldwork' (Wolcott 1999). The primary forms of data collection in ethnography are participant observation within the natural setting and interviews with people in the cultural group. The researcher's fieldnotes and diary are important elements of the data.

Data analysis within ethnography typically results in a number of themes that describe the daily lives of a culture-sharing group. Some typical themes that emerge from ethnographic studies include enculturation, inequalities, life cycles, and empowerment. An example of a qualitative study that used an ethnographic approach concerns the shared experiences of young people with physical impairments during the transition to adulthood (Stewart et al 2001). Interviews with 34 young people, aged 19 to 30, parents, and service providers revealed many common experiences along this developmental journey and the young people's identified needs to build their own bridges into the adult world with appropriate support.

PHENOMENOLOGY

Phenomenology has strong philosophical roots about human lived experience. The focus of a phenomenological enquiry is to understand the meaning of people's lived experiences in relation to a particular phenomenon. Phenomena can include experiences related to growing up (e.g. starting school), interacting with others (e.g. belonging to a club or team), and receiving services (e.g. those provided in rehabilitation). Attention is paid to the common experiences shared by a group of people, often referred to as the 'essence' of the experience (Cresswell 2007).

There are different types of phenomenology, and a researcher must decide on the appropriate type to guide data collection and analysis. In general, the types of issue that are best explored by phenomenology are common experiences of a phenomenon of interest. For example, the phenomenon of using a Youth KIT (Keeping It Together, Youth Version)

(Stewart et al 2010) was explored with young people with developmental impairments and their parents through interviews (Freeman et al 2010). A common experience that arose from the first set of interviews was the importance of a mentor to help a young person get started in using the Youth KIT; the phenomenon of mentorship was then explored in a subsequent study.

Data collection in phenomenology includes in-depth interviews with people who are experiencing the phenomenon of interest in order to gain a deeper understanding. Analysis of the data is conducted by the systematic approach of reading through all the textual data and forming a description of the essence of the experience. Significant statements, in the form of quotes from different participants, are provided to understand the phenomenon from their perspective. For example, in a study about the mobility experiences of adolescents with cerebral palsy, quotes from adolescents with physical impairments supported themes about self-sufficiency, making choices, safety and efficiency, adapting, and constantly planning ahead (Palisano et al 2009).

GROUNDED THEORY

The underlying assumption of grounded theory is that reality is socially constructed. The focus of grounded theory enquiry is on processes and change over time. The goal is to develop a theory to describe the various concepts involved in a process or situation and to explore the relationships among the concepts.

There are different approaches used within a grounded theory tradition of enquiry, but all seek to answer the question 'What's going on here?' (Richards and Morse 2007: 60). The researcher explores the participants' perceptions of change and process in order to develop a theory to explain social processes (Richards and Morse 2007: 62).

Another important criterion for choosing a grounded theory approach is the lack of an available theory, or an incomplete theory, to explain the process or situation of interest. For example, Garth et al (2009) noted that previous understandings of partnership were not sufficient to explain the relationship among children with impairments, their parents, and physicians. The lack of theory about partnership led these researchers to select a grounded theory approach to explore the complex processes involved in a partnership among children with cerebral palsy, aged 8 to 11, their parents, and paediatricians. Although they found variability in the children's involvement in this partnership, the results refuted the idea that children were not regarded as contributors to family–doctor partnerships (Garth et al 2009).

Grounded theory uses specific techniques of data collection and analysis to create 'theoretical sensitivity', which ensures that theory is grounded in the data (Richards and Morse 2007: 59). This means that the data must provide detailed information about the process from the participants' perspectives.

Data analysis in grounded theory results in the emergence of concepts; these in turn lead the researcher to develop a theory about relationships among the various concepts and processes. For example, grounded theory analysis methods were used in a study of an experiential learning module involving medical residents visiting the homes of families of children with impairments. The analysis of the residents' written narrative descriptions of the experience resulted in the authors concluding that a home visit offered important insights about these families that could not be attained through a hospital-based training programme (Sharma et al 2006).

CASE STUDY

Case study enquiry is intended to explore one or more 'cases' within a bounded system of a setting or context (Denzin and Lincoln 2005). It is a suitable form of enquiry when the research has identifiable cases that can be studied to gain an in-depth understanding about the situation of interest. Cases can be singular, such as a single setting of a person's home, school, or workplace, or there can be multiple cases. In one study of family responses to community perceptions about their child's impairment, 45 parents of children with autism, cerebral palsy, Down syndrome, and sickle cell disease formed four 'cases' of different types of impairments (Neely-Barnes et al 2010). The parents participated in focus groups to discuss how they and their family addressed community perceptions.

Data collection must be extensive in a case study, as the researcher needs to explore the cases through multiple sources of information (Cresswell 2007). Sources can include documents, observations within the setting of interest, and interviews with participants. Data analysis focuses on gaining an understanding of the meaning of the case within the context or setting under study. The result is an in-depth case description that increases our understanding of an issue. In the study about community perceptions, outlined in the previous paragraph, researchers described an interactive and circular relationship between families and communities that was common to all cases (meaning that a child's diagnosis alone did not influence this relationship) (Neely-Barnes et al 2010).

PARTICIPATORY ACTION RESEARCH

This form of research is used in situations that require social change and/or community development (Kemmis and McTaggart 2005). There are different types of participatory research, and the choice is dependent on the research question and desired outcome, as with other types of research. However, all types of PAR are based on the assumption that the people who experience a phenomenon are the best people to investigate and explore it (Depoy and Gitlin 2005). The purpose of PAR is to learn about a phenomenon or situation in order to take action towards social transformation.

Kemmis and McTaggart (2005) describe seven features that are necessary for any type of PAR:

- It is a social process.
- It is participatory.
- It is practical and collaborative.
- It is emancipatory.
- It is critical.
- It is reflexive.
- It aims to transform both theory and practice.

Because of the wide variety of PAR designs, different methods of data collection and analysis can be used. In most situations, qualitative methodology is suitable, as the participatory process usually involves people acting, observing, and reflecting in a cyclical manner. PAR is consistent with the principles of naturalistic enquiry, as it takes place in natural settings, similar to qualitative research. The example below demonstrates this type of participatory action research. However, qualitative methods can be combined with quantitative methods if the research question calls for a mixed-methods approach.

As an example: a team of participatory researchers was formed with adolescents, parents, educators, healthcare providers, employers, and policy makers to explore the transition to adulthood for young people with chronic illness and impairments (Depoy et al 2000). The researchers chose focus groups as the method of data collection, and they analysed the transcripts for common themes. Their analysis led to a number of recommendations for community action and social change, which were implemented and evaluated by the participatory team (Depoy et al 2000). The choice of qualitative methods ensured that multiple perspectives were explored in the natural setting of the community.

Conclusion

Qualitative research addresses important questions about the meanings of phenomena, complex issues, and biopsychosocial outcomes by studying the experiences and perceptions of people in their natural environments. Qualitative research is a good choice when our knowledge level is relatively low, or we do not have theories available to explain the complexity of situations that confront us in our work with children and young adults with neurodevelopmental conditions, their families, and their communities.

REFERENCES

*Key references

Bedell GM, Khetani MA, Cousins MA, Coster WJ, Law M (2011) Parent perspectives to inform development of measures of children's participation and environment. *Arch Phys Med Rehab* 92: 765–773.

Berg K (2011) Sustainable transition process for young people with chronic conditions: a narrative summary on achieved cooperation between paediatric and adult medical teams. *Child Care Health Dev* 37: 800–805.

Cairney J, Hay J, Veldhuizen S, Missiuna C, Faught B (2009) Developmental coordination disorder, sex, and activity deficit over time: a longitudinal analysis of participation trajectories in children with and without coordination difficulties. *Dev Med Child Neurol* 52: e67–e72.

Cairney J, Veldhuizen S, Hay J, Faught B, Missiuna C (2010) Trajectories of relative weight and waist circumference in children with and without developmental coordination disorder. *Can Med Assoc J* 182: 1167–1172.

*Cresswell JW (2007) *Qualitative Inquiry and Research Design, Choosing Among Five Approaches*, 2nd edition. Thousand Oaks, CA: Sage.

Davis E, Shelly A, Waters E, et al (2008) Quality of life of adolescents with cerebral palsy: perspectives of adolescents and parents. *Dev Med Child Neurol* 51: 193–199.

*Denzin NK, Lincoln YS (2005) *The Sage Handbook of Qualitative Research*, 3rd edition. Thousand Oaks, CA: Sage.

*Depoy E, Gitlin LN (2005) *Introduction to Research. Understanding and Applying Multiple Strategies*, 3rd edition. St Louis, MO: Elsevier Mosby.

Depoy E, Gilmer D, Martzial E (2000) Adolescents with disabilities and chronic illness in transition: a community action needs assessment. *Dis Stud Quart* 20: 34–57.

Doyle Y, Moffat P, Corlett S (1994) Coping with disabilities: the perspective of young adults from different ethnic backgrounds in inner London. *Soc Sci Med* 38: 1491–1498.

Fraser M (1996) Exploring the needs, expectations and capacities of young adults with physical disabilities. Hamilton, ON: Social Planning and Research Council of Hamilton-Wentworth.

Freeman M, Stewart D, Missiuna C, Burke-Gaffney J, Law M, Jaffer S (2010) Development and evaluation of the Youth KIT to assist youth with disabilities in managing information. Unpublished report. Hamilton, ON: *CanChild* Centre for Childhood Disability Research.

Garth B, Murphy GC, Reddihough DS (2009) Perceptions of participation: child patients with a disability in doctor–parent–child partnership. *Patient Educ Counsel* 74: 45–52.

Gorter JW, Stewart D, Woodbury-Smith M (2011) Youth in transition: care, health and development. *Child Care Health Dev* 37: 757–763.

Harding J, Harding K, Jamieson P, et al (2009) Children with disabilities' perceptions of activity participation and environments: a pilot study. *Can J Occup Ther* 76: 133–144.

Heah T, Case T, McGuire B, Law M (2007) Successful participation: the lived experience among children with disabilities. *Can J Occup Ther* 74: 38–47.

*Kemmis S, McTaggart R (2005) Participatory action research. Communicative action and the public sphere. In: Denzin NK, Lincoln YS, editors. *The Sage Handbook of Qualitative Research*, 3rd edition. Thousand Oaks, CA: Sage, pp. 559–603.

King G, Law M, Hanna S, et al (2006) Predictors of the leisure and recreation participation of children with physical disabilities: a structural equation modeling analysis. *Child Health Care* 35: 209–234.

Law M, King G, King S, et al (2006) Patterns of participation in recreational and leisure activities among children with complex physical disabilities. *Dev Med Child Neurol* 48: 337–342.

Law M, Petrenchik T, King G, Hurley P (2007) Perceived barriers to recreational, community and school participation for children and youth with physical disabilities. *Arch Phys Med Rehab* 88: 1636–1642.

*Miller WL, Crabtree BF (2005) Clinical research. In: Denzin NK, Lincoln YS, editors. *The Sage Handbook of Qualitative Research*, 3rd edition. Thousand Oaks, CA: Sage, pp. 605–639.

Missiuna C, Moll S, Law M, King S, King G (2006) Mysteries and mazes: parents' experiences of children with developmental coordination disorder. *Can J Occup Ther* 73: 7–17.

Missiuna C, Moll S, King S, King G, Law M (2007) A trajectory of troubles: parents' impressions of the impact of developmental coordination disorder. *Phys Occup Ther Pediatr* 27: 81–101.

Missiuna C, Cairney J, Pollock N, et al (2011) A staged approach for identifying children with developmental coordination disorder from the population. *Res Dev Dis* 32: 549–559.

Missiuna M, Moll S, King G, Stewart D, Macdonald K (2008) Life experiences of young adults who have coordination difficulties. *Can J Occup Ther* 75: 157–166.

Morris C, Liabo K, Wright P, Fitzpatrick R (2007) Development of the Oxford Ankle Foot Questionnaire: finding out how children are affected by foot and ankle problems. *Child Care Health Dev* 33: 559–568.

Morris C, Doll H, Davies N, et al (2009) The Oxford Ankle Foot Questionnaire for children: responsiveness and longitudinal validity. *Qual Life Res* 18: 1367–1376.

Neely-Barnes SL, Graff C, Roberts RJ, Hall HR, Hawkins JS (2010) 'It's our job': qualitative study of family responses to ableism. *Int Dev Disabil* 48: 245–258.

Palisano R, Shimmel L, Stewart D, Lawless J, Rosenbaum P, Russell D (2009) Mobility experiences of adolescents with cerebral palsy. *Phys Occup Ther Pediatr* 29: 133–153.

Parkinson KN, Rice H, Young B (2011) Incorporating children's and their parents' perspectives into condition-specific quality-of-life instruments for children with cerebral palsy: a qualitative study. *Value Health Care* 14: 705–711.

Petrenchik T, King G (2011) Pathways to positive development: childhood participation in everyday places and activities. In: Bazyk S, editor. *Mental Health Promotion, Prevention, and Intervention with Children And Youth. A Guiding Framework for Occupational Therapy*. Bethesda, MD: AOTA Press.

Powers LE (2001) *Take Charge for the Future*. Portland, OR: Center on Self-Determination, Oregon Health Sciences University.

Renwick R, Schormans AF, Zekovic B (2003) Quality of life for children with developmental disabilities: a new conceptual framework. *J Dev Disabil* 10: 107–114.

*Richards L, Morse JM (2007) *Readme First for a User's Guide to Qualitative Methods*, 2nd edition. Thousand Oaks, CA: Sage.

Ronen GM, Rosenbaum P, Law M, Streiner DL (1999) Health-related quality of life in childhood epilepsy: the results of children's participation in identifying the components. *Dev Med Child Neurol* 41: 554–559.

Ronen GM, Rosenbaum P, Law M, Streiner DL (2001) Health-related quality of life in childhood disorders: a modified focus group technique to involve children. *Qual Life Res* 10: 71–79.

Ronen GM, Streiner DL, Rosenbaum P, Canadian Pediatric Epilepsy Network (2003) Health-related quality of life in children with epilepsy: development and validation of self-report and parent proxy measures. *Epilepsia* 44: 598.

Sharma N, Lalinde PS, Brosco JP (2006) What do residents learn by meeting with families of children with disabilities? A qualitative analysis of an experiential learning module. *Pediatr Rehabil* 9: 185–189.

Stewart D, Law M, Rosenbaum P, Willms D (2001) A qualitative study of the transition to adulthood for youth with disabilities. *Phys Occup Ther Pediatr* 21: 3–22.

Stewart D, Freeman M, Law M, et al (2009) *The Best Journey to Adult Life. An Evidence-based Model and Best Practice Guidelines for the Transition to Adulthood for Youth with Disabilities.* Hamilton, ON: McMaster University and *CanChild* Centre for Childhood Disability Research.

Stewart D, Freeman M, Missiuna C, et al (2010) *The KIT – Keeping It Together. Youth Version.* Hamilton, ON: McMaster University and *CanChild* Centre for Childhood Disability Research.

Stewart D, Lawless J, Shimmell LJ, et al (2012) Social participation of adolescents with cerebral palsy: experiences, trade-offs and choices. *Phys Occup Ther Pediatr* 32: 167–179.

Turnbull AP, Turnbull R (2006) Self-determination: is a rose by any other name still a rose? *Res Prac Pers Sev Disabil* 31: 83–88.

Vander Laenen F (2009) 'I don't trust you, you are going to tell', adolescents with emotional and behavioural disorders participating in qualitative research. *Child Care Health Dev* 35: 323–329.

Waters E, Maher E, Salmon L, Reddihough D, Boyd R (2005) Development of a condition-specific measure of quality of life for children with cerebral palsy: empirical data reported by parents. *Child Care Health Dev* 31: 127–135.

Wolcott HF (1999) *Ethnography: A Way of Seeing.* Walnut Creek, CA: AltaMira.

World Health Organization (2001) *International Classification of Functioning, Disability and Health.* Geneva: WHO Press.

17

SELF- AND PROXY-RATED VALUATIONS OF OUTCOMES

Gabriel M. Ronen and David L. Streiner

Overview

This chapter assesses factors associated with self-report and proxy ratings of instruments measuring health and patient-reported outcomes (PROs) of children and young people with chronic neurological and developmental conditions. We first discuss the concepts of self- and proxy reports, as well as the rationale and available data on the application of such ratings. Next we review the literature on self- and proxy reports of adults with dementia and other neurological impairments to provide a more complete picture of the research on the topic. Third, we examine the potential sources of variation in self- versus proxy respondents' reports – factors within patients (e.g. age, sex, disability status, mental health, etc.) and similar or other issues within proxies (e.g. level of demand, sense of burden, etc.). Finally, we critically appraise the methodological challenges associated with these approaches and conclude with practical recommendations for the clinician and researcher.

Introduction

Many adult self-report health questionnaires provide important information that can be used in clinical decision making and research. The issue becomes more complicated, however, when evaluating non-literate populations, such as young children and adults with dementing disorders. With these groups, it is necessary to use proxy reports. However, the literature is confusing regarding the correlations between self- and proxy-reported quality of life (QOL). Anticipating our conclusions, we believe that studies that combine qualitative with quantitative approaches can be far more informative than those that simply report correlations. Later in this chapter we demonstrate that awareness of particular patient proxy issues identified in the adult population with specific neurological conditions helps to explain the difficulties of studying similar questions in young populations with neurological and developmental conditions.

Although proxy report is somewhat inconsistent with the concepts of PROs and QOL that are defined as being a patient's own perceptions, proxy accounts have been used as either a

234

complementary or an alternative source of information about patients. The rationale behind this practice is that proxy raters may be effective sources either for obtaining information that might otherwise be unavailable (for example, when patients are unable or unwilling to provide the information) or to complement and expand on patients' own accounts (Banerjee et al 2008). The expectations are that proxy-reported data may provide additional important information in clinical decision making for patients, whether they are children or adults. Tackett (2011) comments that parents do possess the attributes of 'good informants' as they have access to an extensive breadth and depth of information about their child. However, parental informants might have limitations as good judges in that they might be motivated to cast the child in a positive light. On the other hand, parents also show features of good judges by being motivated to respond thoughtfully and carefully. It is a reality that parents' perceptions of their children's health and QOL already influence healthcare utilization (Varni et al 2007).

Reviewers have repeatedly suggested that parents or caregivers would have sufficient objectivity to evaluate the individual's own perceptions and have recommended their use as proxies when a respondent is too young or too cognitively impaired, immature, ill, distressed, or fatigued to respond. Furthermore, it has been recommended that proxies are used for people with communication disorders, those with limited social experience, or people with continued dependency (Eiser et al 2000, Varni et al 2007).

The Rashomon effect of multirealities

The term 'Rashomon effect' has been used in social sciences to describe multiple realities (Roth and Mehta 2002). In this Japanese crime tale set in the twelfth century, written by Akutagawa in 1915 and made into a classic film in 1950, a single event, the murder of a samurai and the rape of his wife, is retold from the perspectives of different characters, including the ghost of the samurai, who are witnesses to the event. Ultimately, when the tale is over, the reader is left with the realization that, while none of the versions are a truthful objective account, all must be true at least from the character's own awareness and perspective. It is not just their version; it is their unique personal reality as each perceives it.

The Rashomon effect illustrates the difficulty of examining the constructs and validity of standardized health evaluations by different sources that include the patients themselves, physicians, nurses, therapists, psychologists, social workers, teachers, caregivers, and family members. Within the International Classification of Functioning, Disability and Health (ICF) model (World Health Organization 2001) (see Chapter 4), one may expect physicians to be competent to evaluate the level of *impairment*; patients, physicians, therapists, and nurses to evaluate the level of *activity*; patients, family members, and teachers to evaluate *participation*; patients, family members, therapists, and social workers to assess *contextual environmental* factors; and the patients to evaluate *contextual personal* factors. But when personal experiences and perceptions such as satisfaction, QOL, expectations, or pain are evaluated, those reported directly by the population of interest, namely patients themselves (even if they are children) are able to provide either the only or the most valid information (Sneeuw et al 2002, Ronen et al 2003, Cremeens et al 2006).

Parents, caregivers, or other proxies can respond in a number of ways. They may: (1) report their perceptions and the personal expressed opinions of the patient's internal life and well-being (*observer informant*); (2) respond the way they believe the patients would answer themselves (*surrogate informant*); (3) answer as if they were the patient themselves, envisaging themselves in the situation of the patient's disability (*substitute informant*); or (4) respond as an advocate for the patient (*advocacy informant*). Proxies including parents make their valuations with one or more of these perspectives in mind, and some are able to respond differentially from any of these approaches when specifically instructed to do so (Davis et al 2007). For example, caregivers were asked to rate the global QOL of patients with Alzheimer disease using two questions: 'How would you rate the overall QOL of your relative's life at present' (*observer proxy*) and 'How do think your relative would rate his or her overall QOL at present?' (*surrogate proxy*) (Karlawish et al 2001). In the *observer* role, a lower QOL rating was associated only with the Caregiver Burden Screening scale (Vitaliano et al 1991), predominantly with the item 'I have little control over my relative's behaviour', whereas in the *surrogate* role a lower QOL rating was associated only with a lower caregiver rating of the patient's mental health. Most significantly, half of the respondents did not differ using the two perspectives, raising the possibility that they were not acting as reliable proxies. We were unable to identify similar proxy studies using multidimensional QOL measures.

The Rashomon effect of multiple realities has consistently been shown to exist among different responders such as physicians, nurses, therapists, teachers, and caregivers (Boyer et al 2004, Janse et al 2005, White-Koning et al 2008); among different caregivers such as spouses, sons, or daughters (Conde-Sala et al 2010); between parents in assessing their child's personality (Tackett 2011); and within a single person. It is obvious that proxy reports are guided and influenced by a multitude of factors (see also below). Consequently, we strongly suggest instructing proxy responders on which specific approach to take and detailing the specific approach in any subsequent reports.

The theoretical constructs of patients and proxies

Studies have almost consistently reported that ratings obtained from proxies are not identical to those provided by the patients themselves. Whenever self- and proxy ratings have been compared, the level of agreement is highest on visible performance and function questions with a median intraclass correlation coefficient (ICC) of about 0.6 to 0.7 and lower ICCs (around 0.5) on other health status components (Sneeuw et al 2002). The correlations are typically below 0.5 when patients' own perceptions are rated. Within QOL domains, correlations tend to be lower the more abstract the domain is; for example, the child–parent ICCs on the CHEQOL-25, a specific health-related QOL measure for children with epilepsy, are 0.32 for the domain of 'current worries' and 0.24 for the domain of 'concealment' of epilepsy (Verhey et al 2009). Proxy scores tend to deviate from patient scores in either direction. As a case in point, in assessing the QOL scores in young people with epilepsy, children's and mothers' mean scores on a forced response scale (avoiding potential biases associated with multiple response types) deviated from each other in both positive and negative directions in studies from both Canada and Hong Kong (Ronen et al 2003, Yam et al 2008); similar findings were obtained from a Dutch study of adolescents with somatic chronic conditions (Sattoe et al 2012). Independent observers are inclined to rate performance and function scales more accurately than the patient (Gotay 1996).

There are many possible explanations for the discordance in scoring. Our interpretation is that, when patient and proxy evaluate a theoretical concept such as QOL, their perceptions, although related, represent different realities that from a measurement theory perspective embody unique constructs. The following arguments may support this contention.

The *disability paradox* is an important theoretical explanation for differences in perception. It has been shown that some patients with chronic health conditions are satisfied with at least some aspects of their life, apparently against all odds (at least as judged from the 'outside'). Some of these individuals consider their life trajectories to be as satisfactory and fulfilling as those of healthy people, in apparent discordance with their externally perceived health status. For example, patients mildly to moderately affected with amyotrophic lateral sclerosis (ALS) score their QOL equal to that of non-impaired individuals (Lulé et al 2008). Albrecht and Devlieger (1999: 977) explored this paradigm and raised the question: 'Why do many people with serious and persistent disabilities report that they experience a good or excellent quality of life when to most external observers these people seem to live an undesirable daily existence?' How is it that in some patients with ALS, the more severe the physical impairment the better is the experienced QOL? And why do some ventilated patients with ALS show significantly better QOL scores than non-ventilated patients (Lulé et al 2008)?

Ratings of the perceived health and the biomedical impairments from the patients' perspectives have been found to be distinct concepts, demonstrating that perceptions of outcomes cannot be explained by biomedical variables alone. This has been illustrated in young people with cerebral palsy (CP) (Rosenbaum et al 2007) and with spinal muscular atrophy (de Oliveira and Araújo 2011). In contrast to a purely medical approach, life issues are highly individual. They differ from person to person, highlighting the fact that an apparently similar medical condition or even comparable levels of functioning can be valued or perceived by individuals in many different ways. It is obvious that proxies can hardly have insight into patients' 'positive psychology' attributes and style of coping with a chronic health condition or the factors that affect how they think about their own QOL and about their ability to develop strategies for taking or restoring control (Manassis et al 1997, Barbosa et al 2002, Velissaris et al 2007) (see Chapter 10 for more on positive psychology). Therefore, proxy evaluations of QOL have been consistently more closely related to health status than to patients' own assessments. In addition, the constant adaptation of the patient to his or her impairment means continuously setting new expectations and goals that are attainable but are not clearly apparent to the proxy. Albrecht and Devlieger (1999) interpreted their results by suggesting that, among people with disabilities, one dimension of the self may compensate for the poorer function in another dimension so that the relative balance of self is maintained whereby good outcomes may result. (The disability paradox is discussed in more detail in Chapter 2.)

Proxies may score similar items very differently as a result of their different reasoning and valuations of the patients' QOL – reasoning and valuations that can be worlds apart. For example, while exploring the variables that explain the expression of QOL in childhood epilepsy, we have identified that different variables often explain the variance of the child self-report and parent surrogate responses. More specifically, regression analyses showed that the most significant variables associated with the *interpersonal social consequence of epilepsy* subscale were *social support* for the children but *perceived victimization* for the parents

(Ronen et al 2010). Likewise, patients with ALS are more likely than those without obvious impairments to name friends, family, and social environment as determinants of their QOL (Lulé et al 2008). Other probable causes for lower proxy ratings in the evaluation of patients' QOL are the particular stresses and burdens experienced by parents and caregivers, associated with chronic and prolonged neurological and developmental conditions, that are not likely to be cured, or have an extremely poor prognosis (Banerjee et al 2009).

Assessment of the *factor structure* of patient and proxy ratings can be used to identify the dimensions that underlie a construct. When factor structures were derived for both patient and proxy responses on the QOL measure for children with epilepsy (CHEQOL-25), we identified similar but not identical patterns. Four of the five factors identified by the children were also identified by the parents, but the parents' responses did not correspond to the factor of children's 'quest for normality'. Furthermore, the children's assessments of their concerns centred only on worries about present issues, whereas the parents focused on both present and future concerns (Ronen et al 2003). The latter difference can be explained by the reality that the life experiences of parents enable them to think also about how their child might adapt to life with a chronic condition throughout his or her lifespan and by the fact that for children 'the future' may mean tomorrow.

Similarly, the Dementia QOL questionnaire (Brod et al 1999) is a self-report measure with five intended domains: aesthetics or enjoyment; positive affect; negative affect; self-esteem; and feeling of belonging. The factor structure analysis was performed only several years after the scale was published. The caregivers' responses aggregated into only three factors, shown from highest to lowest loading: *positive affect*; *negative affect*; and *aesthetics*. The patients' responses aggregated to four factors out of the five subscales, *negative affect*, *positive affect*, *self-esteem*, and *aesthetics*, suggesting that the caregivers were oblivious to the presence of self-esteem in patients with dementia (Ready et al 2007). As we see, proxies, including parents, are often unaware of important personal facilitators for enhanced coping skills and better QOL of patients, factors such as self-esteem, quest for normality, and the overwhelming need for social support.

Self-responders to standardized measures

With self-report we expect the population of interest to complete the questionnaire without external influence by either parents or others regarding their responses. The value of information obtained directly from specific patient groups, such as those with attention deficit disorder, or with motor, communication, or cognitive impairment, can be enhanced by the participation of an independent interviewer who can check the questions for accuracy and completeness, follow up on particular responses, and provide clarification or answer respondents' questions (Cella and Tulski 1993, Matza et al 2004).

Empirical data show that children aged 8 years and older, including those with an IQ of 70 and above, are able and willing to give unique and reliable information by responding to specifically constructed health and QOL questionnaires (Ronen et al 2003, 2010). Data from studies in adults show that mild or moderate cognitive impairment does not stop patients providing consistent and reliable responses to questions about QOL within and across domains and over time (Feinburg and Whitlatch 2001, Sands et al 2004, Trigg et al 2007). Furthermore, studies on self-reports of patients with dementia consistently fail to show convincing evidence that lower cognitive ability, greater activity limitation, poor degree of insight (at least in early dementia), behaviour, age, sex, or education are related to QOL scores (Sands et al 2004, Banerjee et al 2009).

On the one hand, perceptions of suffering arising from depression or pain are consistently associated with poorer QOL scores irrespective of the age of the person or the primary biomedical condition, whether it is CP (White-Koning et al 2007), ALS (Lulé et al 2008), or dementia (Banerjee et al 2009). Indeed, patients with mild to moderate dementia do recognize when they are depressed (Sands et al 2004). On the other hand, persons with dementia tend to score their QOL higher with lower levels of awareness of memory function, better daily activity functioning levels, or when experiencing enjoyable activities. These last independent factors imply that the better perception of QOL is not simply the result of the 'blissful ignorance' one might assume as an explanation for the reported better QOL (Trigg et al 2010).

Understanding caregivers and how they respond as proxies to standardized measures
Given that most proxy responders are also caregivers (often parents or children) of the patients, it is imperative to understand what factors guide their responses (Davis et al 2011). In a large population-based study (Lach et al 2009), caregivers who reported having children with dual diagnoses of neurological/developmental and behavioural conditions were least likely to describe their general health as excellent or very good compared with other caregivers. This group frequently reported chronic conditions such as asthma, arthritis, back problems, headaches, and limitation of activities. They also displayed higher depression scores, experienced more problematic family functioning, reported lower social support, and had lower income than other caregivers. Caregivers of persons with only neurological/developmental or only externalizing behaviour conditions scored in between the dual diagnosis group and the group without these conditions. This means that parents of children with the dual conditions are 3.7 times more likely to have elevated depressive symptoms than the 'neither' group. These differences are clinically important. The regression analysis in this study shows that the impact of caring for a child with both conditions affects the health of caregivers in an additive manner, which explains the extraordinary level of distress of many of these parents.

Not surprisingly, data show that parental and caregiver stress, depression, and sense of burden are mediating factors in proxies reporting poorer QOL than the patients' own ratings. Most examples from the literature are from parents or caregivers of persons with CP or dementia (Sands et al 2004, White-Koning et al 2007, Davis et al 2011). A case in point is a study on people with dementia, where the difference between self- and proxy reports of the same measure correlate closely with the depression score of the proxy (Schiffczyk et al 2010).

In self- and parent proxy evaluations of QOL in adolescents with somatic conditions, larger discrepancies in scoring occurred when the adolescents had a lower educational level, attended special education, had physical limitations, or had a higher number of hospital admissions (leading to school absences), and also with higher surrogate proxy-perceived burden of their child (Sattoe 2012). As expected, disruptive behaviour of the patients is also associated with poorer QOL ratings by caregivers but not by the patients themselves (Banerjee et al 2009).

Evaluation of pain by caregivers or other proxies provides another example of the challenges of interpreting people's responses. Facial expression of pain is far more consistent in infants than in adults and is perhaps the most useful indication when judging pain in children (Schiavenato 2008). Nevertheless, it is unclear whether the observed expression of pain in children with neurological impairments is different from that of other children. This question creates concerns if parents are asked to rate their child's pain. For example, when parents rate their child's pain as a basis for postoperative treatment decisions, 67% of the children would have been appropriately treated, 25% would have been overtreated, and 8% would have been undertreated compared with ratings by experienced nurses (Voeple-Lewis et al 2005). Parents' ratings of their children's pain may reflect their own anxiety and expressed opinions about the pain their child experiences and their intention to ensure effective treatment. Upwardly skewed proxy pain scores can potentially be corrected by preoperative training using structured and individualized observational pain measures (Voeple-Lewis et al 2005). In comparing agreement levels of pain between adolescents with juvenile idiopathic arthritis and their parents, 71% of dyads agreed, 13% of proxies underestimated, and 16% of proxies overestimated the level of pain (Lal et al 2011). Results from this and other studies should be used with caution because the individual correlations can be highly variable (Zhou et al 2008).

Data on caregiver reports of dementia patients' QOL show no evidence that the reporters' age, sex, or number of hours spent each week caring for the patient (a measure of increased demand) have any influence on their ratings. Furthermore, the caregiver's sense of his or her own burden is not associated with the patient's activity level, dementia severity, level of daily living activity, duration of illness, memory problems, or attention-seeking behaviour (Sands et al 2004).

Both higher and lower parental education levels were separately reported to be associated with higher odds of disagreement with their child (White-Koning et al 2007, Sattoe et al 2012). Caregivers score QOL lower when depression is present in patients with mild to moderate dementia or ALS, and the same is likely to be the case for caregivers of patients with other types of impairments (Lulé et al 2008, Banerjee et al 2009). Caregiver proxy ratings of functioning (but not QOL) decrease with increased severity of patients' dementia. For example, the differences between self- and proxy report of the same measure correlate with the Mini-Mental Status score of the patient (Schiffczyk et al 2010).

Measure-related perspectives
At this juncture, before examining the validity issues of patient–proxy correlations, we focus on measure-related issues that play a role in how people respond to questionnaires.

Scale developers and users have to try to ensure that all the items in a questionnaire are answered truthfully, non-judgementally, and without ulterior motives. Scale developers and users also need to choose whether the items can be better assessed by the patients themselves or by another source, because, as discussed earlier, each potential respondent may perceive the situation from another perspective (Streiner and Norman 2008).

There are several cognitive steps involved in responding to questions in which errors in accurate responses may turn up. These biases can add up and, at their worst, can render findings useless (Streiner and Norman 2008). These include:

1 *Understanding the question* A study that assessed children's comprehension of health-related terms found that among 5-year-olds only 50% of the children had a clear understanding of the terms, 6-year-olds understood 75%, and 7-year-olds 81%, while by age 8 participants understood nearly 97% of the terms. There were no significant differences in understanding between the chronically ill and community samples (Rebok et al 2001). Another study showed that 8 years appears to be the lowest age for children to be able to respond with acceptable test–retest results on their QOL questionnaire (Ronen et al 2003). The general impression is that younger children can often provide some information on concrete aspects of their health status but not on complex and abstract perceptions (Juniper et al 1996). The lower age limit varies according to the children's cognitive abilities and grasp of the various components of health status (Matza et al 2004). Children and parents may interpret the wording of items differently: for example, 'paying attention' may mean 'understanding' for the child (Davis et al 2007). This problem may be encountered less in measures in which the children's own phrasings are used in the scale development. Parents can play a positive role by helping their child understand questions about which they are otherwise unsure (Ungar et al 2006). Our experience is that independent facilitators may be more reliable for this task than parents.

2 *Recall* Younger children may have difficulty comprehending time frames for recalling events accurately (Ungar et al 2006). Eight-year-old children have been shown to use a 4-week recall period with reasonably accuracy, but younger children may have difficulty with the concept of even 1 week (Rebok et al 2001). In these situations parents can often enhance or prompt their child's ability to recall by providing cues from specific past events (Ungar et al 2006). In addition, child and parent may think of different events as the basis for their responses (Jokovic et al 2004). Besides, children tend to base their response on a single event, whereas parents tend to cite several examples (Davis et al 2007). Above and beyond this, children tend to relate the questions asked to the context of the setting first and to the question afterwards (Tammivaara and Enright 1986). However, even adults may have difficulty in this regard, as memory is organized by life events (e.g. 'when we lived in that house', 'when we owned that car', 'when I worked at that job') rather than by calendar time; a recall beyond 2 or 3 months is often quite poor (Streiner and Norman 2008). Some children (and parents as well) may attribute aspects of memory and learning problems to poor attention and concentration (Elliott et al 2005).

3 *Framing the answer* Children tend to differ from their parents in their reasoning (or by their inability to express their reasoning) behind giving a specific response to an item. In addition, children tend to rate their item prior to providing their explanations, whereas parents tend to discuss and verbalize the content of the item and then select the answer (Davis et al 2007). Extra problems occur in adult patients with frontal lobe impairments who may lack awareness in relation to specific cognitive deficits, social functioning behaviour, or general life circumstances (Aalten et al 2005). In these populations the items that show most disagreement between patient and proxy are: lack of insight and concern, lack of concern for social rules, distractibility, decision-making ability, and other emotional regulation problems such as aggression and euphoria (Burges and Robertson 2002).

4   *Mapping the answers into the response alternative and editing the answer* In this context, *optimizing* means devising and answering the question as truthfully as is possible. *Satisficing* means giving an answer that satisfies the requirements of the task (i.e. giving a response) but not the optimal answer, and is therefore biased or incorrect. For example, the respondent may check the first or last alternative, or say 'No opinion', because little thought is required. This often happens if the question exceeds the cognitive ability of the person, or the respondent is not invested in the task (Streiner and Norman 2008). Children and parents tend to use different response styles when mapping their answers on to Likert-style scales. Children, especially younger ones, often provide extreme scores (Rebok et al 2001), whereas parents avoid extreme scores, often with the reasoning that they do not know everything about their child's life (Davis et al 2007).

5   *Editing the answer* In search of the 'right' answer, both children and adults may search for socially acceptable responses, and answer in a way that presents them positively (Ungar et al 2006). Response bias may also depend on how a questionnaire is constructed. Parents accompanying their child while responding to health-related QOL issues may coerce, intimidate, influence, bully, or override their child's answer in order that the child does not appear in an unfavourable light (Ungar et al 2006).

6   *Attribution and disposition* Qualitative data show that parents often ask themselves whether a particular behaviour is attributed to the biomedical condition or to unrelated factors in the patient's life (Ronen et al 1999). In addition, parents tend to think about and refer to their child's general disposition rather than to a specific time frame such as 'last week' (Davis et al 2007).

7   *Attrition may occur at any of the above steps* Children and some parents feel frustrated and lose motivation when the questions seem irrelevant to them, particularly when they are asked to complete numerous questionnaires (Ungar et al 2006).

Is there any validity to the practice of measuring patient proxy level of agreement?
Patient- and proxy-reported questionnaires are a relatively low-cost and efficient way of collecting information. The guiding assumption from studies examining the degree of agreement between patient and caregiver is that a high level of agreement would indicate that either the patient or the caregiver could be used as the respondent without compromising the validity of the QOL assessment. Researchers have therefore suggested that, when possible, one should obtain ratings from both patient and caregiver (Matza et al 2004). Yet, the foremost critical question is: how valid is the practice of measuring the level of agreement if patients and proxy measures are tapping different constructs and where scores should not be expected to correlate or correlate despite different allocated determinants or reasoning behind the scoring (Davis et al 2007)? This key question has major implications for a number of other important questions, chiefly whether parents' or other caregivers' reports of outcomes measures can or should be used in clinical decision making and choice of treatments.

There are additional related questions: (1) Are proxies capable of making clear distinctions between various aspects of the patients' perceptions of QOL? (2) What does a 'good' or 'poor' correlation mean? (3) Do proxy reports truly complement self-reported information from children or young adults, specifically those with cognitive, developmental, or psychiatric conditions, or are they only as meaningful as either report alone? (4) Should one pool both self- and proxy data together or interpret the data separately? (5) How should we interpret findings when patient and caregiver scores diverge? (6) How can the variation in the proxy ratings from self-reported ratings be balanced against the total absence of important information for specific subpopulations of patients whose voices would otherwise be excluded?

It remains unclear whether, and how, we should incorporate both patient and proxy ratings when assessing the perceived (subjective) components of QOL. We are not in any position to answer these questions in an informed manner, and distrust hasty conclusions based on incomplete empirical data. On the one hand, one may argue that the patient–proxy level of agreement is the closest validity assessment currently available (Ready et al 2006). On the other hand, one should question the practice of comparing level of agreement which often relies on different reasoning just because we have the means to do so. These issues are multifaceted, as nothing can be understood in isolation and everything must be studied in connection to everything else. For example, it is important to keep in mind that the perceptions of health and functioning held by parents and teachers can have important impacts on their attitudes, expectations, and behaviour responses, which in turn could have developmental consequences for children. Therefore, parent rating, whether reflecting their own valuations or their understanding of the child's perceptions, may supplement our understanding of the child's QOL by adding another dimension to take into consideration both empirically and clinically (Ronen et al 2010).

We do not believe that there is currently a clear answer to the question of the degree of usefulness for proxies' assessments of the QOL of patients. We join in the recommendation for researchers and clinicians to bear in mind that, even when they are children, patients' responses probably have more validity, even if the parent's or caregiver's responses have better test–retest reliability (Matza et al 2004), when evaluating or planning research studies.

Technical aspects on correlating levels of agreement

Which statistical indices should be used to measure the level of agreement? The Pearson correlation (r) provides information on the covariation (i.e. association) between scores but does not indicate absolute agreement (Ottenbacher 1995). That means it is insensitive to biases in which one party answers consistently higher or lower than the other. On the other hand, the ICC based on absolute agreement provides an index that does take into account systematic differences (De Civita et al 2005). It should be noted, however, that the default option in most statistical analysis packages, such as SPSS, is consistency (i.e. association) rather than absolute agreement. Because scores are usually continuous rather than discrete, kappa (and weighted kappa when there are more than two categories) is rarely used. Even when the results are categorical rather than continuous, however, the ICC yields the same results as weighted kappa, when quadratic weights are used (Streiner and Norman 2008).

Summary

In this chapter we have explored theoretical, practical, and measurement-related issues and highlighted specific elements that should assist scale developers and users to recognize the intricacies of the topic and the complex interrelationship of a multitude of factors. We believe that self- and proxy-related issues are in many ways more complicated in patients with neurological and psychiatric conditions than in other individuals but that many aspects are similar across ages once child developmental perspectives are accounted for. Future scientific explorations are badly needed to identify the precise role of self- and proxy raters in assessing different outcomes in both cross-sectional and longitudinal studies. At the moment we recommend making the effort and applying self-reported measures that reflect what is important to the patient when intrinsic perceptions are pursued. Complementary views will convey awareness of the multiple realities and the interrelationships among the players involved.

REFERENCES

Key references

Aalten P, Van Valen E, Clare L, Kenny G, Verhey F (2005) Awareness in dementia: a review of clinical correlates. *Aging Ment Health* 9: 414–422. http://dx.doi.org/10.1080/13607860500143075

*Albrecht GL, Devlieger PJ (1999) The disability paradox: high quality of life against all odds. *Soc Sci Med* 48: 977–988. http://dx.doi.org/10.1016/S0277-9536(98)00411-0

*Banerjee S, Samsi K, Petrie CD, et al (2009) What do we know about quality of life in dementia? A review of the emerging evidence on the predictive and explanatory value of disease specific measures of health related quality of life in people with dementia. *Int J Geriatr Psychiatry* 24: 15–24. http://dx.doi.org/10.1002/gps.2090

Barbosa J, Tannock R, Manassis K (2002) Measuring anxiety: parent–child reporting differences in clinical samples. *Depress Anxiety* 15: 61–65. http://dx.doi.org/10.1002/da.10022

Boyer F, Novella JR, Morrone I, Jolly D, Blanchard F (2004) Agreement between dementia patients report and proxy reports using the Nottingham Health Profile. *Int J Geriatr Psychiatry* 19: 1026–1034. http://dx.doi.org/10.1002/gps.1191

Brod M, Stewart AL, Sands L, Walton P (1999) Conceptualization and measurement of quality of life in dementia: the dementia quality of life instrument (DQoL). *Gerontologist* 39: 25–35. http://dx.doi.org/10.1093/geront/39.1.25

Burgess PW, Robertson IH (2002) Principles of the rehabilitation of frontal lobe function. In: Stuss DT, Knight RT, editors. *Principles of Frontal Lobe Function*. New York: Oxford University Press, pp. 557–572. http://dx.doi.org/10.1093/acprof:oso/9780195134971.003.0033

Cella DR, Tulski DS (1993) Quality of life in cancer: definition, purpose, and method of measurement. *Cancer Invest* 11: 327–336. http://dx.doi.org/10.3109/07357909309024860

Conde-Sala JL, Garre-Olmo J, Turró-Garriga O, Vilalta-Franch J, López-Pousa S (2010) Quality of life of patients with Alzheimer's disease: differential perceptions between spouse and adult child caregivers. *Dement Geriatr Cogn Disord* 29: 97–108. http://dx.doi.org/10.1159/000272423

Cremeens J, Eiser C, Blades M (2006) Factors influencing agreement between child self-report and parent proxy-reports on the pediatric quality of life inventory TM 4.0 (PedsQLTM) generic core scales. *Health Qual Life Outcomes* 4: 58. http://dx.doi.org/10.1186/1477-7525-4-58

*Davis E, Nicolas C, Waters E, et al (2007) Parent proxy and child self-reported health-related quality of life: using qualitative methods to explain the discordance. *Qual Life Res* 16: 863–871. http://dx.doi.org/10.1007/s11136-007-9187-3

Davis E, Mackinnon A, Waters E (2012) Parent proxy-reported quality of life for children with cerebral palsy: is it related to parental psychosocial distress? *Child Care Health Dev* 38: 553–560. http://dx.doi.org/10.1111/j.1365-2214.2011.01267.x

De Civita M, Regier D, Alamgir AH, Anis AH, Fitzgerald MJ, Marra CA (2005) Evaluating health-related quality of life studies in pediatric populations. *Pharmacoeconomics* 23: 659–685. http://dx.doi.org/10.2165/00019053-200523070-00003

Eiser C, Mohay H, Morse R (2000) The measurement of quality of life in young children. *Child Care Health Dev* 26: 401–414. http://dx.doi.org/10.1046/j.1365-2214.2000.00154.x

Elliot IM, Lach L, Smith ML (2005) I just want to be normal: a qualitative study exploring how children and adolescents view the impact of intractable epilepsy on their quality of life. *Epilepsy Behav* 7: 664–678. http://dx.doi.org/10.1016/j.yebeh.2005.07.004

Feinburg LF, Whitlatch CJ (2001) Are persons with cognitive impairment able to state consistent choices? *Gerontologist* 41: 374–382. http://dx.doi.org/10.1093/geront/41.3.374

Gotay CC (1996) Patient-reported assessments versus performance-based tests. In: Spilker B, editor. *Quality of Life and Pharmacoeconomics in Clinical Trials*, 2nd edition. Philadelphia, PA: Lippincott-Raven, pp. 413–420.

Harter S (1982) The perceived competence scale for children. *Child Dev* 53: 87–97. http://dx.doi.org/10.2307/1129640

Janse AJ, Uiterwaal CSPM, Gemke RJ, Kimpen JLL, Sinnema G (2005) A difference in perception of quality of life in chronically ill children was found between parents and pediatricians. *J Clin Epidemiol* 58: 495–502. http://dx.doi.org/10.1016/j.jclinepi.2004.09.010

Jocovic A, Locker D, Guyatt GH (2004) How well do parents know their children? Implications for proxy responding of child health-related quality of life. *Qual Life Res* 13: 1297–1307. http://dx.doi.org/10.1023/B:QURE.0000037480.65972.eb

Juniper EF, Guyatt GH, Feeny DH, Ferrie PJ, Griffith LE, Townsend M (1996) Measuring quality of life in children with asthma. *Qual Life Res* 5: 35–46. http://dx.doi.org/10.1007/BF00435967

Karlawish JHT, Casarett D, Klocinski J, Clark CM (2001) The relationship between caregivers' global ratings of Alzheimer's disease patients' quality of life, disease severity, and the caregiving experience. *J Am Geriatr Soc* 49: 1066–1070. http://dx.doi.org/10.1046/j.1532-5415.2001.49210.x

*Lach LM, Kohen DE, Garner RE, et al (2009) The health and psychosocial functioning of caregivers of children with neurodevelopmental disorders. *Disabil Rehabil* 31: 741–752. http://dx.doi.org/10.1080/08916930802354948

Lal SD, McDonagh, Baildam E, et al (2011) Agreement between proxy and adolescence assessment of disability, pain, and well-being in juvenile idiopathic arthritis. *J Pediatr* 158: 307–312. http://dx.doi.org/10.1016/j.jpeds.2010.08.003

Lulé D, Häcker S, Ludolph A, Birbaumer N, Kübler A (2008) Depression and quality of life in patients with amyotrophic lateral sclerosis. *Dtsch Arztebl Int* 105: 397–403.

Manassis K, Mendlowitz S, Menna R (1997) Child and parent reports on childhood anxiety: differences in coping styles. *Depress Anxiety* 6: 62–69. http://dx.doi.org/10.1002/(SICI)1520-6394(1997)6:2<62::AID-DA2>3.0.CO;2-7

Matza LS, Swensen AR, Flood EM, Secnik K, Leidy NK (2004) Assessment of health-related quality of life in children: a review of conceptual, methodological, and regulatory issues. *Value Health* 7: 79–92.

de Oliveira CM, Araújo CA (2011) Self-reported quality of life is not correlated with functional status in children and adolescents with spinal muscular atrophy. *Eur J Paediatr Neurol* 15: 36–39.

Ottenbacher KJ (1995) An examination of reliability in developmental research. *J Dev Behav Pediatr* 16: 177–182. http://dx.doi.org/10.1097/00004703-199506000-00005

Ready RE, Ott BR, Grace J (2006) Insight and cognitive impairment: effect on quality-of-life reports from mild cognitive impaired and Alzheimer patients. *Am J Alzheimers Dis Other Demen* 21: 242–248. http://dx.doi.org/10.1177/1533317506290589

Ready RE, Ott BR, Grace J (2007) Factor structure of patient and caregiver ratings on the dementia quality of life instrument. *Neuropsychol Dev Cogn B Aging Neuropsychol Cogn* 14: 144–154. http://dx.doi.org/10.1080/138255891007056

Rebok G, Riley A, Forrest C, et al (2001) Elementary school aged children reports on their health: a cognitive interviewing study. *Qual Life Res* 10: 59–70. http://dx.doi.org/10.1023/A:1016693417166

Ronen GM, Rosenbaum P, Law M, Streiner DL (1999) Health-related quality of life in childhood epilepsy: the results of children's participation in identifying the components. *Dev Med Child Neurol* 41: 554–559. http://dx.doi.org/10.1017/S0012162299001176

Ronen GM, Streiner DL, Rosenbaum P, Canadian pediatric Epilepsy Network (2003) Health-related quality of life in children with epilepsy: development and validation of self-report and parent proxy measures. *Epilepsia* 44: 598–612. http://dx.doi.org/10.1046/j.1528–1157.2003.46302.x

Ronen GM, Streiner DL, Verhey LH, et al (2010) Disease characteristics and psychosocial factors: explaining the expression of quality of life in childhood epilepsy. *Epilepsy Behav* 18: 88–93. http://dx.doi.org/10.1016/j.yebeh.2010.02.023

Rosenbaum PL, Livingston MH, Palisano RJ, Galuppi B, Russell DJ (2007) Quality of life and health-related quality of life of adolescents with cerebral palsy. *Dev Med Child Neurol* 49: 516–521. http://dx.doi.org/10.1111/j.1469-8749.2007.00516.x

Roth WD, Mehta JD (2002) The Rashomon effect: combining positivist and interpretivist approaches in the analysis of contested events. *Soc Method Res* 31: 131–173.

*Sands LP, Ferreira P, Stewart LA, Brod M, Yaffe K (2004) What explains differences between dementia patients' and their caregivers' ratings of patients' quality of life. *Am J Geriat Psychiatry* 12: 272–280. http://dx.doi.org/10.1097/00019442-200405000-00006

Sattoe JNT, van Sta A, Moll HA, On Your Feet Research Group (2012) The proxy problem anatomized: child-parent disagreement in health related quality of life reports in chronically ill adolescents. *Health Qual Life Outcomes* 10: 10. http://dx.doi.org/10.1186/1477-7525-10-10

Schiavenato M (2008) Facial expression and pain assessment in pediatric patients: the primal face of pain. *J Spec Pediatr Nurs* 13: 89–97. http://dx.doi.org/10.1111/j.1744-6155.2008.00140.x

Schiffczyk C, Romero B, Jonas C, Lahmeyer C, Müller F, Riepe MW (2010) Generic quality of life assessment in dementia patients: a prospective cohort study. *BMC Neurol* 10: 48. http://dx.doi.org/10.1186/1471-2377-10-48

Sneeuw KCA, Sprangers MAG, Aaronson NK (2002) The role of health care providers and significant others in evaluating quality of life of patients with chronic disease. *J Clin Epid* 55: 1130–1143. http://dx.doi.org/10.1016/S0895-4356(02)00479-1

Streiner D, Norman G (2008) *Health Measurement Scales. A Practical Guide to their Development and Use*, 4th edition. Oxford: Oxford University Press.

Tackett JL (2011) Parent informants for child personality: agreement, discrepancies and clinical utility. *J Pers Assess* 93: 539–544. http://dx.doi.org/10.1080/00223891.2011.608763

Tammivaara J, Enright D (1986) On eliciting information: dialogues with child informants. *Anthrop Ed Quart* 17: 218–238. http://dx.doi.org/10.1525/aeq.1986.17.4.04x0616r

Trigg R, Jones RW, Skevington SM (2007) Can people with mild to moderate dementia provide reliable answers to self-report QoL items? *Age Ageing* 36: 663–669. http://dx.doi.org/10.1093/ageing/afm077

Trigg R, Watts S, Jones R, Tod A (2010) Predictors of quality of life ratings from persons with dementia: the role of insight. *Int J Geriat Psychiatry* 26: 83–91. http://dx.doi.org/10.1002/gps.2494

*Ungar WJ, Mirabelli C, Cousins M, Boydell KM (2006) A qualitative analysis of a dyad approach to health-related quality of life measurement in children with asthma. *Soc Sci Med* 63: 2354–2366. http://dx.doi.org/10.1016/j.socscimed.2006.06.016

Varni JW, Limbers CA, Burwinkle TM (2007) Parent proxy-report of their children's health-related quality of life: an analysis of 13,878 parents' reliability and validity across age subgroups using the PedsQL 4.0 generic core scales. *Health Qual Life Outcomes* 5: 2. http://dx.doi.org/10.1186/1477-7525-5-2

Velissaris S, Wilson S, Saling M (2007) The psychological impact of a newly diagnosed seizure: losing and restoring perceived control. *Epilepsy Behav* 10: 223–233. http://dx.doi.org/10.1016/j.yebeh.2006.12.008

Verhey LH, Kulik DM, Ronen GM, Rosenbaum P, Lach L, Streiner DL (2009) Quality of life in childhood epilepsy: what is the level of agreement between youth and their parents? *Epilepsy Behav* 14: 407–410. http://dx.doi.org/10.1016/j.yebeh.2008.12.008

Vitaliano PP, Russo J, Young HM, Becker J, Maiuro RD (1991) The screen for caregiver burden. *Gerontologist* 31: 76–83. http://dx.doi.org/10.1093/geront/31.1.76

Voepel-Lewis T, Malviya S, Tait AR (2005) Validity of parent ratings as proxy measures of pain in children with cognitive impairment. *Pain Manag Nurs* 6: 168–174. http://dx.doi.org/10.1016/j.pmn.2005.08.004

*White-Koning M, Arnaud C, Dickinson HO, et al (2007) Determinants of child–parent agreement in quality-of-life reports: a European study of children with cerebral palsy. *Pediatrics* 120: e804–e814. http://dx.doi.org/10.1542/peds.2006-3272

White-Koning M, Grandjean H, Colver A, Arnaud C (2008) Parent and professional reports of the quality of life of children with cerebral palsy and associated intellectual impairment. *Dev Med Child Neurol* 50: 618–624. http://dx.doi.org/10.1111/j.1469–8749.2008.03026.x

World Health Organization (2001) *International Classification of Functioning, Disability and Health*. Geneva: WHO Press.

Yam WK, Ronen GM, Cherk SW, et al (2008) Health-related quality of life of children with epilepsy in Hong Kong: how does it compare with youth with epilepsy in Canada? *Epilepsy Behav* 12: 419–426. http://dx.doi.org/10.1016/j.yebeh.2007.11.007

Zhou H, Roberts P, Horgan L (2008) Association between self-report pain ratings of child and parent, child and nurse and parent and nurse dyads meta-analysis. *J Adv Nurs* 63: 334–342. http://dx.doi.org/10.1111/j.1365-2648.2008.04694.x

Appendix: checklist recommendations for patient self-reports

- Use self-report questionnaires whenever possible and do not overextend the use of proxy report simply for the sake of convenience in young people who may not be the easiest source to tap.
- Self-assessment is less expensive and may also empower the patient (Gotay 1996).
- Arrange for strategies to help children or adults with impairments respond without external influence or coercion and offer neutral guidance to complete the questionnaire when required.
- Look for questionnaires that minimize the impact of response style, such as Harter's forced response style (Harter 1982), or incorporate leading cartoons (Rebok et al 2001, Matza et al 2004).
- Check for measures with neutral phrasing (neither positive nor negative) to minimize emotional distress and bias.
- Items that incorporate phrasing from the population of interest, for example children's own wording for child self-questionnaires, tend to decrease misunderstanding and cognitive burden.
- Add measures for depression or pain once these impairments are suspected in the patients as they may influence the perception of their health and QOL.
- Larger sample sizes are required to overcome potential measurement errors for studies involving children's self-evaluations (Matza et al 2004).
- Be cautious when the responders' cognitive development is under 8 years.

RECOMMENDATIONS FOR PROXY REPORTS

- Clarify the specific circumstances in which proxy reports are warranted.
- Hypothesize how the results may lead to improvement in health outcomes.
- Identify what type of proxy perspective is desired (i.e. surrogate, substitute, etc.).
- Add measures of the proxy's levels of stress and depression to explain potential poor ratings where appropriate.

RECOMMENDATIONS FOR COMBINED SELF- AND PARENT PROXY REPORT

- Use when both perspectives may be independently related to healthcare utilization.
- Use when both perspectives may be important to risk factors.
- Use when both perspectives may be needed for quality of care.
- Include measures of depression and stress for all raters. Note that constructs that promote positive adaptive attitude such as hope have a positive relationship with satisfaction and well-being and a negative relationship with depression and stress. Additional measurements of these constructs may clarify some of the discrepancies between self- and proxy reports (Chapter 10 describes the positive adaptive attitude in detail).
- Include a measure of behaviour for the patient.
- Keep in mind that strong correlations between respondents do not mean that respondents rely on the same reasoning or determinants.
- Individual patient–proxy correlation may hold significant variability despite relatively good total correlation statistics.

18
ETHICAL ISSUES IN MEASUREMENT STUDIES

David L. Streiner

Overview

At first glance, it might appear as if the ethical problems involved in measuring traits, attitudes, beliefs, and feelings would be minimal, especially when contrasted with the issues present in studies that administer drugs, have placebo control groups, or use deception. While it is true that there are few threats to a person's physical integrity due to filling out questionnaires, there are still many ethical issues that must be considered in any study that involves measurement. Fortunately, studies involving measurement do not present the same level of ethical challenge as do those involving invasive medical procedures. However, this does not mean that there are no ethical problems at all. Issues of truth-telling, confidentiality, consent, coercion, processes used in developing a measure, and misinterpretation of findings can exist. It is incumbent on the researcher to be aware of possible problems and to take steps to eliminate or minimize them as much as it is possible to do so.

Introduction

Consider the following scenarios:

Scenario 1

A validation study of a scale measuring self-esteem involves giving the measure to children after they complete an exam. One group is told that it did very well and another group told that it did poorly, irrespective of the actual performance. After completing the self-esteem scale, the students are told about the study and that they actually all had done very well.

Scenario 2

In order to validate a scale of social interaction, it is necessary to video record a class of 8-year-olds during recess. Although all of the children assent to the procedure, the parents of one child refuse to give consent. It would be impossible to eliminate the one child from the recording.

Scenario 3
On a scale measuring children's mood, one child scores in a range indicating a significant degree of depression. Complicating the picture, the scale is still in its developmental stages and has not been thoroughly validated.

Scenario 4
A study involves administering scales to children and their parents. As part of the consent process, the participants are promised anonymity and that any reports will include only summary information. Two years after the study ends, the parents of one child are involved in divorce proceedings and one party subpoenas the researcher to release the data, which will be used in court proceedings.

Scenario 5
A new scale developed to measure positive parenting shows that families from a particular minority group have much poorer skills.

The first four situations describe a number of ethical issues: deception, consent, confidentiality, duty to warn, and so forth. They arise in all types of research, not just in those involving measurement in children, but come to the fore when testing is involved. The fifth situation, in which one group of individuals scores lower than others, is a particular problem in measurement. In this chapter, we will discuss these concerns, focusing mainly (although not exclusively) on research with children. What will be missing are definitive solutions to these problems, because there are none. There are no right or wrong answers for many ethical dilemmas; they are highly situationally dependent and may vary from one study to the next, or even, in multicentre studies, be interpreted differently from one ethics board to another. However, there are some answers that are better than others and, whenever possible, these will be emphasized.

Concern about ethics in research is a relatively recent phenomenon, dating back only to the end of World War II. After the revelations of the horrific 'experiments' done on inmates of the concentration camps in Nazi Germany, the Nuremberg Code of 1947 (Trials of War Criminals before the Nuremberg Military Tribunals 1949) was adopted and later formalized in the Declaration of Helsinki of 1964 (World Medical Association, undated). Although the Declaration has been revised six times since then, the central tenets have remained unchanged. These involve respect for the individual and his or her ability to make a *free* and *informed* decision about participating in a specific research study.

Freedom to consent

Undue Influence
Let us take a closer look at those two components – free and informed. Free means that the person is able to refuse an invitation to participate in a specific study. A number of factors

can limit this ability to say 'No'. In clinical research settings, one of the primary reasons is that the person requesting consent is a clinician who is involved in the care of the potential participant or a relative. Despite all written or oral assurances that refusal to participate will not jeopardize the person's or relative's care, we have to question the degree to which this will be believed and will happen. It is natural to assume that patients or relatives of patients would not want to alienate staff, out of justifiable concern that one does not want to be in the care of an unhappy or resentful clinician.

The other side of this coin, however, is that patients or their families may be very grateful for the care they have received, and wish to thank the clinician by enrolling in the study. There is considerable debate whether this is a subtle form of undue influence, capitalizing on the person's perceived sense of obligation, or a legitimate quid pro quo when the person is unable to thank the staff in other ways (especially in Canada, where health care is free and there is no exchange of money).

The seemingly obvious way out of this bind is to forbid clinicians from enrolling their own patients into a study, and, indeed, this is the position taken by most research ethics boards (REBs; usually referred to as Institutional Review Boards, or IRBs, in the USA). There are times, however, when this injunction comes into conflict with the concept of informed consent, which we will discuss shortly. If the clinician is the principal investigator of the project, then he or she is the person who is in the best position to explain the study and to answer any questions about it. When situations like this arise, the most prudent approach would be for the clinician to discuss the project with the prospective participant, but then to state that the actual consent will be gathered by someone else – e.g. a research assistant, a resident, or a colleague not associated with the study – who will not discuss with the clinician whether or not the person has been enrolled.

Another threat to freedom to consent seems unique to psychology, and that is the use of undergraduate students as research subjects. They are often asked to participate in studies to validate scales, and receive course credit for doing so. Sometimes there is a course requirement that students must enrol in a minimum number of studies. Leaving aside the question of whether students are an appropriate sample for validational studies of scales that will be used clinically – and, indeed, Quinn McNemar (1946) once defined psychology as the study of the college sophomore – we can question the ethics of mandating participation in a study, even if it is as innocuous as completing some questionnaires. Following a revision to the ethical principles of the American Psychological Association (1992), most universities in the USA have banned this practice outright, or allow the student to replace participation with some other task, such as writing a paper. However, not all universities in Canada have followed suit.

FREEDOM TO WITHDRAW

Another aspect of freedom is that granting consent is not an iron-clad contract. The person should be told that he or she is free to withdraw from the study at any time without penalty. In measurement studies, this also means that participants should be told that they are free to skip any item that they find to be troublesome – too intrusive, too personal, too upsetting, and so on. This is not much of a problem with paper-and-pencil questionnaires, as respondents can always ignore an item, even if they have not been explicitly told they could do so. However, as scales are administered more and more often by computer, special consideration must be given to the response options to allow people to move forward and respond. One available answer should be 'I prefer not to answer' or words to that effect, even on questions that may be considered to be relatively innocuous, such as age or sex. This is particularly important if the computer has been programmed so that it will not advance to the next item until the current one has been answered.

Related to the issue of being able to withdraw from a study is the question of how often a person can be contacted requesting participation. To some degree, this depends on the intrusiveness of the mode of request, and there are few guidelines. If it is by mail, Dillman (2000) advocates three follow-up letters; the rationales against more are ones of pragmatism and the law of diminishing returns rather than being based on ethical considerations. Telephone calls are generally viewed as more annoying, and one 'Thanks but no thanks' should be sufficient.

PAYMENTS TO PARTICIPANTS

Finally, the question of the absence of coercion in obtaining consent raises the question of remuneration. Historically, Canada has had a stronger tradition of volunteering for altruistic purposes than the USA. For example, it is expected that people in Canada donate blood rather than sell it. Notwithstanding that, study participants in both countries are often given something for participating. Wendler et al (2002) differentiate among four different types of payments used in research: (1) reimbursement for out-of-pocket expenses (e.g. bus fare, parking, meals); (2) compensation for time or inconvenience; (3) appreciation for participating; and (4) incentives, which go beyond the first three and are meant to induce people to participate. The first category is obviously a given; people are donating their time (and sometimes their bodies) to assist the researcher. They should not also be expected to underwrite the cost of the study by paying to get to it. The last three categories of remuneration, however, present increasingly more problematic situations.

Again, filling out questionnaires is rarely as uncomfortable or dangerous as participating in studies that involve invasive procedures, such as drugs, tissue biopsies, or ionizing radiation from brain scans. However, projects sometimes require the person to complete many scales, and may include questions asking about personal or controversial topics, such as sexual experiences, episodes of physical or sexual abuse, having engaged in illegal or illicit activities, and so forth. The issues are: how much participants should be paid; for which of Wendler et al's last three categories they should be paid; and when they should be paid?

Compensation for time and inconvenience is not too controversial, although it is possibly inequitable. The inequity stems from the fact that patients are rarely remunerated. This is usually justified by the fact that they may benefit from the study. However, the 'benefit' is often more abstract than real, in that the increased knowledge may help future patients with the same condition, rather than be of immediate help to the participants themselves. The potential problem arises from the amount of compensation, and concern that paying for time and inconvenience may shade into the fourth category, incentives. The IRB of one institution has published a schedule of suggested compensations for various procedures (Partners Human Research Committee, undated). It recommends between $5 and $30 per hour for completing psychological scales and tests; $20 to $75 for participating in focus groups ranging between

1 hour and 3 hours; and $30 to $70 for an outpatient visit, depending on what else the person must do (e.g. bring a 24-hour urine sample or complete a diary).

Similarly, tokens of appreciation are rarely controversial, because they are often symbolic in nature – a concrete expression of thanks, rather than a payment. Indeed, their monetary value, balanced against the time spent in the study, would often qualify the participant for welfare payments. For children, the token can consist of a tee-shirt with the study's logo, a gift certificate for a toy store or book store, pizza, tickets to a movie, and so forth. For adults, tokens can consist of lottery tickets (where legal), chances to win a prize (e.g. money, an electronic gadget), or course credit for university students.

The trade-off is that the amount should be sufficient to serve as a thank you for having participated, but not so much that the person feels coerced into doing something that he or she would otherwise not have done. The dividing line between what is unduly coercive and what is merely inviting is a fuzzy one, and depends on the person's age and circumstances, the amount of time required by the project, and so on. Indeed, there is a concern that even modest incentives, which would be seen as tokens of appreciation by middle class participants, may be coercive for those in lower socio-economic circumstances (a category that includes many students).

There is one other aspect to remuneration to participants, and that is the issue of when they are paid. This is not an issue if there is only one assessment session, but it may be a problem if multiple sessions are required. From the researcher's perspective, a person who does not show up for subsequent sessions represents a loss of time, data, and sample size. After all, it is impossible to determine the test–retest reliability of a scale if people miss the follow-up session. The researcher may be tempted to adopt a policy by which people would be paid only on completion of the entire study. However, most REBs and IRBs would view this as unduly coercive, in that participants who do not want to continue feel compelled to do so in order to protect their 'investment' from the earlier sessions.

This means that a lump sum payment of the entire amount at the end is frowned upon, and people should be paid for each session they attend. However, most REBs are comfortable with either a sliding scale of increasing amounts for each session, or a bonus for appearing for all sessions, as long as the final amount itself is not unduly coercive. For example, in a study of the test–retest reliability of a scale, a participant could be paid one-third of the total amount for the first session, and the remaining two-thirds after the second.

Informed consent

Freedom to consent is meaningless unless the person is fully informed regarding what he or she is consenting to. Needless to say, this is not as problematic in studies involving measurement as in intervention studies, in which participants may or may not be given medications or other experimental forms of treatment. However, this does not obviate the researcher's need to tell people what will be expected of them.

INFORMING THE PARTICIPANT

At a minimum, potential participants should be told how long the sessions will last and how many sessions there will be. If the study takes place in a clinical setting, and especially with patients, the researcher must clearly differentiate between what is expected from the person for purposes of clinical care and what is for research, and thus discretionary. So, if a person must complete some forms as part of the intake or follow-up, and other forms for a research study, the latter must be clearly labelled as such, with clear instructions that they are voluntary and failure to complete them will not jeopardize clinical care. Also, as mentioned previously, the participants must be told that they can omit any items they find too intrusive or personal, and response options should be provided for this.

THE USE OF DECEPTION

There are times, however, when it is not possible to honestly describe the nature of the scale or the study to the respondent. For example, if the researcher were interested in measuring social desirability bias, putting the name of the scale prominently on the top may in itself produce social desirability bias, jeopardizing the validity of the study. The scale name could be omitted entirely, or replaced with an innocuous one, such as 'A Scale of Beliefs'. In other situations, it may be necessary to deceive the respondent more completely regarding the nature of the study itself. If a scale developer were interested in constructing a measure of social anxiety, for instance, a validational study could consist of administering it under conditions of low and high stress. In order to induce stress, the researcher may have participants give an oral presentation in class and tell them, falsely, that their performance will constitute 50% of their final grade (Scenario A). Again, were the scale developer to be completely honest about the nature of the study, the stress-induction manoeuvre would be completely vitiated.

There are some who argue that deception should never be used, because it 'can strongly affect the reputation of individual labs and the profession, thus contaminating the participant pool' (Ortman and Hertwig 1997, 1998: 806). Others, however, state that deception is sometimes necessary and often defensible (e.g. Bröder 1998, Kimmel 1998). In Canada, research ethics is guided by the second edition of a document called *Ethical Conduct for Research Involving Humans*, issued by the three federal funding agencies, the Canadian Institutes of Health Research, the Natural Sciences and Engineering Research Council, and the Social Sciences and Humanities Research Council (TCPS2; Tri-Council Policy Statement 2010). It states that an REB may allow deception to be used if certain conditions are met: (1) there is no more than minimal risk to the participants; (2) it is impractical to carry out the research without deception; and, most importantly, (3) the participants are debriefed as soon as feasible after the study. When children are involved, it may be best to debrief the parents, instead of or in addition to the children. Regarding the nature of the debriefing, the document states:

> Often, debriefing can be a simple and straightforward candid disclosure. In sensitive cases, researchers should also provide a full explanation of why participants were temporarily led to believe that the research, or some aspect of it, had a different purpose, or why participants received less than full disclosure. The researchers should give details about the importance of the research, the necessity of having to use partial disclosure or deception, and express their concern about the welfare of the participants. They should seek to remove any misconceptions that may have

arisen and to re-establish any trust that might have been lost, by explaining why these research procedures were necessary to obtain scientifically valid findings.

(Tri-Council Policy Statement 2010: 38)

Most professional organizations whose members are engaged in research, such as the American Psychological Association (2010), have adopted similar policies with regard to both deception and debriefing.

GAINING CONSENT FROM VULNERABLE POPULATIONS

The essence of informed consent is that the person understands what he or she is being asked to do. There are some groups, however, whose ability to understand fully is compromised because of their age (i.e. children) or some cognitive limitation due to intellectual impairment, a mental disorder, dementia, or some other factor. This is not too much of an issue when the aim of the study is to develop a self-report scale, because if the participant is unable to comprehend the nature of the research, it is unlikely that he or she could understand the content of the items, even if they are read aloud. However, problems may arise if the scale being developed is based on observation of the participant by a rater, such as the Conners Rating Scale (Conners 1997) or the Brief Psychiatric Rating Scale (Overall and Gorham 1962). The issue is whether such people should be enrolled in studies and, if so, how.

Some have advocated that vulnerable people should not be used as research participants unless they benefit directly from the project. However, such injunctions usually pertain to therapeutic research where there is the possibility of harm, as from a medication or injection – conditions that are rarely obtain in psychometric research. However, it must still be recognized that those with a compromised ability to comprehend, and especially children, lack the capacity to make mature decisions and may defer to adults even if they are not comfortable with the study (Roth-Cline et al 2011). Accepted practice is to get consent from the parents or guardians, and to get assent from the participant, where 'assent' means that the child agrees to be in the study (Alderson 1995). In fact, though, this may better be seen as 'informed dissent', allowing the child's refusal to trump the parent's consent (Boyden and Ennew 1997).

There are legal definitions regarding the age at which children can give their own consent, and these vary from one jurisdiction to another. From the researcher's perspective, however, Thompson (1992) suggests that looking for a minimum age at which children can give consent is asking the wrong question. He states that:

Depending on the question and the complexity of the judgment, children at most ages are capable of making decisions concerning what they want to do, so perhaps the child's competency to consent to research participation should not be regarded as an inflexible limitation deriving from the child's age, but rather as an interaction of the child, the context, and the nature of the (decision-making) task. Children from a surprisingly early age can understand basic elements of the research process and their role within it if this information is presented in an age-appropriate manner.

(Thompson 1992: 60)

CONSENT IN GROUP SITUATIONS

Scenario B in the introduction involved recording a group of children to validate a scale of social interaction, in which one parent refused to give consent. It is not always possible simply to exclude that child's data, because removing him or her from the session may both distort the situation and expose the child to unwanted scrutiny: 'Why is he or she being asked to leave the room?' Under such circumstances, the only ethical course of action would be not to record the group at all. This may result in a loss of data and the possibility of bias, but to do otherwise would subvert the notion of freedom of consent, i.e. the ethics of consent trump the quality of the data.

WHEN CONSENT IS NOT NEEDED

There are times when it is necessary to validate a scale using data taken from hospital charts or school records (e.g. McGrath et al 2002, Green et al 2006). The issue is whether the individual (or the parents) need to give consent in order for the information to be used. The answer, in most cases, is 'Yes'.

According to the Tri-Council Policy Statement (2010), consent can be waived only under a fairly strict set of circumstances: (1) the data are essential for the research; (2) the use of the data is unlikely to harm the individual; (3) the researchers have obtained REB approval for all aspects of the study; and (4) it is impossible or impractical to seek consent from all of the individuals concerned. The Policy emphasizes that 'impossible or impractical' means 'undue hardship or onerousness that jeopardizes the conduct of the research; it does not mean mere inconvenience' (Tri-Council Policy Statement 2010: 63). Examples of 'impossible or impractical' include very large or geographically dispersed groups or where state or provincial privacy rules prohibit a researcher from using personal information to contact the individual in order to obtain consent.

Another circumstance in which consent is not required is when the data are anonymous or anonymized (i.e. identifying information has been stripped off). Because it is usually necessary to link a person's scale results with his or her personal information (as opposed to using group data), anonymity is rarely possible in measurement research. One possible way around this is to use anonymized data. For example, the researcher can assign a code number to each participant, and then remove the name and any other identifying information from the data. The researcher would give a list of names and code numbers to the school or hospital, which would then return the information using only the code numbers. In this way, the researcher would not be privy to identifiable person-specific data. However, it is an individual REB's decision whether this would be considered adequate, or if consent is necessary.

My experience of sitting on a number of REBs is that most would not approve this work-around. They would insist that the consent for the study should include a statement that participants' results will be linked with other information. There could be two separate consents, one regarding completion of the scale and the other for the release of information. In that way, the potential participant could agree to both parts of the study, or only the first.

WRITTEN CONSENT

In most studies, the participant signs a consent form that documents what has been discussed so far: what the study is about, what the person is being asked to do, the right of refusal and withdrawal, confidentiality of the individual's responses, and so on. The researcher keeps this form, and the participant is often given a copy. However, bear in mind that the form is not synonymous with consent. The most important aspect is that the person understands the study, not that he or she signs a form. This has two implications. The first is that the form by itself is not enough; the researcher must ensure that the participants (and their guardians, in the case of children and others who may not be able to fully comprehend the description) understand what is being asked of them. The second implication is that the form is not always necessary.

Leaving aside the issues involved with written consent in non-Western or aboriginal cultures (these are spelled out in the TCPS2), it may not be required in many measurement studies. Consent may be implied by the actions of the participant. This is most obvious when a questionnaire is mailed or emailed to a person; the very fact that the person returns it, rather than throwing it in the waste basket or hitting the delete key, signals implicit consent. Signing a separate consent form (as I have been asked to do innumerable times) is probably ethical overkill, required by university lawyers or 'risk management' people, designed more to protect the collective rear-ends of the institution against the rather unlikely event of a court case rather than guaranteeing the rights of the participant, which is the intended purpose of consent.

Even when consent is gained face to face rather than through correspondence, it is often sufficient to explain the voluntary nature of the study and the rights of refusal and withdrawal. If one wants to be extra cautious, these can be written out at the top of the questionnaire. Again, having the person sign the form is superfluous, but the researcher should document the fact that the person gave consent in the research and/or clinical record.

The limits of confidentiality

One of the pledges given to participants is that of confidentiality: that their individual results will not be made public, and that any resulting publication will use only aggregate data. However much the researcher may believe this, there are in fact at least two situations in which this blanket assurance may be compromised: when the test reveals information that may affect the health, life, or safety of the participant or another person, or when there has been a subpoena to release the results as part of legal proceedings.

Situations like these are, fortunately, quite rare, but researchers must be aware of provincial or state laws mandating the reporting of children in need of protection (e.g. at risk of physical or sexual abuse). It is relatively straightforward if the participants state outright that they have been abused or are contemplating harming themselves or someone else. In the former case (abuse), law trumps ethical principles of confidentiality; if there are provincial or state laws or regulations mandating the reporting of abuse, then it must be reported to the appropriate agencies (e.g. the Children's Aid Society). If the study involves a high-risk group where there is 'a reasonably foreseeable prospect that researchers may acquire information that a child is being abused' (Tri-Council Policy Statement 2010: 59), then the REB should be advised ahead of time that confidentiality may have to be breached and the prospective participants told about the possibility of compelled disclosure.

In the latter case (danger to self or others), there is a 'duty to warn,' which was established in the case of *Tarasoff* v. *Regents of the University of California* (1976), in which the court ruled that 'the right to confidentiality ends when the public peril begins'. This case involved a person who, while in therapy, stated his intention to kill his girlfriend. Although campus police were notified, he did in fact kill her, and the issue was whether others should have been informed or if this violated confidentiality. This and subsequent cases applied to therapeutic relationships. According to Appelbaum and Rosenbaum (1989), the Tarasoff case may affect researchers if they have a 'special relationship' with the participant: that is, they are able to predict danger because of their training or the validity of the scale; and they are in a position in which they can 'with little effort, prevent serious harm from occurring to another person or group of persons' (Appelbaum and Rosenbaum 1989: 885). In this unlikely event, it would be prudent to assume that the Tarasoff case similarly applies to information obtained during research studies.

It is more problematic if the researcher suspects that the participant may be suicidal or dangerous to others based on a scale that has not yet been validated (Scenario C). Strictly speaking, there is no conclusive evidence to support these suppositions. However, prudence again would obligate researchers to do something: to interview the person in greater depth (if there is a qualified clinician on the team) and then to notify someone – the parent or family physician – of their suspicions, emphasizing the fact that the scale is still in its development phase.

Finally, there may be situations in which research records are subpoenaed by the court (Scenario D). The Tri-Council Policy Statement (2010) states that:

> Researchers shall maintain their promise of confidentiality to participants within the extent permitted by ethical principles and/or law. This may involve resisting requests for access, such as opposing court applications seeking disclosure. Researchers' conduct in such situations should be assessed on a case-by-case basis and guided by consultation with colleagues, any relevant professional body, the REB and/or legal counsel.
>
> (Tri-Council Policy Statement 2010: 58)

So, if research records are requested by a lawyer for use in a domestic case, for example, confidentiality must remain paramount. However, if there is a court subpoena for records, the researcher should protest as much as possible and seek guidance, but, if it is decided that the information must be released, then so be it.

Reporting results

A research project may result in the development of a new scale, either as the main objective of the study or as a by-product. The sad fate of most such scales is that they then disappear from view, never to be seen again. Indeed, Goldman and Mitchell (2008) have now published their ninth volume listing unpublished scales, which must number close to 15 000. Despite that, it is still incumbent on the author to report the process and results of the scale development in sufficient detail that others who may use the measure do not misinterpret the scores.

There are a number of standards and guidelines that outline what should be reported, especially for tests that may be used diagnostically. These include the *Standards for Educational and Psychological Testing* (American Educational Research Association, American Psychological Association, and the National Council on Measurement in Education 1999), the *Standards for Reporting of Diagnostic Accuracy* (STARD; Bossuyt et al 2003), a modification of STARD for psychological tests (Meyer 2003), and the *Guidelines for Reporting Reliability and Agreement Studies* (Kottner et al 2011), and these are summarized in a chapter of *Health Measurement Scales: A Practical Guide to Their Development and Use* (Streiner and Norman 2008).

There are a few points to bear in mind from an ethical perspective. First, especially for scales that will be used to diagnose individuals, the processes used in developing the measure – e.g. sample selection, the choice of the 'criterion standard', blinding, and so forth – must be fully described, as outlined in the STARD initiative. This is required so that others using the instrument can determine if it was adequately evaluated and if the people in the reliability and validity studies are representative of those to whom the scale will be administered. Without this information, it is possible that erroneous conclusions will be drawn about the people taking the test.

Second, there may be problems if different ethnic or marginalized groups have scores that deviate significantly from those of middle class, white respondents (Scenario E). There can be many reasons for this:

- Differing interpretations of the items. One of my colleagues, Dr Michael Phillips, found that an item commonly used in activities of daily living questionnaires, 'I am able to climb a flight of stairs', was understood in China to reflect wealth: 'I am rich enough to afford a second story on my house.'
- Differing manifestations of the construct. In some cultures, depression is experienced more in terms of physical complaints rather than emotional difficulties.
- Differing cultural norms regarding what is acceptable behaviour. Corporal punishment, for example, is a more acceptable method of disciplining children among some groups than it is in dominant North American culture (e.g. Aracena et al 1999), and having conversations with dead relatives is common among some First Nations cultures (SL Kahgee, personal communication, 1983).
- Differing educational levels, leading to problems with written English.

The test developer should ensure that these and other factors are not distorting the interpretation of scale scores, and that differences in scores actually reflect differences in the underlying construct. Whenever possible, norms should be reported for individual subgroups if differences are present.

Summary

Fortunately, studies involving measurement do not present the same level of ethical challenge as do those involving invasive medical procedures. However, this does not mean that there are no ethical problems at all. Issues of truth telling, confidentiality, consent, coercion, and misinterpretation of findings can exist. It is incumbent on the researcher to be aware of possible problems, and to take steps to eliminate or minimize them as much as it is possible to do so.

REFERENCES

Key references

*Alderson P (1995) *Listening to Children: Children, Ethics, and Social Research*. London: Barnardo's.

American Educational Research Association, American Psychological Association, and the National Council on Measurement in Education (1999) *Standards for Educational and Psychological Testing*. Washington, DC: AERA, APA, and NCME.

American Psychological Association (1992) Ethical principles of psychologists and code of conduct. *Am Psychol* 47: 1597–1611. http://dx.doi.org/10.1037/0003-066X.47.12.1597

American Psychological Association (2010) Ethical principles of psychologists and code of conduct: 2010 amendments. Available at: http://www.apa.org/ethics/code/index.aspx?item=11#802 (accessed 5 August 2011).

*Appelbaum PS, Rosenbaum A (1989) Tarasoff and the researcher: does the duty to protect apply in the research setting? *Am Psychol* 44: 885–894.

Aracena M, Haz AM, Román F, Muñoz S, Bustos L (1999) Pesquisa de maltrato físico infantil: una dificultad metodológica o conceptual. *Psykhe* 8: 117–124.

Bossuyt PM, Reitsma JB, Bruns DE, et al (2003) Toward complete and accurate reporting of studies of diagnostic accuracy: the STARD initiative. *BMJ* 326: 41–44. http://dx.doi.org/10.1136/bmj.326.7379.41

*Boyden J, Ennew J (1997) *Children in Focus: A Training Manual on Research With Children*. Stockholm: Radda Bamen.

Bröder A (1998) Deception can be acceptable. *Am Psychol* 53: 805–806. http://dx.doi.org/10.1037/h0092168

Conners CK (1997) *Technical Manual – Conners Rating Scales, Revised*. San Antonio, TX: Pearson.

Dillman DA (2000) *Mail and Internet Surveys: The Total Design Method*, 2nd edition. New York, NY: John Wiley & Sons.

Goldman BA, Mitchell DF (2008) *Directory of Unpublished Experimental Measures*. Washington, DC: American Psychological Association.

Green BA, Handel RW, Archer RP (2006) External correlates of the MMPI-2 content component scales in mental health inpatients. *Assessment* 13: 80–97. http://dx.doi.org/10.1177/1073191105284432

Kimmel AJ (1998) In defense of deception. *Am Psychol* 53: 803–805. http://dx.doi.org/10.1037/0003-066X.53.7.803

Kottner J, Audigé L, Brorson S, et al (2011) Guidelines for reporting reliability and agreement studies (GRRAS) were proposed. *J Clin Epidemiol* 64: 96–106. http://dx.doi.org/10.1016/j.jclinepi.2010.03.002

McGrath RE, Pogge DL, Stokes JM (2002) Incremental validity of selected MMPI-A content scales in an inpatient setting. *Psychol Assess* 14: 401–409. http://dx.doi.org/10.1037/1040-3590.14.4.401

McNemar Q (1946) Opinion–attitude methodology. *Psychol Bull* 43: 289–374. http://dx.doi.org/10.1037/h0060985

Meyer GJ (2003) Guidelines for reporting information in studies of diagnostic accuracy: the STARD initiative. *J Pers Assess* 81: 191–193. http://dx.doi.org/10.1207/S15327752JPA8103_01

Ortmann A, Hertwig R (1997) Is deception acceptable? *Am Psychol* 52: 746–747. http://dx.doi.org/10.1037/0003-066X.52.7.746

Ortmann A, Hertwig R (1998) The question remains: is deception acceptable? *Am Psychol* 53: 806–807. http://dx.doi.org/10.1037/0003-066X.53.7.806

Overall JE, Gorham DR (1962) The Brief Psychiatric Rating Scale. *Psychol Rep* 10: 799–812. http://dx.doi.org/10.2466/pr0.1962.10.3.799

Partners Human Research Committee (undated) Remuneration for research subjects. Available at: http://healthcare.partners.org/phsirb/remun.htm (accessed 29 July 2011).

*Roth-Cline MD, Gerson J, Bright P, Lee CS, Nelson RM (2011) Ethical considerations in conducting pediatric research. *Handb Exp Pharmacol* 205: 219–244.

Streiner DL, Norman GR (2008) *Health Measurement Scales: A Practical Guide to Their Development and Use*, 4th edition. Oxford: Oxford University Press.

Tarasoff v. *Regents of the University of California* (1976) 17 Cal. 3d 425; 551 P.2d 334; 131 Cal. Rptr. 14.

Thompson RA (1992) Developmental changes in research risk and benefit: a changing calculus of concerns. In: Stanley B, Sieber JE, editors. *Social Research on Children and Adolescents: Ethical Issues*. Newbury Park, CA: Sage, pp. 31–65.

Tri-council Policy Statement (2010) *Ethical Conduct for Research Involving Humans*. Available at: www.pre.ethics.gc.ca (accessed 5 August 2011).

Trials of War Criminals before the Nuremberg Military Tribunals under Control Council Law No. 10, Vol. 2 (1949) Washington, DC: US Government Printing Office. Available at: http://ohsr.od.nih.gov/guidelines/nuremberg.html (accessed 21 July 2011).

Wendler D, Rackoff JE, Emanuel EJ, Grady C (2002) The ethics of paying for children's participation in research. *J Pediatr* 141: 166–171. http://dx.doi.org/10.1067/mpd.2002.124381

World Medical Association (undated) *Declaration of Helsinki: Ethical Principles for Medical Research Involving Human Subjects*. Available at: http://www.wma.net/en/30publications/10policies/b3/17c.pdf (accessed 21 July 2011).

Section C Opportunities for Interventions

19
CAN TRANSLATION OF RESEARCH INFORMATION IMPROVE OUTCOMES?

Iona Novak, Dianne J. Russell, and Marjolijn Ketelaar

Overview

This chapter introduces and explores the imperative, the challenges, and the practicalities of using research to inform decision making when providing care to children and young people with impairments and their families. In an ideal world, effective and realistic interventions will do no harm, will improve quality of life, and will meet the expectations of parents and children regarding meaningful and clinically important outcomes. This chapter defines knowledge translation (KT) and presents relevant models for understanding how KT relates to evidence-informed decision making. Also described is where to locate evidence, followed by an in-depth summary of what KT strategies actually work and what tools are available for measuring the outcomes of these KT interventions. By the end of this chapter, readers should have an overview of the process involved in providing evidence-informed answers to questions that families and clinicians ask.

Case scenario

John is a 5-year-old with GMFCS level II cerebral palsy. This means that he can walk independently and unaided on level surfaces but has limited capacity on uneven or slippery surfaces (Palisano et al 1997). John is attending clinic with his mother, Kim. He has recently started school and is having difficulty participating in playground games with friends. Kim has recently read on a parent web forum about strength training and asks if strengthening John's muscles would help. How do you proceed?

Introduction

'Do no harm' speaks plainly to the crux of good health care. There are professional, ethical, and social obligations to do no harm to John or his mother. However, in any clinical decision-making situation there are several potential sources of harm, which may include: (1) use of interventions with harmful effects; (2) the use of ineffective interventions; (3) providing interventions that do not reflect families' needs and goals; and (4) making claims about successful outcomes from interventions without objective evidence based on appropriate outcome measurement.

In the context of childhood impairment and disability Palisano et al (2012) have discussed evidence-informed decision making as it relates to paediatric practice. The process involves: (1) identifying the child's and the family's strengths and needs; (2) understanding the research evidence for each of the possible intervention options; (3) considering child and family preferences; and (4) integrating the service providers' practice knowledge and expertise to reach an evidence-informed recommendation. John and Kim require relevant up-to-date evidence-based information to guide their decision making.

We believe that the ideas articulated by Palisano et al (2012) are relevant to people with neurological and developmental conditions across the entire age spectrum. In helping to achieve effective and meaningful interventions professionals may play a variety of KT roles. They may be 'research users' who provide research-informed intervention to people with impairments and their families or use such information to plan effective programmes or policies. They may be 'research translators' in roles as clinical leaders, managers, or educators, acting as 'knowledge brokers' and helping clinicians to access, understand, and use research to inform intervention. They may be 'research producers' who contribute new knowledge and wish to communicate and translate this information effectively to a variety of audiences (e.g. clinicians, families, administrators, policy makers, other researchers, and knowledge translators, as well as to the media for communication to the community and funders) in order to inform intervention and to improve services. This chapter explores the challenges and the practicalities of using research to inform decision making when providing services to people with disabilities and their families.

Knowledge translation: definition and purpose

WHAT IS KNOWLEDGE TRANSLATION?
KT has been defined as 'a dynamic and iterative process that includes the synthesis, dissemination, exchange, and ethically sound application of knowledge to improve health, provide more effective health services and products and strengthen the healthcare system'(Canadian Institutes of Health Research 2009). While McKibbon et al (2010) identified over 100 terms used in the literature to describe the process of getting research knowledge integrated into decision making, including research transfer, knowledge mobilization, KT, KT and exchange, in this chapter we will use the term KT to refer to these many ideas. We believe that KT involves an interactive exchange with end users and that it should be integrated along the continuum of research, from identifying important research questions, methods, and measures to the interpretation and implementation of the results.

WHY IS KNOWLEDGE TRANSLATION IMPORTANT AND HOW DOES IT RELATE TO EVIDENCE-INFORMED DECISION MAKING?
Routine clinical practice is known to lag a staggering 10 to 20 years behind current research evidence (Bates et al 2003, Gilbert et al 2005). The phenomenon is known as the 'research–practice gap'. Healthcare research indicates that 10% to 40% of patients *do not* receive proven

effective treatments, and more than 20% of patients receive ineffective or harmful treatments (Flores-Mateo and Argimon 2007).

Perhaps the most shocking example of harm caused by the research–practice gap comes from the sudden infant death syndrome (SIDS) field. The risk of SIDS associated with putting infants to sleep on their belly was known for 20 years before professionals revised advice about safe infant positioning (the 'Back to Sleep' movement). In the time lag between identifying and closing the SIDS research–practice gap, it is estimated that 50 000 infants in Australia, the USA, and the UK died (Gilbert et al 2005).

Recent evidence indicates that, despite numerous systematic reviews available to provide guidance about what does and does not work in cerebral palsy, many children are still provided with ineffectual interventions (Rodger et al 2005, Saleh et al 2008). This seems remarkable when professionals aim to help, families want and need the most effective interventions, and the health system demands timely and cost-efficient services. Why then is it so hard to change health professionals' behaviour when it comes to integrating the most up-to-date research evidence into routine practice?

Recent advances in the impairment and disability evidence base have meant that some mainstay treatments have been proven ineffective and new more effective interventions have emerged as viable treatment options. It is difficult for parents and clinicians to keep abreast of new evidence as it emerges and to determine the best course of intervention for an individual child. For example, 15 years ago, strengthening muscles was thought to be harmful for children with cerebral palsy, but this approach is now a proven effective intervention for certain indications (Damiano and Abel 1998, Dodd et al 2003, Scianni et al 2009).

Theories and models of knowledge translation

There are many models of KT in the literature (Sudsawad 2007, Ward et al 2009) but the knowledge to action (KTA) framework (Fig. 19.1), proposed by Graham et al (2006) is built upon a review of many theories and draws together commonalities between KT approaches.

The KTA framework breaks the process into two parts: (1) knowledge creation, depicted in the upside-down triangle; and (2) knowledge application, depicted in the boxes and arrows surrounding the triangle.

Knowledge creation relates to the process of gathering individual research until there is enough evidence to believe that a change in practice is needed. This usually requires more than one study and often takes the form of a synthesis of knowledge through a systematic review of available research on the topic. Ideally, the knowledge creation process ends with specific tools or products in user-friendly formats to help meet the needs of those who wish to use the research.

Knowledge application refers to all of the stages of implementing the knowledge by understanding barriers in the user's context and tailoring the knowledge mobilization intervention based on that understanding. Once evidence has been accepted as valid, the implementation must be monitored and evaluated to determine whether the knowledge makes a difference in terms of health service provider behaviour and client outcomes.

The final phase of this model highlights the importance of ensuring sustained use of knowledge in practice. It is not sufficient to 'transfer' knowledge to service providers. Rather,

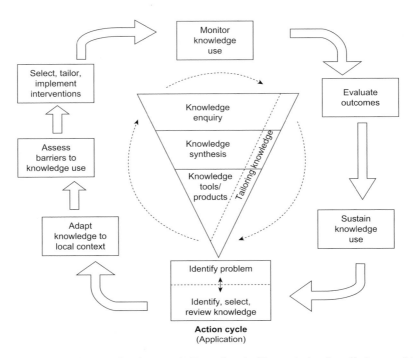

Fig. 19.1 The knowledge to action framework. Reproduced with permission from Graham et al (2006). Copyright © 2006. The Alliance for Continuing Medical Education, the Society for Academic Continuing Medical Education, and the Association for Hospital Medical Education.

it is necessary to know whether the knowledge has made a difference to practitioners (and of course to patients) such that service delivery will be changed on a long-term basis, for improved outcomes for patients and their families.

Research and experiences have shown that one of the most difficult phases in the model is the step referred to as '*Select, tailor, implement*' (Ketelaar et al 2008). Implementing evidence as it refers to the use of outcome measures or the application of an intervention requires a change in behaviour and in routines of service providers. A 10-step model for inducing change in professional behaviour has been devised to provide guidance (Grol and Wensing 2004, Grol et al 2007). The steps include: (1) promote awareness of the innovation; (2) stimulate interest and involvement; (3) create understanding; (4) develop insight into own routines; (5) develop positive attitude to change; (6) create positive intention/decision to change; (7) try out change in practice; (8) confirm value of change; (9) integrate new practice into routines; and (10) embed new practice in organization. The model provides a framework to plan strategies in the implementation phase of the KTA model and to focus on specific incentives and barriers at each stage.

Current use of evidence: where to find evidence

It is difficult for clinicians to remain up to date because the volume of research published is increasing exponentially each year (Egger et al 2001, Moseley et al 2002). In order to find the best evidence for better patient outcomes, it is imperative to know how to search for high-quality research evidence. One of the simplest ways is to search within trustworthy databases acknowledged to produce effective information gathering and quality assessments. These are known as secondary source databases, containing systematic reviews that provide evidence summaries, clinical trials with an assigned quality score, or clinical guidelines describing what to do. Some of the best-known examples in the field of childhood disability have been included within the Appendix.

Sometimes there is very little published evidence to provide guidance, and being an evidence-based professional takes on even greater importance. Here it is essential that the outcomes of care be validly measured to determine whether the intervention being used is helping to achieve the individual patient's or family's goals. Note, however, that under these circumstances it may be inappropriate to generalize the findings to other people without further careful assessment of the effectiveness of that intervention.

Effective knowledge translation strategies

IMPLEMENTATION BARRIERS

There are many barriers to KT (Sitzia 2002, Peach 2003, Haines et al 2004, Mitton et al 2007). In a systematic review by Cochrane et al (2007) the following barriers to moving evidence into practice were identified: (1) organizational supports/resources (e.g. time, funding, resources); (2) system/process factors (e.g. workload, team structure, referral process); (3) service provider cognitive/behavioural factors (e.g. knowledge, awareness, skills); (4) healthcare professional characteristics (e.g. age/maturity of practice, peer influence); (5) attitudinal/rational–emotive factors (e.g. perceived competence, perceived outcome expectancy, authority); (6) patient factors (e.g. patient characteristics, adherence); and (7) clinical practice guidelines/evidence (e.g. utility, access, local applicability).

In the field of childhood neurodevelopmental conditions we work with families, and it is important to realize that children and families may unintentionally create barriers to evidence implementation by professionals. Families may demand ineffective services or out-of-date, unproven approaches with which they are familiar, or have pre-set perceptions or cultural beliefs about (Haines et al 2004). Parents find information about diagnoses and treatments on the Internet, and it is a challenge for both service providers and parents to ensure that the information is evidence based and that they feel comfortable to communicate and share the information with each other (Jadad 1999). It is important to recognize that complex relationships may exist between being family centred and being evidence based. It is neither family centred nor evidence based simply to provide children or families with an intervention because they request it. Family-centred care requires collaboration and partnership (Bamm and Rosenbaum 2008), and thus involves supporting families to increase their knowledge and asking for their thoughts, aspirations, and concerns.

In the KTA framework (Fig. 19.1), an understanding of the specific barriers and supports within one's institution will help guide the strategies one would use to make change. The 10-step stages of change model (Grol and Wensing 2004) aids in the understanding of specific challenges professionals might meet in changing their behaviour and routines.

IMPLEMENTATION FACILITATORS

Given the many barriers to knowledge uptake, it follows that numerous strategies have been recommended to bridge the research–practice gap, including education and intervention for professionals (Sitzia 2002, Haines et al 2004, Flores-Mateo and Argimon 2007, Mitton et al 2007), information technology supports (Haynes and Haines 1998, Sitzia 2002, Haines et al 2004, Flores-Mateo and Argimon 2007), workplace alterations (Haynes and Haines 1998, Sitzia 2002, Haines et al 2004, Ketelaar et al 2008, Novak and McIntyre 2010, Russell et al 2010), and patient-mediated interventions (Haines et al 2004).

EFFECTIVE STRATEGIES

We have summarized the evidence about the effectiveness of KT by drawing data from KT systematic reviews (Table 19.1). Evidence was appraised using a traffic colour-coding system developed by Novak and McIntyre (2010). The codes provide a simple common language among professionals, researchers, managers, and families for understanding the implications of evidence. Green = 'Go', i.e. high-quality evidence exists supporting the effectiveness of this intervention – therefore use this approach. Yellow = 'Measure', i.e. low-quality or conflicting evidence exists supporting the effectiveness of this intervention – therefore measure the outcomes of intervention carefully when using this approach to ensure that the goal is met. Red = 'Stop', i.e. high-quality evidence exists demonstrating that this intervention is ineffective – therefore do not use this approach (Novak and McIntyre 2010: 389).

Multiple KT strategies have been proposed and implemented but not all have been shown to lead to changes in professionals' behaviour (Grimshaw et al 2001, 2004). Somewhat alarmingly, systematic reviews have consistently shown that the majority of KT strategies used in isolation induce 6% improvement in professionals' knowledge of evidence-based practice but have very little influence on how they practice (Grimshaw et al 2001, Haines et al 2004, Forsetlund et al 2009). Evidence suggests that stand-alone strategies are insufficient for inducing change in professionals' evidence-based practice decision making because 'one-size does not fit all' (Dizon et al 2011). For this reason, tailored, multifaceted interventions are recommended that seek to redress the unique workplace barriers to research utilization and are specific to the stage and outcome of interest (Haines et al 2004, Cheater et al 2005, Menon et al 2009, Baker et al 2010).

What is known about the effectiveness of these KT strategies in the childhood disability field? There is an emerging body of evidence about the use of a multifaceted strategy using 'knowledge brokers' to move evidence-based measures into practice. Knowledge brokering involves supporting a local champion within the workplace to collaborate with both the clinical and administrative teams within an organization on research translation, outcome measurement, and research implementation (Lomas 2007, Ketelaar et al 2008, Russell et al 2010). Knowledge brokering is a promising strategy to bridge the research–practice gap because it

TABLE 19.1
Effectiveness of knowledge translation strategies

Strategy	Outcome of interest		Evidence alert traffic code	References
Audit and feedback of clinical performance in evidence use	Behaviour change	G	Gains are small–moderate. Unlikely to work in isolation	Mugford et al 1991, Bero et al 1998, Thomson et al 1998a,b, Haines et al 2004, Jamtvedt et al 2006
Clinical guidelines	Behaviour change	G	If simple, written in precise behavioural terms (describing the 'ideal' behaviour in specific terms – what, who, when, where, and how), accounts for local factors, disseminated via active education, and uses patient reminders. Gains are small–moderate	Grilli and Lomas 1994, Davis and Taylor-Vaisey 1997, Grimshaw et al 2001, 2004, Michie et al 2004, Thomas et al 2009
		R	If complex, unable to be trialled, or if disseminated without action	Lomas 1991, Grilli and Lomas 1994, Grimshaw et al 2001
	Patient outcomes	Y	Insufficient evidence. Gains are small–moderate	Worrall et al 1997, Thomas et al 2009
Collaboration between professionals	Behaviour change	Y	Insufficient evidence	Zwarenstein et al 1997, Grol and Grimshaw 2003, Haines et al 2004, Zwarenstein and Reeves 2006
Communities of practice to facilitate workplace learning through participation in practice and interaction with colleagues	Behaviour change	Y	Insufficient evidence	Fung-Kee-Fung and Watters 2009, Li et al 2009, Ranmuthugala et al 2010
Consensus building at a local level to ensure agreement on the importance of a clinical problem and the evidence strategy for addressing the problem	Behaviour change	Y	Conflicting evidence	Bero et al 1998
Continuing education about evidence-based practice techniques or explanations of the supporting evidence for a particular intervention approach	Knowledge change	G		Grimshaw et al 2001, Grol and Grimshaw 2003, Haines et al 2004, Pennington et al 2005, Forsetlund et al 2009
	Skill change	Y	Conflicting evidence	Brettle 2003, Taylor et al 2000
	Behaviour change	Y	Conflicting evidence. Small gains more likely if interactive, involves discussion, and is embedded in clinical scenarios	Bero et al 1998, Coomarasamy and Khan 2004, Parkes et al 2001, Pennington et al 2005
		R	If didactic	Bero et al 1998
Continuous quality improvement to target an evidence implementation behaviour at a local level	Behaviour change	G	Gains, however, are very small	Shortell et al 1998, Grimshaw et al 2001, 2003, Grol and Grimshaw 2003, Haines et al 2004

TABLE 19.1
(Continued)

Strategy	Outcome of interest	Evidence alert traffic code		References
Educational materials, including clinical recommendations, audiovisual materials, etc., disseminated in a passive way	Behaviour change	R		Soumerai et al 1989, Lomas 1991, Oxman et al 1995, Fremantle et al 1996, Bero et al 1998, Grimshaw et al 2001, 2004, Grol and Grimshaw 2003, Haines et al 2004
Financial interventions whereby financial incentives are provided to perform an evidenced-based behaviour, or budgets and fund withholding occurs for non-compliance	Behaviour change	G		Haines et al 2004
Journal clubs	Knowledge change	G		Del Mar et al 2001, Deenadayalan et al 2008
	Behaviour change	Y	Insufficient evidence	Deenadayalan et al 2008
Knowledge brokers that have a role dedicated to facilitating the transfer of research evidence between researchers and professionals	Behaviour change	Y	Lower-level supportive evidence and a randomized controlled trial suggesting the gains were small, if any	No systematic review yet available, therefore primary source evidence used: Lomas 2007, Ketelaar et al 2008, Dobbins et al 2009, Russell et al 2010
Librarian assistance to find and interpret literature at the time of decision making	Behaviour change	Y	Insufficient evidence	Winning and Beverly 2003
Mass media to target evidence uptake by professionals and patients	Behaviour change	G		Grilli and Lomas 1998, Grimshaw et al 2001, Grol and Grimshaw 2003, Haines et al 2004
Multifaceted interventions such as a combination of audit, 'gap-analysis', reminders, consensus, e-libraries, policies	Behaviour change	G		Davis et al 1995, Bero et al 1998, Wensing et al 1998, Grimshaw et al 2001, 2004, Grol and Grimshaw 2003, Haines et al 2004, Menon et al 2009
	Attitude change	R	Although attitude does not change from intervention, it is a predictor of behaviour if the clinician is able to make autonomous decisions about whether or not he or she will use evidence	Menon et al 2009, Lizarondo et al 2011
Opinion leaders to influence clinical decision making via persuasive workshop presentations	Behaviour change	Y	Conflicting evidence	Thomson et al 1997b, Bero et al 1998, Grimshaw et al 2001, Grol and Grimshaw 2003, Haines et al 2004, Flodgren et al 2011

Strategy	Outcome of interest	Evidence alert traffic code	References
Outreach visits from a trained person to a health professional in their workplace	Behaviour change	G	Gains are small–moderate	Thomson et al 1997a, Grimshaw et al 2001, 2004, Grol and Grimshaw 2003, Haines et al 2004
Patient communication strategies for helping patients understand evidence and communicate preferences	Patient knowledge	Y	Decision aids exist but lack balance, accuracy, completeness, and adequate patient consultation	Feldman-Stewart et al 2006
	Patient outcomes	G		Trevena et al 2006
Patient-mediated interventions aimed at changing the behaviour of professionals	Behaviour change	Y	Lower-level supportive evidence. Gains are moderate	Bero et al 1998, Grol and Grimshaw 2003, Grimshaw et al 2004, Haines et al 2004
Peer comparison feedback aimed at providing feedback on evidence use	Behaviour change	G	Unlikely to work in isolation	Balas et al 1996, Grimshaw et al 2001
Reminders (either manual or computerized) about diagnostic testing or the most evidence-based option at the time of decision making	Behaviour change	G		Buntinx et al 1993, Austin et al 1994, Sullivan and Mitchell 1995, Yano et al 1995, Balas et al 1996, Shea et al 1996, Bero et al 1998, Hunt et al 1998, Grimshaw et al 2001, Grol and Grimshaw 2003, Haines et al 2004
	Patient outcomes	Y	Insufficient evidence	Sullivan and Mitchell 1995, Grimshaw et al 2001
Research-active or evidence-based practice-active staff in the workplace role modelling evidence-based practice decision making	Behaviour change	G		Lizarondo et al 2011
Small group meetings	Behaviour change	Y	Lower-level supportive evidence	Grol and Grimshaw 2003, Haines et al 2004
Task substitution between team members, whereby a professional's role is expanded to ensure uptake of a new intervention	Behaviour change	Y	Conflicting evidence	Grol and Grimshaw 2003, Haines et al 2004
Tailored interventions to overcome barriers to change unique to the workplace	Behaviour change	G	More effective than guidelines	Cheater et al 2005, Baker et al 2010

G, green (go), denotes use this approach; R, red (stop), denotes do not use this approach; Y, yellow (caution), denotes measure outcome carefully.

not only targets change within individuals but also has a focus on building a network of prac-titioners and researchers to facilitate collaborative problem solving (Barwick 2009, Rivard et al 2010, Russell et al 2010).

A recent randomized controlled trial, carried out in a community-based childhood dis-ability service, has shown that tailored, multifaceted interventions led to complex changes in professionals' research utilization and outcome measurement behaviours (Novak and McIntyre 2010, Campbell et al 2011). The study specifically addressed local barriers to research utilization at both a workplace and an individual level via organizational policy and procedure changes and with the leadership of knowledge brokers. In addition, professionals were provided with a customized e-evidence library, in which the evidence relating to their work was summarized and appraised for them and made available at their desk, colour-coded using the 'traffic light evidence alert' system (Novak and McIntyre 2010). While the field is beginning to accrue evidence for strategies to change practice there is still no evidence that these changes have an impact on client outcomes. This is an important area for future research.

Knowledge translation evaluation tools

With the growing interest in the effectiveness of KT strategies, various tools have been developed to evaluate these effects. Van Eerd and colleagues (2011) published an overview of instruments that have been used in KT research. They found a wide variety of instruments such as questionnaires, interviews, and counting of events from administrative data; however, few articles reported measurement properties, such as reliability and validity. They also noted that almost no studies used patient- or client-level instruments.

We have concluded that there is no single intervention that automatically leads to KT and changes in clinical practice, and have argued that interventions should be tailored to the unique workplace barriers, stage, and outcome of interest. It is also clear that no single instrument can be used to evaluate all KT interventions.

Based on the KTA framework (Fig. 19.1) and the stages of change model (Grol and Wensing 2004) objectives should be defined based on the particular stage, and strategies and evaluations planned accordingly. There are several useful frameworks to help with this planning process (see, for example, Reardon et al 2006, Provincial Centre of Excellence for Child and Youth Mental Health at Children's Hospital of Eastern Ontario 2006, Barwick 2011). In terms of evaluation, if one's aim were to improve familiarity or knowledge one would need to use a questionnaire to test that directly. On the other hand, if one's aim is to change professional behaviour, one would need to evaluate specific behaviours, for example by asking professionals, colleagues, or even children and families. If one aims to understand whether KT has led to changes in the organization one would want to evaluate protocols and procedures.

Two recent studies on the effects of knowledge brokering used mixed methods, collecting both quantitative and qualitative data to gain insight into the accomplishment of the specific aims, as well as into the process. A questionnaire that provided ratings of familiarity with and use of measurement tools was developed and tested for reliability prior to its use, and included questions on organizational supports. Qualitative information was collected by interview to gain insight into the process of knowledge brokering (Ketelaar et al 2010, Russell et al 2010,

Rivard et al 2010, Cameron et al 2011). A second example can be found in a study focusing on research knowledge, attitudes, and practices (Lyons et al 2011). The Knowledge, Attitudes, and Practices of Research Survey was used to assess participants' knowledge of, willingness to engage in, and ability to perform activities related to the conduct and utilization of research.

Thus, selecting the most appropriate tool to evaluate KT activities requires careful definition of the aims and likely outcomes. Precise specification makes implementation more likely, and there is greater certainty about whether it has been accomplished. Moreover, it is also important to recognize that the primary aim of KT should be not only to change professional knowledge or to change attitudes or clinical practice; ultimately KT should lead to improvements in patient and family outcomes.

Evidence for the clinical scenario

Translating evidence into clinical practice is not a simple process, as it requires complex clinical reasoning. Returning to John's mother's goal of increased participation in the playground, before deciding upon strength training as a possible solution one would need to know if muscle weakness was the main explanation for why John was having difficulty participating. Ideally one would want to observe John in the playground as well as conduct assessments to determine whether weakness was a factor limiting John's participation. If weakness were a factor, one would search the literature about the known benefits of strength training using an answerable clinical question in a searchable question format, such as: 'Is strength training effective to improve function and participation in children with cerebral palsy?' We would find that strength training has been shown not to increase spasticity and to be an effective and beneficial intervention for some children with cerebral palsy (Damiano and Abel 1998, Dodd et al 2003), but there is little evidence whether such changes are associated with increased participation.

Is John one of these children? What are the characteristics of the children that benefit? We also discover from the literature that strength training effectively increases muscle strength, which may carry over to improvements in activities (Franki et al 2011), but has not yet been shown to lead to improvements in participation (Scianni et al 2009, Verschuren et al 2011). Remembering that John's desired outcome is increased participation in the playground, how does one respond to Kim when she asks if strengthening John's muscles might help? We share what we found about strength training being a 'green' light intervention (i.e. treatment of choice) for improving muscle strength but a 'yellow' light intervention for improving participation (i.e. an uncertain effect). If strength training were something that John and Kim did want to try, we would need to measure any trial of strength training objectively to see if it helped John achieve his goals. We would also recommend looking at the evidence related to strategies for increasing participation and work on a strategy more directly targeted to the goal of increasing participation in the playground.

Future directions

We are just beginning to understand ways to increase the use of research evidence in practice and policy to support evidence-informed decision making. There is a need for reliable and valid outcome measures, including (in the child health field) a focus on child, young adult, and family outcomes. In addition, we need more research utilizing randomized controlled trials and mixed methods approaches to further the science of KT. Organizations need to value the time and resources it takes to support KT activities and provide opportunities for their service providers to be truly evidence informed. This will ultimately lead to empowering service providers and ensuring that we are giving the most up-to-date care to improve outcomes for people with neurodevelopmental conditions and their families.

Further information

Canadian Medical Association Infobase: Clinical Practice Guidelines: www.cma.ca/index. php/ci_id/54316/la_id/1.htm

- Clinical Evidence: http://clinicalevidence.bmj.com/ceweb/index.jsp
- Cochrane Collaboration Cochrane Reviews: www2.cochrane.org/reviews/
- National Clinical Guideline Clearinghouse: www.guideline.gov/
- National Institute for Health and Clinical Excellence (NICE): www.nice.org.uk/
- New Zealand Guidelines Group: www.nzgg.org.nz/
- OT Seeker – Occupational therapy evidence database: www.otseeker.com/
- Physiotherapy Evidence Database (PEDro): www.pedro.org.au/
- Psychological Database for Brain Impairment Treatment Efficacy (PsycBITE): www. psycbite.com/
- Scottish Intercollegiate Guidelines Network (SIGN): www.sign.ac.uk/
- Speech Pathology Database for Best Interventions and Treatment Efficacy (speechBITE): www.speechbite.com/
- TRIP database: www.tripdatabase.com/
- University of Washington, School of Medicine: www.dme.washington.edu/ebm-uwsom/ index.html

Many groups of researchers and clinicians collaborate to synthesize the evidence on specific diagnostic groups into practice guidelines and recommendations. Some examples include:

- Cerebral palsy – ISPO: http://ispoint.org/images/docs/publications/ispo_cp_report.pdf
- Developmental Coordination Disorder (DCD) EACD Recommendations: www.eacd. org/index.php

Research groups often publish their research findings in plain language summaries and factsheets:

- *CanChild*: www.canchild.ca
- NetChild: www.netchild.nl/
- American Academy for Cerebral Palsy and Developmental Medicine Database of Evidence Reports: www.aacpdm.org/membership/outcome/

REFERENCES

*Key references

Austin SM, Balas EA, Mitchell JA, Ewigman GB (1994) Effect of physician reminders on preventative care: meta-analysis of randomized clinical trials. *Proc Annu Sympt Comput Appl Med Care* 121–124.

*Baker R, Camosso-Stefinovic J, Gillies C, et al (2010) Tailored interventions to overcome identified barriers to change: effects on professional practice and health care outcomes. *Cochrane Database Syst Rev* 3: CD005470. http://dx.doi.org/10.1002/14651858. CD005470.pub2

Balas EA, Boren SA, Brown GD, Ewigman BG, Mitchell JA, Perkoff GT (1996) Effect of physician profiling on utilisation. *J Gen Interm Med* 11: 584–590. http://dx.doi.org/10.1007/BF02599025

Bamm EL, Rosenbaum P (2008) Family-centred theory: origins, development, barriers, and supports to implementation in rehabilitation medicine. *Arch Phys Med Rehabil* 89: 1618–1624. http://dx.doi.org/10.1016/j.apmr.2007.12.034

Barwick M (2011) Knowledge Translation Planning Template™ Hospital for Sick Children, Toronto. Fillable form available online at: www.melaniebarwick.com/training.php (accessed 21 April 2011).

Barwick MA, Peters J, Boydell K (2009) Getting to uptake: do communities of practice support the implementation of evidence-based practice? *J Can Acad Child Adolesc Psychiatry* 18: 16–29.

Bates DW, Kuperman GJ, Wang S, et al (2003) Ten commandments for effective clinical decision support: making the practice of evidence-based medicine a reality. *J Am Med Inform Assoc* 10: 523–530. http://dx.doi.org/10.1197/jamia.M1370

Bero LA, Grilli R, Grimshaw JM, Harvey E, Oxman AD, Thomson MA (1998) Closing the gap between research and practice: an overview of systematic reviews of interventions to promote the implementation of research findings. *BMJ* 317: 465. http://dx.doi.org/10.1136/bmj.317.7156.465

Brettle A (2003) Information skills training: a systematic review of the literature. *Health Info Libr J* 20(Suppl. 1): 3–9. http://dx.doi.org/10.1046/j.1365-2532.20.s1.3.x

Buntinx F, Winkens R, Grol R, Knottnerus JA (1993) Influencing diagnostic and preventative performance in ambulatory care by feedback and reminders: a review. *Fam Pract* 10: 219–228. http://dx.doi.org/10.1093/fampra/10.2.219

Cameron D, Russell DJ, Rivard L, Darrah J, Palisano R (2011) Knowledge brokering in children's rehabilitation organizations: perspectives from administrators. *J Contin Educ Health Prof* 31: 28–33. http://dx.doi.org/10.1002/chp.20098

Campbell L, Novak I, McIntyre S (2011) Effectiveness of providing evidence-based practice education with workplace supports for changing health professionals decision-making and outcomes of care: an evaluator blinded randomised controlled trial. *Aust Occup Ther J* 58(Suppl. 1): 120.

*Canadian Institutes of Health Research. Available at: www.cihr-irsc.gc.ca/e/29418.html (accessed 10 June 2011).

*Cheater F, Baker R, Gillies C, et al (2005) Tailored interventions to overcome identified barriers to change: effects on professional practice and health care outcomes. *Cochrane Database Syst Rev* 3: CD005470. http://dx.doi.org/10.1002/14651858.CD005470

Cochrane LJ, Olson CA, Murray S, Dupuis M, Tooman T, Hayes S (2007) Gaps between knowing and doing: understanding and assessing the barriers to optimal healthcare. *J Contin Educ Health Prof* 27: 94–102. http://dx.doi.org/10.1002/chp.106

Coomarasamy A, Khan KS (2004) What's the evidence that postgraduate teaching in evidence-based medicine changes anything? A systematic review. *BMJ* 329: 1017–1019. http://dx.doi.org/10.1136/bmj.329.7473.1017

Damiano DL, Abel MF (1998) Functional outcomes of strength training in spastic cerebral palsy. *Arch Phys Med Rehabil* 79: 119–125. http://dx.doi.org/10.1016/S0003-9993(98)90287-8

*Davis DA, Taylor-Vaisey A (1997) Translating guidelines into practice. A systematic review of theoretical concepts, practical experience and research evidence in the adoption of clinical practice guidelines. *Can Med Assoc J* 157: 408–416.

Davis DA, Thomson MA, Oxman AD, Haynes RB (1995) Changing physician performance: a systematic review of the effect of continuing medical education strategies. *JAMA* 274: 700–705. http://dx.doi.org/10.1001/jama.1995.03530090032018

Deenadayalan Y, Grimmer-Somers K, Prior M, Kumar S (2008) How to run an effective journal club: a systematic review. *J Eval Clin Pract* 14: 898–911. http://dx.doi.org/10.1111/j.1365-2753.2008.01050.x

Del Mar CB, Glasziou PP (2001) Ways of using evidence-based medicine in general practice. *Med J Aust* 174: 347–350.

Dizon JM, Grimmer-Somers K (2011) Complex interventions required to comprehensively educate allied health practitioners on evidence-based practice. *Adv Med Educ Pract* 2: 105–108. http://dx.doi.org/10.2147/AMEP.S19767

Dobbins M, Robeson P, Ciliska D, et al (2009) A description of a knowledge broker role implemented as part of a randomized controlled trial evaluating three knowledge translation strategies. *Implement Sci* 4: 23. http://dx.doi.org/10.1186/1748-5908-4-2

Dodd KJ, Taylor NF, Graham HK (2003) A randomized clinical trial of strength training in young people with cerebral palsy. *Dev Med Child Neurol* 45: 652–657. http://dx.doi.org/10.1111/j.1469-8749.2003.tb00866.x

Egger M, Davey Smith G, Altman D, editors (2001) *Systematic Reviews in Health Care: Meta-Analysis in Context*, 2nd edition. London: BMJ Publishing Group.

Feldman-Stewart D, Brennenstuhl S, McIssac K, et al (2006) A systematic review of information in decision aids. *Health Expect* 10: 46–61. http://dx.doi.org/10.1111/j.1369-7625.2006.00420.x

Flodgren G, Parmelli E, Doumit G, et al (2011) Local opinion leaders: effects on professional practice and health care outcomes. *Cochrane Database Syst Rev* 8: CD000125. http://dx.doi.org/10.1002/14651858.CD000125.pub4

Flores-Mateo G, Argimon JM (2007) Evidence based practice in postgraduate healthcare education: a systematic review. *BMC Health Serv Res* 7: 119. http://dx.doi.org/10.1186/1472-6963-7-119

*Forsetlund L, Bjorndal A, Rashidian A, et al (2009) Continuing education meetings and workshops: effects on professional practice and health care outcomes. *Cochrane Database Syst Rev* 2: CD003030.

Franki I, Desloovere K, De Cat J, et al (2011) Evidence-based physical therapy in cerebral palsy: a systematic review of literature in an ICF framework. Part A: basic physical therapy techniques. *Dev Med Child Neurol* 53(Suppl. 5): 44–45.

Fremantle N, Harvey EL, Wolf F, et al (1996) Printed educational materials to improve the behaviour of health care professionals and patient outcomes (Cochrane review). *Cochrane Database Syst Rev* 3.

Fung-Kee-Fung M, Watters J, Crossley C, et al (2009) Regional collaborations as a tool for quality improvements in surgery: a systematic review of the literature. *Ann Surg* 249: 565–572. http://dx.doi.org/10.1097/SLA.0b013e31819ec608

Gilbert R, Salanti G, Harden M, See S (2005) Infant sleeping position and the sudden infant death syndrome: systematic review of observational studies and historical review of recommendations from 1940 to 2002. *Int J Epidemiol* 34: 874–887. http://dx.doi.org/10.1093/ije/dyi088

Graham I, Logan J, Harrison M, et al (2006) Lost in translation: time for a map? *J Contin Educ Health Prof* 26: 13–24. http://dx.doi.org/10.1002/chp.47

Grilli R, Lomas J (1994) Evaluating the message: the relationship between compliance rate and the subject of practice guideline. *Med Care* 32: 202–213. http://dx.doi.org/10.1097/00005650-199403000-00002

*Grimshaw JM, Shirran L, Thomas R, et al (2001) Changing provider behavior: an overview of systematic reviews of interventions. *Med Care* 39(Suppl. 2): 112–145.

Grimshaw J, McAuley LM, Bero LA, et al (2003) Systematic reviews of the effectiveness of quality improvement strategies and programmes. *Qual Safe Health Care* 12: 298–303. http://dx.doi.org/10.1136/qhc.12.4.298

*Grimshaw JM, Thomas RE, MacLennan G, et al (2004) Effectiveness and efficiency of guideline dissemination and implementation strategies. *Health Technol Assess* 8(6).

Grol R, Grimshaw J (2003) From best evidence to best practice: effective implementation of change in patient care. *Lancet* 362: 1225–1230. http://dx.doi.org/10.1016/S0140-6736(03)14546-1

Grol R, Wensing M (2004) What drives change? Barriers to and incentives for achieving evidence-based practice. *Med J Aust* 180: S57–S60.

Grol RP, Bosch MC, Hulscher ME, Eccles MP, Wensing M (2007) Planning and studying improvement in patient care: the use of theoretical perspectives. *Milbank Q* 85: 93–138. http://dx.doi. org/10.1111/j.1468-0009.2007.00478.x

Haines A, Kuruvilla S, Borchert M (2004) Bridging the implementation gap between knowledge and action for health. *Bull World Health Org* 82: 724–732.

Haynes B, Haines A (1998) Barriers and bridges to evidence based clinical practice. *BMJ* 317: 273. http:// dx.doi.org/10.1136/bmj.317.7153.273

Hunt DL, Haynes RB, Hanna SE, Smith K (1998) Effects of computer-based clinical decision support systems on physician performance and patient outcomes: a systematic review. *JAMA* 280:1339–1346. http://dx.doi. org/10.1001/jama.280.15.1339

Jadad AR (1999) Promoting partnerships: challenges for the internet age. *BMJ* 319: 761–764. http://dx.doi. org/10.1136/bmj.319.7212.761

Jamtvedt G, Young JM, Kristoffersen DT, O'Brien MA, Oxman AD (2006) Audit and feedback: effects on professional practice and health care outcomes. *Cochrane Database Syst Rev* 2: CD000259. doi:10.1002/14651858.CD000259.pub2.

Ketelaar M, Russell D, Gorter JW (2008) The challenge of moving evidence-based measures into clinical practice: lessons in knowledge translation. *Phys Occup Ther Pediatr* 28: 191–206. http://dx.doi. org/10.1080/01942630802192610

Ketelaar M, Harmer-Bosgoed M, Willems M (2010) Knowledge Brokers PERRIN. Bridging the gap between research and practice: the role of a network of knowledge brokers in the implementation of measurement instruments in pediatric rehabilitation. Newsletter available at: www.perrin.nl/pdf/ NewsletterresultsProjectKBPERRIN2008-2010.pdf (accessed 13 May 2011).

Li LC, Grimshaw JM, Nielsen C, Judd M, Coyte PC, Graham ID (2009) Use of communities of practice in business and health care sectors: a systematic review. *Implement Sci* 4: 27. http://dx.doi.org/10.1186/1748–5908–4–27. Available at: www.implementationscience.com/content/4/1/27 (accessed)

Lizarondo L, Grimmer-Somers K, Kumar S (2011) A systematic review of the individual determinants of research evidence use in allied health. *J Multidiscip Healthcare* 4: 261–272. http://dx.doi.org/10.2147/ JMDH.S23144

Lomas J (1991) Words without action? The production, dissemination, and impact of consensus recommendations. *Annu Rev Public Health* 12: 41–65. http://dx.doi.org/10.1146/annurev.pu.12.050191.000353

Lomas J (2007) The in-between world of knowledge brokering. *BMJ* 334: 129–132. http://dx.doi.org/10.1136/ bmj.39038.593380.AE

Lyons C, Brown T, Tseng MH, Casey J, McDonald R (2011) Evidence-based practice and research utilization: perceived research knowledge, attitudes, practices and barriers among Australian pediatric occupational therapists. *Aust Occup Ther J* 58: 178–186. http://dx.doi.org/10.1111/j.1440-1630.2010.00900.x

McKibbon A, Lokker C, Wilczynski N, et al (2010) A cross-sectional study of the number and frequency of terms used to refer to knowledge translation in a body of health literature in 2006: a Tower of Babel? *Implement Sci* 5: 16. http://dx.doi.org/10.1186/1748-5908-5-16

*Menon A, Korner-Bitensky N, Kastner M, McKibbon KA, Straus S (2009) Strategies for rehabilitation professionals to move evidence-based knowledge into practice: a systematic review. *J Rehabil Med* 41: 1024–1032. http://dx.doi.org/10.2340/16501977-0451

*Michie S, Johnston M (2004) Changing clinical behaviour by making guidelines specific. *BMJ* 328: 343–345. http://dx.doi.org/10.1136/bmj.328.7435.343

Mitton C, Adair CE, McKenzie E, Patten SB, Waye Perry B (2007) Knowledge transfer and exchange: review and synthesis of the literature. *Milbank Q* 85: 729–768. http://dx.doi.org/10.1111/j.1468-0009.2007.00506.x

Moseley AM, Herbert RD, Sherrington C, Maher CG (2002) Evidence for physiotherapy practice: a survey of the Physiotherapy Evidence Database (PEDro). *J Physiother* 48: 43–49.

Mugford M, Banfield P, O'Hanlon M (1991) Effects of feedback of performance on clinical practice: a review. *BMJ* 303: 398–402. http://dx.doi.org/10.1136/bmj.303.6799.398

Novak I, McIntyre S (2010) The effect of education with workplace supports on practitioners' evidence-based practice knowledge and implementation behaviours. *Aust Occup Ther J* 57: 386–393. http://dx.doi.org/10.1111/j.1440-1630.2010.00861.x. Available at: http://onlinelibrary.wiley.com/doi/10.1111/j.1440–1630.2010.00861.x/pdf (accessed)

Oxman AD, Thomson MA, Davis DA, Haynes RB (1995) No magic bullets: a systematic review of 102 trials of interventions to improve professional practice. *Can Med Assoc J* 153: 1423–1431.

Palisano R, Rosenbaum P, Walter S, Russell D, Wood E, Galuppi B (1997) Development and reliability of a system to classify gross motor function in children with cerebral palsy. *Dev Med Child Neurol* 39: 214–223. http://dx.doi.org/10.1111/j.1469-8749.1997.tb07414.x

Palisano RJ, Campbell SK, Harris SR (2012) Evidence-based decision making in pediatric physical therapy. In: Campbell SK, Palisano RJ, Orlin M, editors. *Physical Therapy for Children*, 4th edition. St. Louis, MO: Elsevier Saunders, pp. 1–36.

Parkes J, Hyde C, Deeks J, Milne R (2001) Teaching critical appraisal skills in health care settings. *Cochrane Database Syst Rev* 3: CD001270.

Peach H (2003) Should Australia's hospitals be reviewing the use of research in patient care by nurses, managers and allied health professionals? A systematic review of recent evidence. *Aust Health Rev* 26: 49–62. http://dx.doi.org/10.1071/AH030049

Pennington L, Roddam H, Burton C, Russell I, Godfrey C, Russell D (2005) Promoting research use in speech and language therapy: a cluster randomised controlled trial to compare the clinical effectiveness and costs of two training strategies. *Clin Rehabil* 19: 387–397. http://dx.doi.org/10.1191/0269215505cr878oa

Provincial Centre of Excellence for Child and Youth Mental Health at Children's Hospital of Eastern Ontario (2006) *Doing More with What You Know: A Tool Kit on Knowledge Exchange*. Available at: www.onthepoint.ca/ke/documents/KEtoolkit.pdf (accessed 12 May 2012).

Ranmuthugala G, Plumb J, Cunningham F, Georgiou A, Westbrook J, Braithwaite J (2010) *Communities of Practice in the Health Sector: A Systematic Review of the Peer-reviewed Literature*. Sydney: University of New South Wales, Australian Institute of Health Innovation.

Reardon R, Lavis J, Gibson J (2006) *From Research to Practice: A Knowledge Transfer Planning Guide*. Toronto, ON: Institute for Work & Health. Available at: www.ktecop.ca/wp-content/uploads/2008/01/iwh_kte_workbook.pdf (accessed 28 April 2011).

Rivard LM, Russell DJ, Roxborough L, Ketelaar M, Bartlett DJ, Rosenbaum P (2010) Promoting the use of measurement tools in practice: a mixed-methods study of the activities and experiences of physical therapist knowledge brokers. *Phys Ther* 90: 1580–1590. http://dx.doi.org/10.2522/ptj.20090408

Rodger S, Brown T, Brown A (2005) Profile of paediatric occupational therapy practice in Australia. *Aust Occup Ther J* 52: 311–325. http://dx.doi.org/10.1111/j.1440-1630.2005.00487.x

Russell DJ, Rivard LM, Walter SW, et al (2010) Using knowledge brokers to facilitate the uptake of pediatric measurement tools into clinical practice: a before–after intervention study. *Implement Sci* 5: 92. http://dx.doi.org/10.1186/1748-5908-5-92

Saleh MN, Korner-Bitensky N, Snider L, et al (2008) Actual vs. best practices for young children with cerebral palsy: a survey of paediatric occupational therapists and physiotherapists in Quebec, Canada. *Dev Neurorehabil* 11: 60–80. http://dx.doi.org/10.1080/17518420701544230

Scianni A, Butler JM, Ada L, Teixeira-Salmela LF (2009) Muscle strengthening is not effective in children and adolescents with cerebral palsy: a systematic review. *J Physiother* 55: 81–87. http://dx.doi.org/10.1016/S0004-9514(09)70037-6

Shea S, DuMouchel W, Bahamonde L (1996) A meta-analysis of 16 randomized controlled trails to evaluate computer-based clinical reminder systems for preventative care in the ambulatory setting. *J Am Med Inform Assoc* 3: 399–409. http://dx.doi.org/10.1136/jamia.1996.97084513

Shortell SM, Bennett CL, Byck GR (1998) Assessing the impact of continuous quality improvement on clinical practice: what it will take to accelerate programs. *Milbank Q* 76: 1–37. http://dx.doi.org/10.1111/1468-0009.00107

Sitzia J (2002) Barriers to research utilisation: the clinical setting and nurses themselves. *Intensive Crit Care Nurs* 18: 230–243. http://dx.doi.org/10.1016/S0964339702000125

Soumerai SB, McLaughlin TJ, Avorn J (1989) Improving drug prescribing in primary care: a critical analysis of the experimental literature. *Milbank Q* 67: 268–317. http://dx.doi.org/10.2307/3350142

Sudsawad P (2007) Knowledge Translation: Introduction to Models, Strategies and Measures. Madison, WI: University of Wisconsin-Madison and the National Center for the Dissemination of Disability Research. Available at: www.ncddr.org/kt/products/ktintro/ (accessed 4 August 2011).

Sullivan F, Mitchell E (1995) Has general practitioner computing made a difference to patient care? A systematic review of published reports. *BMJ* 311: 848–852. http://dx.doi.org/10.1136/bmj.311.7009.848

Taylor R, Reeves B, Ewings P, Binns S, Keast J, Mears R (2000) A systematic review of the effectiveness of critical appraisal skills training for clinicians. *Med Educ* 34: 120–125. http://dx.doi.org/10.1046/j.1365-2923.2000.00574.x

Thomas LH, Cullen NA, McColl E, Russeau N, Soutter J, Steen J (2009) Guidelines in professions allied to medicine. *Cochrane Database Syst Rev* 1: CD000349. http://dx.doi.org/10.1002/14651858.CD00349

Thomson MA, Oxman AD, Davis DA, et al (1997a) Outreach visits to improve health professional practice and health care outcomes. *Cochrane Database Syst Rev* 3.

Thomson MA, Oxman AD, Davis DA, et al (1997b) Local opinion leaders to improve health professional practice and health care outcomes. *Cochrane Database Syst Rev* 3.

Thomson MA, Oxman AD, Davis DA, et al (1998a) Audit and feedback to improve health professional practice and health care outcomes. Part I. *Cochrane Database Syst Rev* 3.

Thomson MA, Oxman AD, Davis DA, et al (1998b) Audit and feedback to improve health professional practice and health care outcomes. Part II. *Cochrane Database Syst Rev* 3.

Trevena LJ, Davey HM, Barratt A, Butow P, Caldwell P (2006) A systematic review on communicating with patients about evidence. *J Eval Clin Pract* 12: 13–23. http://dx.doi.org/10.1111/j.1365-2753.2005.00596.x

Van Eerd D, Cole D, Keown K, et al (2011) Report on knowledge transfer and exchange practices: a systematic review of the quality and types of instruments used to assess KTE implementation and impact. Available at: www.iwh.on.ca/sys-reviews/kte-evaluation-tools (accessed 11 August 2011).

Verschuren O, Ada L, Maltais DB, Gorter JW, Scianni A, Ketelaar M (2011) Muscle strengthening in children and adolescents with spastic cerebral palsy: considerations for future resistance training protocols. *Phys Ther* 91: 1–10. http://dx.doi.org/10.2522/ptj.20100356

Ward V, House A, Hamer S (2009) Developing a framework for transferring knowledge into action: a thematic analysis of the literature. *J Health Serv Res Policy* 14: 156–164. http://dx.doi.org/10.1258/jhsrp.2009.008120

Wensing M, van der Weijden T, Grol R (1998) Implementing guidelines and innovations in general practice: which interventions are effective? *Br J Gen Pract* 48: 991–997.

Winning MA, Beverly CA (2003) Clinical librarianship: a systematic review of the literature. *Health Info Libr J* 20(Suppl. 1): 10–21. http://dx.doi.org/10.1046/j.1365-2532.20.s1.2.x

*Worrall G, Chaulk P, Freake D (1997) The effects of clinical practice guidelines on patient outcomes in primary care: a systematic review. *Can Med Assoc J* 156: 1705–1712.

Yano EM, Fink A, Hirsch SH, Robbins AS, Rubenstein LV (1995) Helping practices reach primary care goals. Lessons from the literature. *Arch Intern Med* 155: 1146–1156. http://dx.doi.org/10.1001/archinte.1995.00430110051006

*Zwarenstein M, Reeves S (2006) Knowledge translation and interprofessional collaboration: where the rubber of evidence-based care hits the road of teamwork. *J Contin Educ Health Prof* 26: 46–54. http://dx.doi.org/10.1002/chp.50

Zwarenstein M, Bryant W, Bailie R, Sibthorpe B (1997) Interventions to change collaboration between nurses and doctors. *Cochrane Database Syst Rev* 2.

20
INTERPROFESSIONAL EDUCATION AND COLLABORATION: KEY APPROACHES FOR IMPROVING CARE

Scott Reeves

Overview

Interprofessional education (IPE) aims to provide students and practitioners with opportunities to learn together to develop the attributes and skills required to achieve effective interprofessional collaboration (IPC). Interest in IPE and IPC has grown significantly in the past few decades. From a small number of interprofessional enthusiasts scattered across the world 30 years ago, these activities have grown exponentially, and have now become common across health and social care. This chapter offers an overview of key IPE and IPC developments. Specifically, the chapter focuses on the emergence of IPE and IPC, the different approaches employed, and the growing evidence base, as well as the organizational elements needed to deliver effective IPE and IPC. The chapter also discusses the potential contribution of these interprofessional activities for the delivery of care to children and young people with neurological and developmental conditions. In addition, it discusses the use of theories for informing the development of interprofessional initiatives. Finally, the chapter highlights some key directions for the development of the interprofessional field.

The emergence of interprofessionalism

For over three decades, health policy makers across the globe have identified the key role of IPE in improving healthcare systems and outcomes (World Health Organization 1976, 2010). During the past 10 years, in particular, IPE has been at the forefront of much curricular, research, policy, and regulatory activity on a national and international level. The promotion of IPE stems from the complexity and multifaceted nature of patients' health needs and the health system and research demonstrating that effective IPC among multiple healthcare providers is essential for the provision of effective and comprehensive care.

Critical issues with IPC among healthcare professionals have been well documented, particularly in the patient safety literature. For example, failures of collaboration were found to be at the centre of a number of health and social settings across the globe (Joint Commission

2004, Williams et al 2007, Kvarnstrom 2008). There is a clear need, therefore, for education to provide health and social professions with the requisite attitudes, knowledge, skills, and behaviours to work effectively together to deliver safe, high-quality patient care. It has been argued that the traditional uniprofessional approach to health professions' education is insufficient to support effective IPC, and thus the introduction of IPE is needed (World Health Organization 2010).

Policy documents have delineated the role of IPE in contributing to improved IPC and an improved healthcare system. For example, policy makers in the UK re-emphasized their commitment to IPE in a document that stated that the future of education for healthcare and social care professions needed to support teams working to better coordinate services and deliver enhanced patient care (Department of Health 2000). In Canada, a number of health policy documents have been produced outlining the role of IPE within the Pan-Canadian Health Human Resources Strategy (Health Canada 2006).

Recently, the World Health Organization (WHO) re-endorsed its commitment to IPE with the publication of its *Framework for Action on Interprofessional Education and Collaborative Practice* (World Health Organization 2010). This document highlighted the importance of IPE for the development of skills for effective IPC, patient care, and collaborative practice to improve fragmented and struggling health systems throughout the world. While research is growing in this area, at present the evidence base for the impacts of IPE on IPC and teamwork is limited – as discussed below.

The policy documents on IPE are affecting changes at the educational, professional, and organizational levels, resulting in the incorporation of IPE into education programmes, professional requirements, and organizational policies. IPE programmes have been created in higher education institutions in countries such as the USA, Canada, the UK, continental Europe, and Australia (Barr et al 2005, Reeves et al 2010a). For example, in a study comparing medical students learning about patient safety uniprofessionally versus interprofessionally, it was found that, while all students increased their knowledge, those who participated in the IPE gained added value from these interactions and were better able to position their learning within safe IPC (Anderson et al 2009).

Healthcare organizations are also supporting IPE initiatives. For example, Barr et al (2005) report on programmes occurring in the USA and UK whereby primary care practices and medical centres have made a commitment to support healthcare improvements through interprofessional initiatives that involve elements of IPE and IPC (Barr et al 2005, Freeth et al 2009).

Children and young people with neurological and developmental conditions

Chronic neurological and developmental conditions are complex and present multifaceted challenges for parents and professionals. The need to provide high-quality and safe care for children and young people with chronic neurological and developmental conditions means that effective IPE and IPC are crucial (e.g. Pearson 1983). An important development in helping achieve these goals was the publication by the WHO of a unified, shared language framework to describe health and health-related terminology entitled the International Classification of Functioning, Disability and Health (World Health Organization 2001) (see also Chapter 4).

Importantly this framework adopted a unified terminology that Allan et al (2006) argued can serve as an 'interprofessional' language with which to communicate healthcare information across professional boundaries. For these authors, the use of this framework and its common language are fundamental steps in achieving good-quality IPC. As such, Allan et al (2006) stress that education about the framework and its relevance to IPE is an important step for healthcare professionals. Recently, Rosenbaum and Gorter (2011) provided an illuminating discussion in relation to how this framework can be employed by health professions in the care of children and young people with neurological and developmental conditions.

Encouragingly, there has been an increase in accounts that describe how professionals in this field are developing and implementing a range of interprofessional activities and initiatives. For example, Lagacé and colleagues (2008) describe their use of an interprofessional approach that takes into account a child's auditory, language, learning, and associated characteristics to ensure appropriate interpretation and management. These authors outline how their interprofessional model of intervention has been used to deliver services to school-aged children presenting with auditory processing disorders and associated learning difficulties. The interprofessional team reported in this paper was composed of an audiologist, a speech–language pathologist, and an occupational therapist. It was also reported that this team worked well together and helped to address the children's needs in this setting.

However, given the complexities linked to developing interprofessional activities, as outlined above, it can be difficult to develop, implement, and sustain such initiatives. Indeed, the professions involved in the care of children and young people with neurological and developmental conditions arguably encounter a number of problems that are specific to this field. For example, temporal and geographical separation of professions based in different clinics, departments, and units can result in struggles to coordinate time together to discuss and agree care plans. Differing professional perspectives, generated by traditional socialization processes (e.g. Reeves et al 2010b), can also mean that practitioners working with children and young people with neurological and developmental conditions may not share a common understanding or language. For example, in a study that aimed to explore common understandings of development terminology, Peters et al (2001) found that among the professionals who took part there was some agreement around terms. However, beyond that point there was a distinctive divergence of understanding and interprofessional differences in emphasis emerged.

A study by Thylefors et al (2000) goes on to provide an additional insight into the complexities of working in a collaborative manner when caring for children and young people with neurological and developmental conditions. These authors studied the nature of IPC in a Swedish neuropaediatric habilitation context by analysing a nationwide sample of 202 professionals. The study focused on professional cooperation and interaction during different types of formal team meetings. The basic obstacles for the meetings were lack of time, poor interactions, and too large a group. The professionals appeared to interact on a fairly equal basis, and were able to challenge others' views. While physiotherapists and paediatricians were often perceived as being the most dominant professions, the significance of the contribution from the different team members varied according to the age of the child and to changing needs. The authors concluded that the prerequisites for IPC exist in this setting, as far as meeting structures and a 'democratic' pattern of communication between professions. However, challenges remained, particularly connected to scheduling professionals' time to meet.

An important interprofessional initiative for providing effective care to children and young people with neurological/developmental conditions has been the Leadership Education in Neurodevelopmental and Related Disabilities (LEND) programme. Sponsored in the USA by the Maternal and Child Health Bureau for the past 50 years, the LEND programme aims to improve the health of infants, children, and adolescents with impairments. This is achieved by preparing trainees from diverse professions (e.g. audiology, dentistry, family medicine, health administration, law, nursing, nutrition, occupational therapy, physical therapy, psychology, public health, social work, and speech therapy) to assume leadership roles in their respective fields and by ensuring high levels of interprofessional clinical competence (Association of University Centers on Disabilities 2012).

LEND programmes operate within a single university system and collaborate with local hospitals and/or healthcare centres. This allows them access to expert faculty, facilities, and other resources necessary to support effective IPE and IPC activities. At present, there are 43 LEND programmes in 37 states across the USA (Association of University Centers on Disabilities 2012). Collectively, they form a national network that shares information and resources. They work together to address national issues of importance to children and young people with neurological and developmental conditions and their families, exchange best practices, and develop shared products. LEND programmes also come together regionally to address specific issues and concerns. While this programme provides a range of IPE and IPC activities, little formal evaluative research has been published to provide a rigorous empirical base for the effects of this programme.

The interprofessional evidence base

In the past decade, a number of systematic reviews have been conducted to examine and summarize the evidence for IPE and IPC. The reviews used different criteria for the studies to be included, and, thus, while there was overlap, each examined a different group of studies. Recently, these reviews were synthesized in order to provide an overall understanding of the evidence base (Reeves et al 2010c). Here the main findings from this work are outlined to offer an indication of the current level of evidence for IPE and its effects on IPC.

In total, the synthesis located six systematic reviews of IPE that collectively reported on the effects of over 200 studies spanning 1974 to 2005. Although the synthesis found that these six reviews reported on studies that differed in methodological quality, and reported a range of different outcomes, all shared similar interprofessional definitions. The synthesis revealed that IPE was delivered in a variety of acute, primary, and community care settings and addressed a range of health conditions (e.g. asthma, arthritis) or acute conditions (e.g. cardiac care). While different combinations of professional groups participated in the programmes, medicine and nursing were consistent participants across learning groups.

The synthesis found that most studies report that interprofessional programmes can result in positive reactions, where participants 'enjoyed' their interprofessional experiences. It was also found that such programmes reported positive changes in perceptions/attitudes in relation to changes in views of other professional groups, changes in views of IPC, and/or changes in views of the value attached to working on a collaborative basis. In addition, the synthesis indicated that these types of programmes reported positive changes in learner knowledge and skills of interprofessional collaboration, usually related to an enhanced understanding of roles and responsibilities of other professional groups, improved knowledge of the nature of interprofessional collaboration, and/or the development of collaboration/communication skills.

It was found that few programmes reported outcomes related to changes in individual behaviour (e.g. working in a more collaborative manner with colleagues from other professional groups). Of those programmes that did provide this type of evidence, positive change in individual practitioners' interactions was usually cited. A small number of studies did report positive changes to organizational practices resulting from the delivery of IPE, as defined by changes to interprofessional referral practices/working patterns or improved documentation (i.e. guidelines, protocols, use of shared records) related to the organization of care. A smaller number of studies reported changes to the delivery of care to patients. These studies typically reported positive changes to clinical outcomes (e.g. infection rates, clinical error rates), patient satisfaction scores, and/or length of patient stay.

The synthesis revealed that the majority of studies provided little discussion of methodological limitations associated with their research. As a result, it was difficult to understand the nature of biases and the overall quality of a research study. Most IPE programmes also paid little or no attention to sampling techniques in their work or issues relating to study attrition. Across the studies, there was a propensity to report the short-term outcomes linked to IPE. As a result there was little idea of the longer-term impact of this type of education. It was also found that there was a widespread use of non-validated instruments to try to detect impact of IPE on learner and/or patient satisfaction. While the use of such tools can provide helpful data for local quality assurance issues, it limits the quality of the research as it is difficult to assess the tools' validity or reliability.

Importantly, the synthesis indicated that the evidence for the effects of IPE rests upon a variety of programme elements (e.g. duration, balance of professional participation) and methods (e.g. quantitative, qualitative studies) of variable quality, as well as a range of outcomes (e.g. reports of learner satisfaction to changes in the delivery of care) (Reeves et al 2010c).

Interprofessionalism and theory

Social science theory can inform the development and evaluation of IPE and IPC initiatives, yet to date most interprofessional programmes draw upon little theory. Barr et al (2005) identified three foci in which a number of social science theories could be situated for interprofessional activities: preparing individuals for collaborative practice; cultivating collaboration in groups and teams; and improving services and the quality of care.

Preparing Individuals for Collaborative Practice

Social exchange theory (Challis et al 1988) explains social change and stability as a process of negotiated exchanges between parties. According to this theory, all human relationships are formed according to a subjective cost–benefit analysis and the comparison of alternatives. This theory can be used to provide insight into the nature of relationships among different professionals during an interprofessional programme and help in developing individuals' understandings of their relationships with others in a work setting (Barr et al 2005).

Negotiation theory was developed by Strauss (1978) to help explain how formal roles are often transgressed by informal trade-offs between individuals' own goals and those of others. This theory can be used to explain how negotiations shape the nature of interprofessional relations between health providers and also how negotiations affect the development and delivery of an interprofessional initiative. This theory becomes more complex within the context of interprofessional education when negotiations are interprofessional and/or interorganizational as well as interpersonal.

CULTIVATING GROUP/TEAM COLLABORATION

Workgroup mentality theory (Bion 1961) is based in a psychodynamic perspective that aims to explain the unconscious processes involved in a group unable to deal with its 'primary task'. According to this theory, groups will often avoid making decisions to prevent members from addressing potentially difficult group issues. Stokes (1994) and others have extended this theory to interprofessional relations. Stokes suggested that interprofessional team meetings can frequently be non-productive, as a false sense of collaboration prevents members from dealing with potentially difficult issues. Interprofessional initiatives with a group dynamic format can enable participants to reflect on unconscious forces that shape interprofessional relations within the group, with the aim of increasing their understanding of such forces in their workplace.

The concept of the learning team was developed from that of the learning organization (Senge 1990). Team learning is an approach developed to support the development of high-performance teams. Typically, in a team, members do not necessarily trust one another or share collective goals, but, if a learning team develops, the members begin to develop a shared commitment, have mutually agreed goals, and share a concern for the well-being of the team. In relation to interprofessional education, team learning can help transform a loosely affiliated work 'group' of healthcare professionals into a more effective interprofessional 'team' in which members trust one another and share a commitment to collective goals and the welfare of their colleagues (Barr et al 2005).

IMPROVING SERVICES AND THE QUALITY OF CARE

For Von Bertalanffy (1971), the concept of 'system' was developed as a response to the limitations of specialist disciplines in addressing complex problems. It could be applied across all disciplines from physics and biology to the social and behavioural sciences, seeing wholes as more than the sum of their parts, interactions between parties as purposeful, boundaries between them as permeable, and cause and effect as interdependent rather than linear. The underlying philosophy of systems theory is the unity of nature, governed by the same fundamental laws in all its realms. Intervention by one profession at one point in the system affects the whole in ways that can only be anticipated from multiple professional perspectives.

Systems theory has multiple applications in interprofessional education. It offers a unifying and dynamic framework within which all the participant professions can relate to person, family, community, and environment, one or more of which may be points of intervention interacting with the whole. It can also be used to understand relationships within and among professions, service agencies, education, and practice, as well as stakeholders, planning and managing programmes.

According to Foucault (1972) discourse helps to define a particular culture, its language, and the behaviour of individuals who belong to that culture. Lessa (2006) helpfully summarizes Foucault's approach, as he states that discourses are knowledge systems made up of ideas, attitudes, actions, beliefs, and practices that influence how individuals think, see, and speak.

Activity theory provides a means of understanding and intervening in relations at micro- and macro-levels in order to effect change in interpersonal, interprofessional, and interagency relations (Engestrom et al 1999). An analysis of activity involves an understanding of individual relationships and how they relate to the macro-level of collective and community. An important component of this approach is the notion of *knotworking* – a concept that helps describe the nature of collaborative work in which individuals connect – through tying, untying, and retying separate threads of activity during their interactions.

Implementing interprofessional initiatives

Organizational support is crucial to developing successful interprofessional programmes. It is critical to have senior leadership with interest, knowledge, and experience to champion and forward the interprofessional initiative as a priority activity. The organization and specific academic/clinical faculty supportive of IPE and IPC are needed to instil within students and practising professionals a positive attitude to interprofessional approaches (Wilhelmsson et al 2009). Institutional policies and leadership commitment at all levels are also crucial given the resources required to develop and implement IPE and IPC.

The particular type of organizational support required is often dependent on the stage of education. Planning and implementing pre-qualification IPE is challenging given the high number of organizational barriers, such as large numbers of students, professional accreditation requirements, and inflexible curricula that exist. Obtaining approval from each participating profession's regulatory bodies, as well as agreeing on issues of accountability, often adds additional complications. While postqualification IPE can be less problematic to plan because of the smaller number of organizational/logistical barriers, senior faculty support is still required to ensure that providers have sufficient time and resources to attend the IPE programme. Furthermore, this type of support is critical if any knowledge gains from IPE are going to be translated successfully into collaborative changes in practice.

In addition, the issue of finance needs careful consideration during the planning of any interprofessional initiative. As the cost of this form of education tends to span a number of different professional or departmental budgets (Reeves 2008), agreement over financial arrangements can often be a considerable hurdle for IPE. As a result, senior faculty often need to be convinced of the feasibility and acceptability of any proposed interprofessional programme before supporting its implementation.

Developing any interprofessional activity is a complex process and may involve healthcare workers and educators from different departments, work settings, and locations. Indeed, involving faculty from the different programmes interested in the initiative is crucial, and all programmes involved should have a sense of ownership. This can be challenging with smaller faculty/staff. Equal representation ensures that no one group can dominate the planning process and skew the initiative in any one direction. Engaging faculty/staff in the development of an evaluation plan for the initiative is also crucial to increase the probability that the evaluation findings will be useful to programme development.

Developing an interprofessional programme can take considerable time and energy; as a result group members need to have dedication and enthusiasm. However, when programmes are dependent on the input of a few key enthusiasts, their long-term sustainability can be threatened when these individuals move to other organizations (Reeves 2008).

The election of an IPE project leader is important to coordinate the group activities and ensure that progress is achieved. Organizers need to arrange regular meetings and consider all perspectives, which also requires interprofessional skills (Wihelmsson et al 2009). Group members need to share their aims and assumptions about the initiative to ensure that all members are working towards a common goal. Where differences are identified, these need to be discussed and resolved. Regular planning meetings allow group members to update one another and jointly resolve any difficulties they encounter in the planning process.

Sustaining any IPE and IPC activity can be equally complex and requires good communication among participants, enthusiasm for the work being done, and a shared vision and understanding of the benefits of introducing new activities. Organizations need constantly to evaluate and modify their interprofessional initiatives (where needed) to remind all members about the general goals of the activity (Wihelmsson et al 2009).

Faculty/staff development is needed for those involved in developing, delivering, and evaluating an interprofessional initiative. For most faculty/staff, engaging in new (and often untested) interprofessional activities can be a challenging experience. For example, the increasing emphasis on IPC and practice may challenge traditional professional identities. Faculty/staff development may reduce feelings of isolation and help to create more collaborative approaches to sharing knowledge, experiences, and ideas (Rees and Johnson 2007).

There is a growing number of interprofessional faculty/staff development programmes. In general, these programmes focus on offering a similar range of preparatory activities, such as understanding the roles and responsibilities of different professionals, exploring issues of professionalism, and planning learning strategies for interprofessional groups. There is also a need for such programmes to enable individuals to promote change at the individual and organizational level, and thus they should also target diverse stakeholders and address leadership and organizational change (Steinert 2005, Silver and Leslie 2009).

Where formal support cannot be obtained, it is advisable to seek informal input from a colleague more experienced in IPE and IPC. For any interprofessional programme to be successfully implemented, the early experiences of faculty/staff must be positive. This will ensure continued involvement and a willingness to further develop these activities.

Implications

Accumulating evidence of the critical need for interprofessional approaches among different healthcare providers, and the resulting impact on the quality and safety of health care, have together stimulated decision makers to invest in such approaches. As a result, over the past

30 years, there has been a continued expansion in the IPE and IPC initiatives being developed and implemented across the world.

Research has provided an increasingly robust insight into the effects of different interprofessional programmes, as discussed above. We now have knowledge of the value of IPE and its effects on IPC. However, as noted above, at the macro-level attention must be given to programmes that work at the interface of IPE and IPC and to organizational sponsorship and leadership. Also, faculty and professional development will need to occur in parallel with curriculum and practice developments. Ongoing organizational engagement, support, and commitment remain critical to address the extensive logistical and resource issues for IPE and IPC to support faculty/staff development and to develop a culture that endorses interprofessionalism. Leadership from professional associations, universities, and clinical organizations will also be essential to encourage and support students and practitioners fully engaging in interprofessional activities and programmes. A key area for these developments is in the care of children and young people with neurological or developmental conditions that, as noted above, require effective IPE and IPC approaches to ensure that care can be optimal.

This investment in interprofessional activities must, however, be based on rigorous evidence that is underpinned by theoretical perspectives. It is encouraging that the evidence base for interprofessionalism is growing. Indeed, reviews have shown that IPE can have positive outcomes in relation to IPC attitudes, knowledge/skills, and behaviours, as well as practice. With the expanding number of studies, it is to be hoped that the evidence in this field will, over time, become increasingly more rigorous and demonstrate impact and sustainability.

REFERENCES

Key references

*Allan C, Campbell W, Guptill C, Stephenson F, Campbell K (2006) A conceptual model for interprofessional education: the International Classification of Functioning, Disability and Health (ICF). *J Interprof Care* 20: 235–245. http://dx.doi.org/10.1080/13561820600718139

Anderson E, Thorpe L, Heney D, Petersen S (2009) Medical students benefit from learning about patient safety in an interprofessional team. *Med Educ* 43: 542–552. http://dx.doi.org/10.1111/j.1365-2923.2009.03328.x

Association of University Centers on Disabilities (2012) About LEND. Available at: www.aucd.org/template/page.cfm?id=473 (accessed 1 December 2012).

*Barr H, Koppel I, Reeves S, Hammick M, Freeth D (2005) *Effective Interprofessional Education: Argument, Assumption and Evidence*. Oxford: Blackwell. http://dx.doi.org/10.1002/9780470776445

Bion WR (1961) *Experiences in Groups and Other Papers*. London: Tavistock Publications. http://dx.doi.org/10.4324/9780203359075

Challis L, Fuller S, Henwood M, et al (1988) *Joint Approaches to Social Policy*. Cambridge: Cambridge University Press.

Department of Health (2000) *A Health Service of all the Talents: Developing the NHS Workforce*. London: HMSO.

Engestrom Y, Engestrom R, Vahaaho T (1999) When the center does not hold: the importance of knotworking. In: Chaklin S, Hedegaard M, Jensen UJ, editors. *Activity Theory and Social Practice*. Aarhus: Aarhus University Press, pp. 345–374.

Foucault M (1972) *The Archeology of Knowledge*. London: Tavistock.

Freeth D, Ayida G, Berridge EJ, et al (2009) Multidisciplinary obstetric simulated emergency scenarios (MOSES): promoting patient safety in obstetrics with teamwork-focused interprofessional simulations. *J Contin Educ Health Prof* 29: 98–104. http://dx.doi.org/10.1002/chp.20018

Health Canada (2006) Pan-Canadian Health Human Resource Strategy. Available at: www.hc-sc.gc.ca/hcs-sss/pubs/system-regime/2006-wait-attente/hhr-rhs/index-eng.php (accessed 1 December 2012).

Joint Commission (2004) Sentinel Event Alert: Preventing infant death and injury during delivery. Available at: www.aap.org/nrp/simulation/JCAHOSentinelEvent.pdf (accessed 1 December 2012).

*Kvarnstrom S (2008) Difficulties in collaboration: a critical incident study of interprofessional healthcare teamwork. *J Interprof Care* 22: 191–203. http://dx.doi.org/10.1080/13561820701760600

Lagacé J, Bélanger-Schaadt M, Savard J, Dubouloz CJ (2008) Interprofessional approach to auditory processing disorders. *Perspect School Based Issues* 9: 140–150.

Lessa I (2006) Discursive struggles within social welfare: restaging teen motherhood. *Br J Soc Work* 36: 283–298. http://dx.doi.org/10.1093/bjsw/bch256

Pearson P (1983) The interdisciplinary team process, or the professionals' 'Tower of Babel'. *Dev Med Child Neurol* 25: 390–395. http://dx.doi.org/10.1111/j.1469-8749.1983.tb13779.x

*Peters J, Barnett A, Henderson S (2001) Clumsiness, dyspraxia and developmental coordination disorder: how do health and educational professionals in the UK define the terms? *Child Care Health Dev* 27: 399–412. http://dx.doi.org/10.1046/j.1365-2214.2001.00217.x

Rees D, Johnson R (2007) All together now? Staff views and experiences of a pre-qualifying interprofessional curriculum. *J Interprof Care* 21: 543–555. http://dx.doi.org/10.1080/13561820701507878

Reeves S (2008) *Developing and Delivering Practice-Based Interprofessional Education*. Munich: VDM Publications.

*Reeves S, Lewin S, Espin S, Zwarenstein M (2010a) *Interprofessional Teamwork for Health and Social Care*. Oxford: Wiley-Blackwell.

Reeves S, MacMillan K, van Soeren M (2010b) Leadership within interprofessional health and social care teams: a socio-historical overview of some key trials and tribulations. *J Nurs Manage* 18: 258–264. http://dx.doi.org/10.1111/j.1365-2834.2010.01077.x

*Reeves S, Goldman J, Sawatzky-Girling B, Burton A (2010c) A synthesis of systematic reviews of interprofessional education. *J Allied Health* 39: S198–S203.

*Rosenbaum P, Gorter J (2012) The 'F-words' in childhood disability: I swear this is how we should think. *Child Care Health Dev* 38: 457– 463. http://dx.doi.org/10.1111/j.1365-2214.2011.01338.x

Senge PM (1990) *The Fifth Discipline the Art and Practice of the Learning Organization*. New York, NY: Doubleday/Currency.

Silver I, Leslie K (2009) Faculty development for continuing interprofessional education and collaborative practice. *J Contin Educ Health Prof* 29: 172–177. http://dx.doi.org/10.1002/chp.20032

*Steinert Y (2005) Learning together to teach together: interprofessional education and faculty development. *J Interprof Care* 19: S60–S75. http://dx.doi.org/10.1080/13561820500081778

Stokes J (1994) Problems in multidisciplinary teams: the unconscious at work. *J Soc Work Practice* 8: 161–167. http://dx.doi.org/10.1080/02650539408413977

Strauss A (1978) *Negotiations: Varieties, Contexts, Processes and Social Order*. San Francisco, CA: Jossey-Bass.

*Thylefors I, Price E, Persson O, von Wendt L (2000) Teamwork in Swedish neuropaediatric habilitation. *Child Care Health Dev* 26: 515–532. http://dx.doi.org/10.1046/j.1365-2214.2000.00162.x

Von Bertalanffy L (1971) *General Systems Theory*. London: Allen Lane.

Wilhelmsson M, Pelling S, Ludvigsson J, Hammar M, Dahlgren LO, Faresjö T (2009) Twenty years experience of interprofessional education in Linköping – ground-breaking and sustainable. *J Interprofessional Care* 23: 121–133. http://dx.doi.org/10.1080/13561820902728984

Williams R, Silverman R, Schwind C, et al (2007) Surgeon information transfer and communication: factors affecting quality and efficiency of inpatient care. *Ann Surg* 245: 159–169. http://dx.doi.org/10.1097/01.sla.0000242709.28760.56

World Health Organization (1976) *Continuing Education of Health Personnel*. Copenhagen: WHO Regional Office for Europe.

*World Health Organization (2001) *International Classification of Functioning, Disability and Health*. Geneva: WHO Press.

*World Health Organization (2010) Framework for Action on Interprofessional Education and Collaborative Practice. Available at: http://whqlibdoc.who.int/hq/2010/WHO_HRH_HPN_10.3_eng.pdf (accessed 1 December 2012).

21

THE EFFECTIVENESS OF A SPECIALIZED LEARNING ENVIRONMENT TO ENHANCE OUTCOMES OF CHILDREN WITH COGNITIVE IMPAIRMENT

Elizabeth N. Kerr and Miriam Riches

Overview

Within the International Classification of Functioning, Disability and Health (ICF) conceptual framework, education is distinctively represented in two domains: 'Activities and Participation' and 'Environment'. For students with neurological and developmental conditions, education is a major health determinant. Unfortunately, meeting these students' needs presents a challenge to educators. Understanding and addressing neurobiological, cognitive, behavioural, and psychosocial issues, as well as environmental factors, is critical to assist struggling students to learn and acquire basic and complex skills and to strengthen their psychosocial well-being. This chapter highlights the burdens faced by students with neurodevelopmental conditions and their families and emphasizes the types of remedial programming and support required. The plan of care should be based on the needs of the whole child and must encompass both social–emotional and cognitive functions if the child is to develop the tools, self-confidence, and resilience to reach his or her academic potential. A specialized learning environment is effective in producing positive, possibly life-altering, changes in health and quality of life.

Introduction

The ICF framework (World Health Organization 2001) and its Children and Youth version (ICF-CY; World Health Organization 2007) describe health and disability according to an individual's functional capacity within a certain environment. When considering children with neurological and developmental conditions, cognitive functions (i.e. body function) and school education and learning (i.e. activities and participation), as well as the educational and training services/systems and support provided (i.e. environment), represent the primary interactive biopsychosocial components associated with their health outcomes. Specifically, a neurodevelopmental condition places an individual at risk for numerous weaknesses in cognitive functions. These may include intellectual and higher-level cognitive deficits such as executive skills (e.g. abstraction, organization, planning, flexibility, problem solving, etc.)

that are necessary for attaining higher education, functioning independently, and performing well in daily life as an adult. Other possible challenges include various attention problems (e.g. sustaining, shifting, and dividing attention, impulse control); memory limitations; language impairments; and psychomotor restrictions; as well as numerous psychosocial issues (e.g. optimism, confidence, experience of self, and emotional functions). Learning and applying knowledge obtained through education is a major life activity. Whether an individual is successful or displays limitations in activities and restrictions in participation depends largely on his or her health condition and specific environmental factors, including the attitudes of others, the support received, and the approach to education.

'Education for all' assumes that all students, regardless of their learning, behavioural, or social–emotional needs, have the right to receive the most appropriate education to reach their potential. In reality, addressing the health needs of students with neurological and developmental conditions is fraught with difficulties. Within developed countries, one issue pertaining to this human right is the type of programming available to students whose needs are not being met through an ordinary classroom setting. Programmes fall on a continuum, with full integration at one end and complete segregation at the other. Along this continuum students may receive resource support with inclusion, or may spend part of a day or a full day in a self-contained classroom. Our objective is not to challenge prior research pertaining to the benefits of inclusion but rather to acknowledge that segregated special education settings – whether government- or independently funded – exist for students with various neurodevelopmental conditions (e.g. epilepsy, autism, cerebral palsy, language-based learning difficulties, communication disorders, early traumatic brain injury, fetal alcohol syndrome, intellectual impairments, children whose overall abilities fall between the 2nd and 9th centiles, and those with hearing and visual impairments). These environments provide opportunities for educators and healthcare practitioners to support and address students' unmet health needs that are directly associated with their current and future quality of life.

The educational challenge

Neurobiology, cognitive abilities, and behavioural and psychosocial issues, as well as environment, all influence academic success (Fletcher et al 2007). Meeting the education needs of students with neurodevelopmental conditions within the confines of an ordinary classroom is not always possible. Most educators have a poor understanding of neurodevelopmental conditions and their co-existing cognitive and social–emotional challenges. Moreover, they have not received the training necessary to assist these students to reach their potential (Garrison-Wade et al 2007). Figure 21.1 illustrates a perceived model of teachers' hierarchy of concerns for students with neurodevelopmental conditions. The highest priority is on physical safety, a need that is not dealt with in the ICF (Fayed and Kerr 2009a) and that conceivably can be addressed through a safety plan. Behavioural management follows closely. Classroom interventions for students with neurodevelopmental conditions (e.g. attention-deficit–hyperactivity disorder [ADHD]) often focus on reducing problematic behaviour (Iseman and Naglieri 2011); however, for students with cognitive impairment, some of the presenting behaviour is due to deficits in skills related to both body function impairments and participation issues rather than defiance. Social–emotional functioning and academic needs (e.g. learning to read, write,

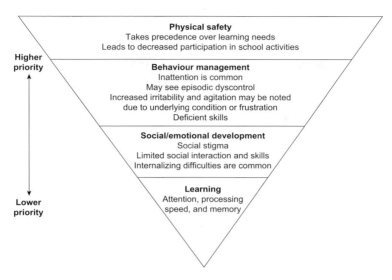

Fig. 21.1 Conceptualization of the hierarchy of educators' concerns for students with neurodevelopemental conditions.

and calculate, acquiring basic and complex skills, applying knowledge) are viewed as less of a priority but should, in fact, be a primary focus.

The cognitive, behavioural, social–emotional, and educational needs of the student, as well as the needs of the family, do not exist within a silo but constantly interact and affect one another. As illustrated by one parent's comments, the resulting scenario can be frustrating:

At the time of diagnosis, [our daughter] was already experiencing challenges in her learning. She had been placed in a small special education classroom the preceding year. She was then placed in a regular classroom with full-time educational assistant (EA) support, which she shared with other students for two years. Despite the engagement of the special education resource teacher, classroom teachers and EA, she continued to struggle. The efforts made to integrate the recommendations from the neuropsychological assessment and her speech and language professional did not materially enhance her learning experiences. In fact, she regressed academically and also started to have emotional and social difficulties; her self confidence deteriorated and our concerns grew.

Characteristically, accepting environments and joyful engagement (Schonert-Reichl and Hymel 2007, Hawn Foundation 2011) as well as targeted, explicit interventions are essential for students with even mild cognitive weaknesses (Minskoff and Allsopp 2003). The ICF-CY framework (see also Chapter 4 on the ICF) can be used as a tool to guide the development of educational goals and processes for students with neurological and developmental conditions (Simeonsson 2003, Hollenweger 2010, 2011, Moretti et al 2012, Rowland et al 2012). From an environment perspective, a segregated special education classroom can provide the opportunity to balance the priorities with the vision of achieving optimal functioning of students and thereby support positive health and life quality outcomes.

Segregated special education

BODY FUNCTIONS AND ACTIVITIES AND PARTICIPATION: EPILEPSY AS A PROTOTYPE

Overview
Epilepsy is one of the most common neurological disorders in children and a frequent cause of disability. The condition is used here to illustrate the complex health needs, activity limitations, and participation restrictions of students with neurodevelopment conditions and to emphasize the importance of educational environmental health determinants on health outcomes and quality of life.

Epilepsy refers to a number of chronic disorders of the central nervous system characterized by recurrent epileptic seizures; however, it is not simply a seizure disorder. Apart from the recurrent seizures, children with epilepsy consistently have much higher rates of cognitive, behavioural, and psychosocial difficulties than those with other chronic health conditions or peers in general (Ronen et al 2003). Young people with epilepsy have lower rates of participation in postsecondary education. As adults, they are more socially isolated, are less likely to be involved in intimate relationships or to have children, and are more likely to work in unskilled mechanical jobs or to be unemployed. Consequently, even major scientific breakthroughs in our understanding of the causes of epilepsy or treatments to improve or arrest seizures are not likely to resolve the multitude of health challenges related to the condition; alternative strategies are required to promote improved well-being and quality of life.

Cognitive and psychosocial comorbidities (see also Chapter 7)
Understanding comorbid issues of any neurodevelopment condition is critical for educational success. Individuals with epilepsy are at increased risk for intellectual deficits (Aldenkamp and Bodde 2005, Cormack et al 2007), with the mean performance of those with intractable epilepsy falling one to two standard deviations (SDs) below the norm (Cormack et al 2007). In practical terms, an individual aged 15 years and 6 months who falls one SD below the norm (16th centile) functions approximately 5 years (SD 2 years) below typically developing peers. Importantly, deficits assessed with intelligence measures fail to capture the complexity of cognitive challenges experienced. Difficulties with memory, processing speed, and attention are the most frequently observed cognitive problems (Aldenkamp and Bodde 2005). In addition, up to 50% perform below grade expectations in some academic domain (McCarthy et al 1995). The academic difficulties cannot be explained by cognitive test scores alone (Berg et al 2011); social–emotional factors are among the most influential factors on any student's learning (Wang et al 1997).

The heightened incidence of mental health issues in children with epilepsy is well established, with rates ranging from 26% to 58% compared with rates of 7% to 9.3% in the general public and 10.6% to 12% in children with non-neurological physical or chronic conditions

(Rutter et al 1970, Davis et al 2003). Difficulties include significantly higher rates of depressive disorders, anxiety disorders, and ADHD than in healthy peers (Caplan et al 2005, Jones et al 2007); however, the psychosocial burden extends beyond diagnosed conditions. Elliot et al (2005) elucidate how intractable epilepsy intrudes on all aspects of a child's quality of life – specifically physical constraints, inertia, emotional distress, and seizure unpredictability create barriers to academic and social engagement. Participation in activities is also a contributing factor (Carpay et al 1996). Parental proxy reports indicate that these children have difficulty completing day-to-day activities related to executive functions (Hermman et al 2007) as well as daily occupations (Fayed and Kerr 2009b). Restrictions on participation, cognitive–developmental level, and self-efficacy related to negative attitudes of others limit social interaction for these children (Austin and Dunn 2000, Elliot et al 2005) and impact their sense of normalcy and belonging (Elliot et al 2005), which in turn is detrimental to other functions (e.g. motivation, optimism, confidence, openness to experience). Social problems represent an enormous concern for children and their parents (Drewel and Caplan 2007); there is both a perceived and an experienced social stigma (see also Chapter 12).

The confounding issues and interactions among body function and activity and participation, highlighted above, are representative of reports of associated disabilities among children with other developmental conditions (e.g. communication and specific language impairment [Campbell et al 2007, Vitkovitch 2008] and cerebral palsy [Beckung and Hagberg 2002]).

A SEGREGATED ENVIRONMENT: THE EPILEPSY CLASSROOM

Overview
The Epilepsy Classroom, a specialized learning environment at Toronto's Hospital for Sick Children, is a Section 23 programme with the Ministry of Education of Ontario and is a partnership between the Centre for Brain and Behaviour at the Hospital and the Toronto District School Board. Like all Section 23 programmes, it is a treatment programme for students whose medical, behavioural, or emotional needs are not being met through the regular school programme. For students who attend our classroom, typically all three conditions are met. Thus, the approaches used in the classroom can be viewed from a non-categorical perspective as an environment for children who have complex neurodevelopmental and neurobehavioural problems who share a commonality of some type of cognitive (e.g. attention, executive function, language function, etc.) or intellectual impairment.

The classroom was established in the early 1990s as a remedial programme for students in grades 1 to 8 with active epilepsy. The programme has continued to evolve based on our understanding of students' health needs, the availability of empirically based remedial strategies, and advances in technology. Our objectives are to assist students to overcome or compensate for their personal learning challenges, thereby achieving academic success as independently as possible, as well as building self-confidence and resilience, thus improving their well-being and quality of life.

The classroom is an effective model of the wraparound approach that is recommended for all students with chronic emotional or behavioural conditions (Quinn and Lee 2007). Specifically, there is seamless integration among the members of the multidisciplinary team who provide a collaborative circle of care for each student and family. A special education teacher and two educational assistants are in the classroom daily with six to eight students, offering a maximum student to staff ratio of 8:3. The classroom environment also incorporates extensive health services. There is coordinated input from a social worker, neuropsychologist, and developmental paediatrician. In addition, an occupational therapist, nurse practitioner, neurologist, and psychiatrist consult to the classroom on a need-be basis. Assessment results are integrated into daily programming to offer maximum support. The underlying interests, strengths, and needs of the student and the family are identified and a plan of care is developed accordingly. With respect to education, we are committed to utilizing research-based and scientifically validated approaches. Students previously attended for one term; however, in 2009 the programme became a full academic year to offer students the time to assimilate and integrate new skills, support smoother transition, and increase the likelihood of sustained success.

Knowledge transfer (see also Chapter 19 on knowledge translation), a vital part of the programme, occurs in a number of ways. First, midway through the year, an information seminar is held in which parents of current students and representatives from students' home schools are invited to learn about the complex health needs of students, programming, and outcomes. Second, at the end of the year, a transition meeting is held for each student. The student's parents, representatives of the school to which they will be transitioned, and the multidisciplinary classroom team meet to discuss the student's medical updates and academic and social progress, as well as to offer recommendations to inform the student's future educational plan. The meeting is in keeping with the consensus in the literature that recommends that transition of services should be an individualized and collaborative process between agencies and disciplines (Kraus de Camargo 2011). Finally, the Board of Education sets the teaching contracts at 3 years with the possibility of renewal for a second term. Upon completion of the commitment, the teacher is in a position to educate school board colleagues about the condition and effective educational interventions (in effect, to become a 'knowledge broker').

Educational and technological programming
Explicit, well-organized instructional programmes that provide opportunities for guided practice and cumulative learning are effective for students with special educational needs (Fletcher et al 2007). Direct instruction (Engelmann 1969, Adams and Engelmann 1996), a scientifically validated and structured or systematic approach to instruction, has been proven to be effective in assisting students with disabilities to learn (Carnine 1999) and is the main approach utilized in the classroom. The lessons are presented in a consistent format, using familiar language so that students can focus on the content of the lesson rather than the style of presentation. Much of the curriculum is scripted, which allows for brisk pacing to help hold students' attention and maximize the amount of the curriculum that can be taught. Guided practice and unison responding further increase attention to task and enhance students' success, thereby building self-confidence. There is significant repetition of points, which facilitates retention. Additionally, the teacher is engaged in reciprocal learning with the students and can quickly identify learning gaps and needs. Instruction commences at the child's functional level, with an expectation of skill mastery prior to moving to the next level. Mastering basic skills is a fundamental step in developing higher-order thinking (Fletcher et al 2007). Through mediated

scaffolding, the teacher initially guides students through problem-solving strategies and then gradually fades the support, which leads to independence (Kameenui and Carnine 1998).

By moving to a full-year programme, the classroom has been able to incorporate Empower Reading™ (Lovett et al 2006) for students in grades 2 to 5. Based on rigorous research with over 4000 struggling readers in Canada and the USA, Dr Lovett and her team created the programme to address the core learning problems that prevent struggling readers and spellers from learning and included only those instructional features found to yield the best long-term outcomes. Empower Reading™ teaches specific decoding strategies and guides students to use the strategies effectively and independently. It also builds motivation and confidence.

While the primary instructional focus is on improving basic academic skills, the classroom timetable allows for instruction in both social studies and science. Additionally, augmenting the curriculum with self-regulation strategies, assistive technology, and social–emotional programming is fundamental. Self-regulation strategies provide benefits beyond those gained through systemic explicit instruction (Fletcher et al 2007). Having students acknowledge their effort and success, using reciprocal teaching with corrective feedback, offering learning to learn strategies, and incorporating education about brain function and mindful focus are routinely implemented in the classroom.

Integrating technological advances into special education provides students with access to the curriculum that was not previously available to them (Girgin et al 2011) and leads to improvements in attitude (Jeffs et al 2006) and academic outcomes (Jeffs et al 2006, Mechling et al 2008, Maor et al 2011). Students in our classroom receive instruction through an interactive white board, as well as training in assistive computer software programs (e.g. word prediction, voice to text, and organizational programmes) and the use of touchpads. The intentions are to facilitate on-task engaged behaviour, build on students' strengths, compensate for their learning needs, and optimize their current and future success as confident, capable students.

Empirical evidence demonstrates that social–emotional learning programmes not only improve typically developing students' social–emotional skills but also their attitudes, behaviours, and academic performance (Durlak et al 2011). Within our segregated classroom, one afternoon a week is set aside for social–emotional group programming with three foci: (1) psychosocial functioning with the purpose of advancing students' knowledge about their neurological condition and increasing their ability to self-advocate; (2) social skills training to enable students to participate more fully in social situations (e.g. developing skills related to understanding social cues, forming relationships, interacting according to social rules, maintaining social space, regulating behaviour, etc.); and (3) MindUp™, a curriculum based on research in cognitive neuroscience, mindful education, social–emotional learning, and positive psychology, which aims to promote self-regulation, resilience, and optimism (Hawn Foundation 2011). Additionally, depending on an individual student's needs, he or she may participate in individual therapy with the social worker. The social worker may also support families in terms of identifying resources to assist them outside of school (e.g. social security and support services). Finally, because of prevailing concerns of physical safety, many of our students have not previously participated in field trips; consequently, during their year in the classroom, special events and trips are scheduled to enhance the educational curriculum and community life experiences.

Case vignette

Sean's early history is much like any other child's. However, unlike most children, his life-course changed when he had his first seizure at 4 years of age. For a few years, he experienced good seizure control on several anticonvulsant medications and his developmental progress was age appropriate. Sean's cognitive and psychosocial developmental trajectories were altered when his seizures returned at the age of 10. By parental report, he experienced an associated decline in cognitive performance. By self-report substantial health challenges emerged:

> When I was 11½ my life changed. I had a prolonged tonic–clonic seizure requiring emergency care... The seizures affected my quality of life, interrupted my sleep, affected my learning and memory, ability to walk and speak, and gave me tremors. I was severely bullied at school regarding my epilepsy; often called 'Seizure Man'. ... The combination of taking several new medications, having multiple seizures a day, along with facing the physical limitations and bullying, forced me into an emotional train-wreck. I became depressed, extremely anxious and had virtually no self-esteem. But one day that all changed: I became a student in the Epilepsy Classroom. The Epilepsy Classroom changed my life in significant ways, both in the short and long term.

Two months into his grade 8 year at age 13, Sean's emotional needs were significant enough that his doctors recommended that he be home schooled. The family found an alternative in a segregated classroom that catered to his needs. At the time of enrolment, Sean experienced different seizure types almost daily and unpredictably. He was taking four anticonvulsant medications daily as well as a fifth for prolonged seizures. The intake psychoeducational assessment revealed average to above average intellectual reasoning abilities along with weaknesses in attention, processing speed, and phonological processing. His academic achievement fell 1 to 2 years below grade expectations.

The social–emotional benefits and reduction in social stigma that Sean experienced during his term in the classroom are captured in a speech he wrote for a fund-raiser 2 years later:

> ... for the first time in months, I did a quite simple but heartfelt thing. I smiled. I felt accepted and was always treated properly by others. One of the teachers took my picture ... and when I brought it home to show my mom and dad, they began to well up with tears. It had been so long since they had seen me happy and this classroom had done what doctors, along with my family and friends, had been trying to do for months in a matter of days!

I greatly appreciate how the Epilepsy Classroom understands the effects epilepsy has on one's life; everything is based on the student's life as a whole.

The learning accommodations still remain unmatched throughout the years of education I have received … The classroom not only focused on the academics of the students, but also on our social and emotional well being.

Not only have I become a successful student, but I have also experienced other successes. Yes, I still have epilepsy. Right now I am on six different medications … I still encounter multiple side effects that are difficult to live with … But, the Epilepsy Classroom taught us that despite the number of hurdles set before us, we should never stop until we reach our goals; people with epilepsy can accomplish anything they set their mind to!

Sean has been accepted to the university programme of his choice and has become a volunteer in the Epilepsy Classroom.

Social–emotional outcomes

The safer students feel, the more they can engage in the learning environment in a meaningful way (Hawn Foundation 2011). The case vignette is a powerful illustration of how a segregated special education classroom can foster stronger psychosocial functions, including belonging and self-confidence. Caregivers also report the transformation described by Sean. A month after being enrolled in the classroom, a grandmother of a 7-year-old girl, who had an academically and emotionally challenging grade 1 year in an ordinary classroom, telephoned the teacher to say, 'It's like we have our old granddaughter back, the one who laughed and had fun with us.' Similarly, several weeks into her daughter's term in the classroom, the mother of a 9-year-old student with social anxiety commented that it was the first time her daughter had met another child with the same neurological condition and that she finally 'felt normal'. The mother stressed that 'feeling normal' had significantly increased her daughter's confidence in social settings. In fact, after years of avoiding social play, her daughter approached other children at the park and joined in on play. Parents also speak about their own relief: 'The opportunity to be included in this unique program was a tremendous relief for us … After years of struggling, intense advocacy and additional support (social skills classes …) we are thrilled to see such significant changes in our daughter … her improved self confidence and academic progress are a joy to us.'

Recognizing the immense value of self- and parent report in understanding the effectiveness of the classroom milieu on life quality outcomes, we recently completed the process of selecting evaluative measures. As part of this process, we conducted a systematic review of quality of life questionnaires (Fayed and Kerr 2009a) and trialled various standardized student self-report surveys. Students' limitations in working memory, sustained attention, and conceptualization of Likert scales limited our options. We are currently completing a prospective study of parents' perspectives of changes in their child's self-competency, social skills, and quality of life, as well as students' self-report of changes in self-esteem.

Academic outcomes

One term of this special education environment is effective in significantly improving academic performance in terms of raw scores (Humphries et al 2005), standard scores, and grade scores (EN Kerr, personal communication, 2011). Here we report on the success of 28 students in five consecutive terms who received direct instruction in basic academic subjects for 12 to 13 weeks. Students were included if at least one indicator of intellectual reasoning (i.e. verbal or performance) fell above the second centile. The mean verbal IQ was 83.4 (SD 12.8, range 63–112) and mean performance IQ was 84.1 (SD 12.6, range 64–109). The mean age at the start of the term was 10.0 (SD 1.9; range 7.1–13.2). Significant raw score improvement was documented on all assessed measures of literacy (i.e. spelling, word reading, word attack, $p<0.001$ and passage comprehension, $p=0.008$) and mathematics (i.e. calculations and quantitative concepts, $p<0.001$ and $p=0.001$, respectively). Figure 21.2 depicts the corresponding improvements in mean grade level, with significant levels of $p<0.001$ for all academic domains except word attack ($p=0.001$) and passage comprehension ($p=0.018$). The gains exhibited exceed those expected for the time period experienced.

Conclusion

Although the movement for inclusive education has been long established, meeting the educational needs of students with neurodevelopmental conditions within the environment of an ordinary classroom is not always achievable. These students carry substantial burdens, including cognitive and mental health comorbidities, social stigma, poor peer relationships, and poor school performance, that drastically set them apart from their typically developing peers. Their inability to participate fully in activities of children their age can further isolate and demoralize them; yet, a strong sense of belonging is necessary for resiliency. Addressing

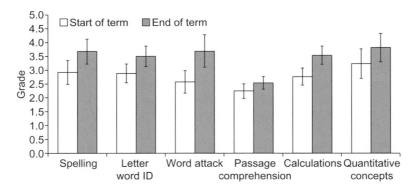

Fig. 21.2 Mean grade increases (±SEM) across academic domains from start to end of term (12–13 weeks) of direct instruction.

these students' physical needs and implementing behavioural management strategies are insufficient to promote their social–emotional well-being and academic success. Students do not detach how they feel about themselves, their social interactions, and their environments from their learning (Schnoret-Reichl and Hymel 2007). How the psychosocial and learning challenges of students with neurodevelopment conditions are supported and addressed can foster or impede academic experience and achievement. Specialized learning environments provide transformative opportunities for enhancing health outcomes and improving quality of life of children with neurodevelopment conditions.

Prevailing positive experiences are reported for education through segregated programmes (Casserly 2011). Moreover, empirical evidence (e.g. Humphries et al 2005, Lovett et al 2006, Fletcher et al 2007, Durlak et al 2011, Iseman and Naglieri 2011, Maor et al 2011) strongly demonstrates the effectiveness of dedicated programming in enhancing outcomes for struggling learners. Scientifically validated interventions aimed at improving students' social–emotional well-being and learning are crucial for students with neurodevelopmental conditions to experience success. Students with chronic and intensive emotional or behavioural disorders (Quinn and Lee 2007), those with cognitive impairment, and those with combinations thereof, benefit from a multidisciplinary team wraparound approach that addresses the individual needs of the student and family. Not only does this approach foster positive social–emotional outcomes and academic success, it can be pivotal in altering students' social and academic trajectories, thus allowing them to reach their potential.

REFERENCES

Key references

*Adams GL, Englemann S (1996) *Research on Direct Instruction: 25 Years Beyond DISTAR*. Seattle, WA: Educational Achievement Systems.

Aldenkamp AP, Bodde N (2005) Behaviour, cognition and epilepsy. *Acta Neurol Scand* 182: 19–25. http://dx.doi.org/10.1111/j.1600-0404.2005.00523.x

Austin JK, Dunn DW (2000) Children with epilepsy: quality of life and psychosocial needs. *Annu Rev Nurs Res* 18: 26–47.

*Beckung E, Hagberg G (2002) Neuroimpairments, activity limitations and participation restriction in children with cerebral palsy. *Dev Med Child Neurol* 44: 309–316. http://dx.doi.org/10.1111/j.1469-8749.2002.tb00816.x

Berg AT, Hesdorffer DC, Zelko FAJ (2011) Special education participation in children with epilepsy: what does it reflect? *Epilepsy Behav* 22: 336–341. http://dx.doi.org/10.1016/j.yebeh.2011.07.014

*Campbell WN, Skarakis-Doyle E (2007) School-aged children with SLI: the ICF as a framework for collaborative service delivery. *J Commun Disord* 40: 513–535.

Caplan R, Siddarth P, Gurbani S, Hanson R, Snakar R, Shields WD (2005) Depression and anxiety disorders in pediatric epilepsy. *Epilepsia* 46: 720–730. http://dx.doi.org/10.1111/j.1528-1167.2005.43604.x

Carnine D (1999) Bridging the research-to-practice gap. *Excep Child* 63: 513–520.

Carpay HA, Vermeulen J, Stronik H, et al (1991) Disability due to restrictions in childhood epilepsy. *Dev Med Child Neurol* 39: 521–526. http://dx.doi.org/10.1111/j.1469-8749.1997.tb07480.x

*Casserly AN (2011) Children's experiences of reading classes and reading school in Ireland. *Support Learning* 26: 17–24.

Cormack F, Cross JH, Isaacs E, et al (2007) The development of intellectual abilities in pediatric temporal lobe epilepsy. *Epilepsia* 44: 944–949.

Davis S, Heyman I, Goodman R (2003) A population survey of mental health problems in children with epilepsy. *Dev Med Child Neurol* 45: 292–295. http://dx.doi.org/10.1111/j.1469-8749.2003.tb00398.x

*Drewel EH, Caplan R (2007) Social difficulties in children with epilepsy: review and treatment recommendations. *Exp Rev Neurotherapeutics* 7: 865–873. http://dx.doi.org/10.1586/14737175.7.7.865

*Durlak JA, Weissberg RP, Dymnicki AB, Taylor RD, Schellinger KB (2011) The impact of enhancing students' social and emotional learning: a meta-analysis of school-based universal interventions. *Child Dev* 82: 405–432. http://dx.doi.org/10.1111/j.1467-8624.2010.01564.x

*Elliot IM, Lach L, Smith ML (2005) I just want to be normal: a qualitative study exploring how children and adolescents view the impact of intractable epilepsy on their quality of life. *Epilepsy Behav* 7: 664–678. http://dx.doi.org/10.1016/j.yebeh.2005.07.004

*Engelmann S (1969) *Conceptual Learning*. Sioux Falls, SD: ADPAT Press.

Fayed N, Kerr EN (2009a) Comparing quality of life scales in childhood epilepsy: what's in the measures? *Int J Disabil Commun Rehabil* 8(3). Available at: www.ijdcr.ca/VOL08_03/articles/fayed.shtml (accesed 28 November 2012).

Fayed N, Kerr EN (2009b) Identifying occupational issues among children with intractable epilepsy: individualized versus norm-referenced approaches. *Can J Occup Ther* 76: 90–96.

*Flectcher JM, Lyon GR, Fuchs L, Barnes MA (2007) *Learning Disabilities: From Identification to Intervention*. New York: Guilford.

Garrison-Wade D, Sobel D, Flumer C (2007) Inclusive leadership: preparing principals for the role that awaits them. *Educ Leadership Admin Teach Program Dev* 19: 117–132.

Girgin U, Kurt AA, Odabasi F (2011) Technology integration issues in a special education school in Turkey. *Cypriot J Educ Sci* 1: 13–21.

*Hawn Foundation (2011) *The MindUP Curriculum*. New York, NY: Scholastic, Inc.

Hermann B, Jones J, Dabbs K, et al (2007) The frequency, complication and aetiology of ADHD in new onset paediatric epilepsy. *Brain* 130: 3135–3148. http://dx.doi.org/10.1093/brain/awm227

Hollenweger J (2010) MHADIE's matrix to analyse the functioning of education systems. *Disabil Rehabil* 32(Suppl. 1): S116–S124. http://dx.doi.org/10.3109/09638288.2010.520809

Hollenweger J (2011) Development of an ICF-based eligibility procedure for education in Switzerland. *BMC Public Health* 11(Suppl. 4): S7. http://dx.doi.org/10.1186/1471-2458-11-S4-S7

Humphries T, Neufel M, Johnson C, Engels K, McKay R (2005) A pilot study of the effect of Direct Instruction programming on the academic performance of students with intractable epilepsy. *Epilepsy Behav* 6: 405–412. http://dx.doi.org/10.1016/j.yebeh.2005.01.015

Iseman JS, Naglieri JA (2011) A cognitive strategy instruction to improve math calculation for children with ADHD and LD: a randomized controlled study. *J Learn Disabil* 44: 184–195. http://dx.doi.org/10.1177/0022219410391190

*Jeffs T (2006) Assistive technology and literacy learning: reflections of parents and children. *J Spec Educ Technol* 21: 37–44.

Jones JE, Watson R, Sheth R, Koehn M, Seidenberg M, Hermann B (2007) Psychiatric comorbidity in children with new onset epilepsy. *Dev Med Child Neurol* 49: 493–497. http://dx.doi.org/10.1111/j.1469-8749.2007.00493.x

*Kameenui EJ, Carnine DW (1998) *Effective Teaching Strategies that Accommodate Diverse Learners*. Upper Saddle River, NJ: Merill.

Kraus de Camargo O (2011) Systems of care: transition from the bio-psycho-social perspective of the International Classification of Functioning, Disability and Health. *Child Care Health Dev* 37: 792–799. http://dx.doi.org/10.1111/j.1365-2214.2011.01323.x

Lovett MW, Lacerenza S, Borden L (2006) *Empower Reading*™. Toronto, ON: The Hospital For Sick Children.

McCarthy AM, Richman LC, Yarbrough D (1995) Memory, attention and school problems in children with seizure disorders. *Dev Neuropsychol* 11: 71–86 http://dx.doi.org/10.1080/87565649509540604

*Maor D, Currie J, Drewry R (2011) The effectiveness of assistive technologies for children with special needs: a review of research based studies. *Eur J Spec Needs Educ* 26: 283–298. http://dx.doi.org/10.1080/08856257.2011.593821

*Mechling L, Gast D, Thompson K (2008) Comparison of the effect of smart board technology and flash card instruction on sight word recognition and observational learning. *J Spec Educ Technol* 23: 34–46.

Minskoff E, Allsopp D (2003) *Academic Success Strategies for Adolescents with Learning Disabilities and ADHD*. Baltimore, MD: Paul H Brookes Publishing Co.

*Moretti M, Alves I, Maxwell G (2012) A systematic literature review of the situation of the International Classification of Functioning, Disability, and Health and the International Classification of Functioning, Disability, and Health-Children and Youth version in education: a useful tool or a flight of fancy. *Am J Phys Med Rehabil* 91(Suppl. 1): S103–S117.

*Quinn KP, Lee V (2007) The wraparound approach for students with emotional and behavioral disorders: opportunities for school psychologist. *Psychol School* 44: 101–111. http://dx.doi.org/10.1002/pits.20209

Ronen GM, Streiner DL, Rosenbaum P (2003) Health-related quality of life in childhood epilepsy: moving beyond 'seizure control with minimal adverse effects'. *Health Qual Life Outcomes* 1: 36–45. http://dx.doi.org/10.1186/1477-7525-1-36

*Rowland C, Fried-Oken M, Steiner SA, et al (2012) Developing the ICF-CY for AAC profile and code set for children who rely on AAC. *Augment Altern Commun* 28: 21–32.

*Rutter M, Grapham P, Yule W (1970) *A Neuropsychiatric Study in Childhood. Clinics in Developmental Medicine Nos. 35/36*. London: William Heineman Medical Books.

Schonert-Reichl KA, Hymel S (2007) Educating the heart as well as the mind. *Educ Can* 47: 20–25

Simeonsson RJ (2003) Classification of communication disabilities in children: contribution of the International Classification on Functioning, Disability and Health. *Int J Audiol* 42(Suppl. 1): S2–S8. http://dx.doi.org/10.3109/14992020309074618

*Vitkovitch J (2008) Speech and language skills: their importance in development. *J Fam Health Care* 18: 93–95.

*Wang MC, Haertel GD, Walberg HJ (1997) Learning influences. In: Walberg HJ, Haertal GD, editors. *Psychology and Educational Proactive*. Berkely, CA: McCatchan, pp. 199–211.

World Health Organization (2001) *International Classification of Functioning, Disability and Health*. Geneva: WHO Press.

World Health Organization (2007) *International Classification of Functioning, Disability and Health, Children and Youth Version*. Geneva: WHO Press.

22

TRANSITION TO ADULTHOOD: ENHANCING HEALTH AND QUALITY OF LIFE FOR EMERGING ADULTS WITH NEUROLOGICAL AND DEVELOPMENTAL CONDITIONS

Jan Willem Gorter and Marij Roebroeck

Overview

Most children with neurological and developmental conditions survive to adulthood. In their journey towards adulthood people with neurological conditions experience many transitions in various life domains. Leaving the family-centred environment of paediatric care for the individual-centred environment of adult services is a difficult challenge for these young people and their families. Poor transition from paediatric to adult health care has been shown to have a negative impact in these conditions with respect to adherence to medical care, health outcomes, and quality of life. This chapter provides the reader with insights into the processes of clinical transition of adolescents with neurological and developmental impairments, as well as with 'points of entry' to improve adult-oriented care using outcomes such as health and quality of life. Future models of care for this specific population are discussed.

Case scenario

I am 47 years old with cerebral palsy. I lead a fairly normal life, married with two children. I work as a manager. As a child 47 years ago, there was very limited information on cerebral palsy. It was something that was diagnosed and then you lived with it the best you could. I am very fortunate to have a mild version of the condition and also to have a loving environment to grow in and flourish in. One thing that I learned from a young age is that cerebral palsy was a stable condition that did not worsen. As I get older I find this to be different. I find my muscles and body in general to be achy and I lack energy (fatigue). When I saw a doctor (I do not have a family doctor) he attributes this to living with cerebral palsy and the impact of years of cerebral palsy on my body.

> The help I am seeking from you is if you would know of any information about adults and ageing with cerebral palsy, what kind of doctor would be best suited for adults with cerebral palsy and what kind of specialist can help me find tools to help my everyday life? I need to have a complete evaluation, information to cope with my premature ageing process and to know what to do to help my condition. I feel alone because I have contacted a few doctors and I have not received much information.

Introduction

Most children with neurological and developmental conditions survive to adulthood. For example, with improved neonatal and paediatric care over the last few decades, life expectancy has changed dramatically for children with cerebral palsy (CP) (Strauss et al 2008, Baird et al 2011). In a report from Sweden, Westbom et al (2011) studied survival in a population of children with CP between 1990 and 2010. In that study virtually all children with good motor abilities, and 96% of the whole population of children with CP, survived into adulthood. Although the risk of death is the highest in fragile children with CP, their estimated survival is 60% at 19 years of age (Westbom et al 2011). The issue of growing up with CP has become a new reality, as it is for children and young people with many other neurological and developmental conditions such as spina bifida (Webb 2010, Oakeshott et al 2011), muscular dystrophy (Gordon et al 2011), and childhood onset epilepsy (Forsgren et al 2005).

In adolescence (derived from the Latin word *adolscere*, which means 'growing up') children transition from one state (childhood) to another (early adulthood). In late adolescence, young people usually, but not always, are able to regulate their own lives (demonstrating autonomy and independence). The term 'emerging adulthood' (Arnett 2004) has been suggested to describe a new stage in the life-course of an individual, one that is typically marked by high school graduation. Many young people in their late teens and early twenties feel that they are neither teenagers nor adults. Adolescence and emerging adulthood is a transition time when adult behaviours become established, and therefore it represents a window of opportunity to promote healthy behaviour.

Our view on transition should not, however, be too narrow. The literature on the unique needs and experiences of young people with neurological and developmental conditions has taught us that health should be broadly conceptualized and include physical, social, cognitive, and emotional aspects, with 'participation' (i.e. involvement in a life situation) as one of the ultimate measures of outcome (World Health Organization 2001). International health experts argued in a 2011 discussion paper for a more dynamic and empowering definition of health: 'health is the ability to adapt and to self manage' (Huber et al 2011). In other words, health of people with neurological and developmental conditions can be seen as a dynamic balance between opportunities and limitations, shifting through life. This balance is affected by external conditions, and the dynamics are most important at transition points, when a young person is dealing with significant changes in personal and environmental changes (Gorter et al 2011). The World Health Organization's International Classification of Functioning, Disability and Health (ICF) (Fig. 22.1) provides both a detailed classification of aspects of people's health

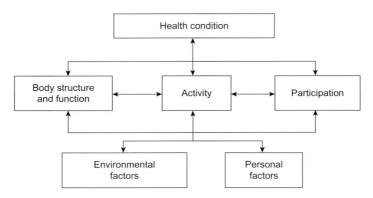

Fig. 22.1 The International Classification of Functioning, Disability and Health framework (World Health Organization 2001).

and function and a pictorial framework that presents the opportunity to consider health issues within a broader social–ecological context. The interconnectedness of the different boxes with aspects of health and contextual factors show that this is a 'dynamic system': changes in any area of the framework may potentially have influences elsewhere in the system (see also Chapters 2 and 4).

Transition in various life domains

For transition planning it is important to understand a young person's functioning by examining the interactions among health condition, environmental factors, and personal characteristics and preferences (Kraus de Camargo 2011). Functional profiles based on the ICF, rather than on the medical diagnosis alone, can be useful in designing transition planning by addressing activities that young people consider important in their daily living. Major life events take place during the process of transition to adulthood, such as finishing education and starting a job, finding a partner, leaving home, and living on one's own. Young adults, whether impaired or not, have to learn a range of new skills to enable them to regulate their own lives. This is a complex process that extends over several years. Transition to adulthood takes place in several domains of participation, including the use of healthcare services. A person's transition does not necessarily follow the same pace in each domain of participation. For example, young adults can have paid work, but still live with their parents. Of a sample of young Dutch adults, between 16 and 22 years of age, with CP but without severe intellectual impairments, almost all were in the transition process or had reached autonomy for specific domains of participation (Donkervoort et al 2009). They organized transportation independently (driving a car, calling a taxi, or using public transportation: 90%), and went out to parties or for nightlife entertainment (80%). About 25% of the young adults with CP lived on their own, and 25% had a job, which is less than the general population of the same age. Over the previous 2 years they had become more independent in all areas, including finances, intimate relationships, and utilization of adult rehabilitation care (Donkervoort et al 2009). In a qualitative study, adults aged 18 to 35 with epilepsy and cognitive impairments spoke clearly of the consequences of epilepsy in terms of education, employment, social life, self-esteem, and hope for the future (Gauffin et al 2011). In young people with neurological and developmental conditions, severity of impairment predicted whether they were employed or enrolled in postsecondary education, which in turn predicted greater participation in leisure activities and greater social interaction. Social interaction, in turn, was identified as a predictor of quality of life (MacCulloch 2012).

Healthcare transition

Although little is known about how young people 'travel' through healthcare services in their adolescence, there are key concerns regarding the 'journey to adult life' in young people with neurological and developmental conditions. Leaving the family-centred environment of paediatric care for the individual-centred environment of adult services (a major component of the medical transition or transfer) is a difficult challenge for young people with neurological and developmental conditions. Indeed, young people in many countries – and their parents/caregivers – have compared their transition experience to 'falling off a cliff'. Poor healthcare transition has been shown to have a negative impact in all chronic conditions with respect to adherence to medical care, health outcomes, and quality of life. For example, 20- to 22-year-olds with CP are twice as likely to rate their health as poor compared with 15- to 16-year-olds (21% vs 9%) (Young et al 2010). In Canada, young people with CP visit physicians on an outpatient basis about twice as often as their age-matched peers. Moreover, annual hospital admission rates for young people and young adults were 11 and 4 times higher, respectively, than those of age-matched peers. Recent surveys in North America, Europe, and Southern Asia showed similar patterns of health care utilization when children with neurological and developmental conditions grow up and become (young) adults (Gorter 2009a).

Not surprisingly, there is a call for comprehensive care models in health care, with a life-course approach filling the gaps in medical and psychosocial care for young people and adults with chronic childhood-onset conditions, including transitional care programmes to promote a planned transition rather than a 'laissez faire' approach (Verhoof et al 2011, Oskoui et al 2012). The reality is that as a consequence of their conditions young people with neurological and developmental impairments are involved in many more 'systems'. For example, healthcare and social services are very different in terms of their expectations of young people and families, and the transition can be highly stressful and requires a great deal of planning and preparation (Gorter 2009b, Young et al 2009, van Staa et al 2011). The transition process within the healthcare system alone is more complex than a simple transfer of care from a paediatric to an adult setting (Kraus de Camargo 2011).

This chapter discusses this subject with a focus on the key factors that must be considered to support the transition of adolescents with neurological and developmental conditions and their families, mainly in the context of health care. Capacity-building in young people, particularly fostering self-determination, problem-solving skills, and relationship building, has been identified as a strategy to empower young people with neurological and developmental conditions (Gorter et al 2011).

The basics of planned transition are simple and are common to all neurological and developmental conditions. The following themes will be addressed in this chapter:

1   Young people and their families need to be prepared well in advance for moving from paediatric to adult services, and they need to have the necessary skill set to thrive there.

2   Healthcare providers have to listen to young people's views about their lives and their needs.

3   It is important to prepare and nurture adult services to receive young people with childhood-onset impairments, with whom those services are often not familiar.

Theme I: Preparation of young people and their families

The transition to adulthood is considered to be a critical journey within an individual's life-course. Staying with the journey analogy, three key phases of the transition process can be distinguished: the preparation; the journey itself; and the landing in the adult world (Stewart et al 2009a). Preparation is critical to every journey. There is convincing evidence that the process of transition should start early with a life-course approach to development and transition, recognizing the chronic nature of childhood illness and impairment (Priestly 2001). While transitional concerns appear to intensify at the age of 17 prior to the transfer of care, children as young as 12 appear to contemplate transition (Moola and Norman 2011). This chapter focuses on the phase that takes place during a young person's late childhood and adolescence as he or she begins to look ahead and prepare for adult life. The process of clinical transition should follow the stages of adolescence, and the preparation should begin when the adolescent is no older than 14 years of age.

Listening to the voices of young people and adults with CP, spina bifida, and acquired brain injuries of childhood in the province of Ontario, Canada, it becomes clear that young people and their families want to be prepared well in advance for moving from paediatric to adult services (Young et al 2009). Young and colleagues (2009) identified early provision of detailed information and extensive support as two possible solutions. For example, adolescents should have the opportunity to meet the paediatric healthcare provider on their own, so that they can practise and learn how to deal with the individualized adult healthcare system. At the same time, the parents can learn to 'let their child go'. Rather than giving extensive support, a strategy to empower young people should be the focus of (paediatric) healthcare providers throughout the transition process. This strategy can be based on the shared management model, a planned systematic approach to a gradual shift in responsibilities from the healthcare provider and parents to the young person, as developmentally appropriate. This approach builds upon a life skills-building programme in which children are encouraged to take responsibility for tasks or household chores from a young age, and parents are required to be active in their parenting style (see Fig. 22.2) (Gall et al 2006). For this model to be effective, however, there will need to be clearly formulated descriptions of the tasks in healthcare transition, and evidence that this model contributes to children's ability to adapt and to self-manage their life. Of course parents can (and, we believe, should) be encouraged to adopt and practise these basic concepts from early in their children's life and to continue their role based on the needs and abilities of the young person. Therefore, parents require ongoing and coordinated support to navigate the complex process of service transition, and an approach fostering family involvement will strengthen them in their roles as care provider, manager, supervisor, and consultant, for example through parent-to-parent support.

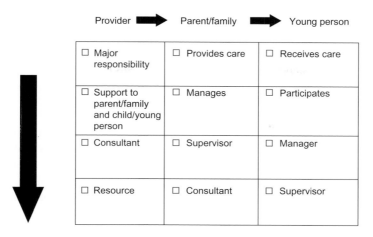

Fig. 22.2 Shared management model (Gall et al 2006).

So far, there are few data evaluating the effectiveness of interventions to improve the preparation of young people for health care transition (Liptak 2008, Grant and Pan 2011). In an outcomes-oriented preparation process one would hope that the young people would have the ability to summarize the main (medical) issues of their condition, for example in the so-called 3-minute summary, at the time that their care is transferred to adult healthcare providers. Another approach to promote partnerships between young adults and service providers is the use of the Youth KIT (Keeping It Together, Youth Version; Stewart et al 2006), a tool developed by researchers at the *CanChild* Centre for Childhood Disability Research at McMaster University, Hamilton, ON, Canada, that recognizes adolescents/young adults as experts on their own needs (Stewart et al 2009b). The Youth KIT promotes information gathering and health self-management and is validated in the paediatric setting and during transition. This tool is being tested in a project together with an Internet-based Transition Coordinator (TRACE) with which young people can interact online (Punthakee and Gorter 2011). The novelty of this approach lies within the way one delivers services to young people and young adults, because it shifts the paradigm from 'doctor knows best' towards an empowered young person who enters the adult world knowing what is important and how to deal with the system.

It is hoped that this presentation of processes and information will promote a new paradigm of patient-driven transition navigation that will enhance self-determination and continuity of care. For young people with neurological and developmental conditions and service providers the Rotterdam Transition Profile can be used to focus attention on developing autonomy in several domains of participation (Donkervoort et al 2009). The profile monitors a young person's transition process in seven areas of life and healthcare management, distinguishing between transition phases that progress from no experience, dependency on adults, the in-between phase (experimenting and orientating to the future), to self-reliance or autonomy. For young people with neurological and developmental conditions the Rotterdam Transition Profile can be introduced early on at age 14. The profile items allow young people to reflect on their development and to talk about mobility (transport), school, employment, finances, relationships and sexual experiences, living situation, and leisure activities. Both an interview version for use in young person–clinician communication and a self-report version for young people are available in English, Dutch, and Norwegian (Rotterdam Transition Profile, 2010) (Table 22.1).

Theme II: Listen to young people's views

Health and quality of life in individuals with neurological and developmental conditions can be enhanced by giving young people a voice. When adolescents were asked to describe their experiences with health care they all greatly appreciated the opportunity to express their opinion (Siebes et al 2007, Gan et al 2008). An inventory among adults with CP revealed a broad spectrum of unmet needs. The most often-mentioned need was for information on their condition (80%), referring to consequences, complications, and causes of CP. This need for information might be due to an inadequate transfer of information to the child as he or she is growing up, or to new questions arising when a child reaches adulthood (Nieuwenhuijsen et al 2008). In a study using the client-centred perspective, young adults with CP, and especially those with lower levels of gross motor functioning, indicated several problems in daily life (Nieuwenhuijsen et al 2009). They identified problems in mobility (using public transport, driving a car), work (seeking employment), preparing meals, housework (e.g. cleaning), and active recreation activities (e.g. sports). Several problems referred to activities that are considered age appropriate and may appear when a child with CP grows older. Therapists and physicians should be aware that new types of problems may arise when a young person with CP reaches adulthood, and these may warrant other approaches or interventions than those that were appropriate in paediatric care (Nieuwenhuijsen et al 2009).

Lessons learned from the experiences and perceptions of older adolescents with CP were that service providers should be encouraged to involve young people actively in making choices on mobility methods, task accommodations, assistive technology, and environmental modifications, rather than therapy with a focus mainly on impairments and activity limitations (Palisano et al 2009). The complexity of the choices and trade-offs made by young people with neurological and developmental conditions supports the importance of considering the dynamic interaction of person and environment, as part of the developmental journey facing all young people, and the need for discussing the trade-offs inherent in the choices that they are making now and for the future. One of the important choices that young people with CP identified was about the amount and type of support they need in order to participate in social activities (Stewart et al 2012). In general, the recommendation for any service provider is to ask clients about the meaning of various experiences in their life, including mobility, health, and their quality of life – all of which should place the focus more on choices and solutions, rather than solely on their problems.

Theme III: Prepare and nurture adult services (see also Chapter 23)

It is clear that individuals with neurological and developmental conditions require ongoing services to decrease morbidity and improve quality of life (Aisen et al 2011, Webb 2010). Adequate routine medical, dental, and specialized care should be provided to all individuals living with neurological and developmental conditions (Liptak 2008, Webb 2010). While in

TABLE 22.1
Rotterdam Transition Profile

Participation domains	Transition phases	0	1	2	3
Education and employment	0. Following no education, no job 1. General education 2. Vocational training, work placement 3. Paid job, volunteer work				
Finances	0. No pocket money 1. Pocket money, clothing allowance 2. Job on the side, student grant 3. Economically independent: job income, benefits				
Housing	1. Living with parents, not responsible for household activities 2. Partly responsible for household activities, domestic training, or seeking housing 3. Living independently				
Leisure (social activities)	1. Young adult arranges leisure activities with peers at home 2. Young adult arranges leisure activities with peers outside the home, during daytime hours 3. Young adult goes out in the evening with peers				
Intimate relationships	0. Young adult has no experience with dating 1. Young adult has experience with dating but not yet with courtship 2. Young adult has experience with courtship 3. Young adult has a current romantic relationship/a partner				
Sexuality	0. Young adult has no experience with French kissing 1. Young adult has experience with French kissing 2. Young adult has experience with caressing under clothes, cuddling nude 3. Young adult has experience with sexual intercourse				
Transport	1. Parents or caregivers transport the adolescent/young adult 2. Parents or caregivers arrange transport, but they do not go with him or her 3. Young adult arranges transportation him-/herself				
Health care					
Care demands	1. Parents formulate care demands 2. Parents and young adults formulate demands together 3. Young adult formulates care demands him-/herself				
Services and aids	1. Parents apply for services and aids 2. Young adult learns the procedures to apply for services and aids 3. Young adult applies for services and aids him-/herself				
Rehabilitation services	In the past year: 1. Young adult consulted paediatric rehabilitation care 2. No consultation of paediatric rehabilitation care 3. Young adult consulted adult rehabilitation services				

Rotterdam Transition Profile, © Department of Rehabilitation Medicine, Erasmus MC – University Medical Centre, Rotterdam:
www.erasmusmc.nl/revalidatie/research/transition/
Source: Donkervoort et al (2009).

theory healthcare providers and policy makers hardly disagree on this human right, in reality young people and adults with CP, spina bifida, and acquired brain injuries of childhood onset identified challenges in transition, including: lack of access to health care; professionals' lack of knowledge; and lack of information and uncertainty regarding the transition process (Young et al 2009). Because most neurological and developmental impairments have traditionally been viewed as disorders of childhood, adult services are not trained to accommodate the needs of these individuals. For example, adult healthcare providers were not taught about management of adults with childhood-onset conditions in their residency training (Aisen et al 2011). Appropriate training (knowledge, attitudes) for medical and dental trainees can help to build capacity at large. Resource centres with transition tools and tips should be established for people with neurological and developmental conditions, including the transition of young people to the adult healthcare system, as well as for their families, their healthcare team, and other service providers. See, for example, http://healthytransitionsny.org and http://www.gottransition.org/. Making the links is essential for overcoming the gap between paediatric and adult specialists and primary healthcare providers (Gorter 2012). At an individual or programme level there is a need to create a network of adult healthcare providers, built around the individual with a neurological or developmental condition and his or her family. Collaboration is also needed at an organizational level to provide healthcare providers with support and resources throughout the individual's lifespan.

For example, a Dutch network of rehabilitation centres (TransitionNet) offers innovate transition and lifespan care for young persons with childhood-onset impairments and disabilities (16–25 years). In young adult teams (YATs), they develop and implement age-appropriate interventions aiming to improve the young people's autonomy in several life areas (Roebroeck et al 2009). YATs typically include a consultant in rehabilitation medicine, a psychologist, therapists, and a social worker. Both health problems and necessary life skills, as indicated above, will determine the goals negotiated with the young person (Chamberlain and Kent 2005). In the UK, YATS have been shown to be cost effective (Bent et al 2002). Building on participation domains of the Rotterdam Transition Profile, the Dutch centres developed a series of eight interventions for young people, focusing on various topics and life areas, including healthy lifestyle and physical fitness. A module for parents is available to encourage them to give their child the room to experience new situations and develop towards independence and autonomy. Studies of the feasibility of some of these interventions suggested preliminary positive findings, with the majority of participants achieving intervention-specific goals, such as increased levels of occupational performance and participation in paid work (work intervention), sexual self-esteem (intimate relationships), everyday physical activity (healthy lifestyle), and a stronger focus of families and professionals on the child's development of autonomy in life areas (skills for growing up) (Buffart et al 2010, Hilberink et al 2013, Verhoef et al 2013). In addition to providing developmentally appropriate transition care, YATs create the opportunity for medical checks and adequate follow-up at adult age, if needed.

Conclusion

The developmental trajectories of young people with neurological or developmental conditions can go in many directions, depending on the interaction of personal risk and protective factors with environmental barriers and supports. These interactions are most important at transition points, when a young person is dealing with significant challenges with personal and environmental changes, including the transition from paediatric healthcare to adult healthcare providers. It is through positive, developmentally appropriate life experiences throughout their childhood and adolescence, and regular opportunities for participation and inclusion, that young people with neurological and developmental conditions can prepare for a healthy, successful, and meaningful adult life.

REFERENCES

Key references

*Aisen ML, Kerkovich D, Mast J, et al (2011) Cerebral palsy: clinical care and neurological rehabilitation. *Lancet Neurol* 9: 844–852. http://dx.doi.org/10.1016/S1474-4422(11)70176-4

Arnett JJ (2004) *Emerging Adulthood. The Winding Road from the Late Teens through the Twenties*. Oxford: Oxford University Press.

Baird G, Allen E, Scrutton D, et al (2011) Mortality from 1 to 16–18 years in bilateral cerebral palsy. *Arch Dis Child* 96: 1077–1081. http://dx.doi.org/10.1136/adc.2009.172841

*Bent N, Tennant A, Swift T, Posnett J, Scuffham P, Chamberlain MA (2002) Team approach versus ad hoc health services for young people with physical disabilities: a retrospective cohort study. *Lancet* 360: 1280–1286. http://dx.doi.org/10.1016/S0140-6736(02)11316-X

Buffart LM, van den Berg-Emons HJG, van Mechelen W, et al (2010) Promoting physical activity in an adolescent and a young adult with physical disabilities. *Disabil Health J* 3: 86–92. http://dx.doi.org/10.1016/j.dhjo.2009.08.005

*Chamberlain MA, Kent RM (2005) The needs of young people with disabilities in transition from paediatric to adult services. *Eur Medicophys* 41: 111–123.

*Donkervoort M, Wiegerink DJHG, van Meeteren J, Stam HJ, Roebroeck ME, Transition Research Group South West Netherlands. (2009) Transition to adulthood: validation of the Rotterdam Transition Profile for young adults with cerebral palsy and normal intelligence. *Dev Med Child Neurol* 51: 53–62. http://dx.doi.org/10.1111/j.1469-8749.2008.03115.x

Forsgren L, Hauser WA, Olafsson E, Sander JW, Sillanpää M, Tomson T (2005) Mortality of epilepsy in developed countries: a review. *Epilepsia* 46(Suppl. 11): 18–27. http://dx.doi.org/10.1111/j.1528-1167.2005.00403.x

*Gall C, Kingsnorth S, Healy H (2006) Growing up ready: a shared management approach. *Phys Occup Ther Pediatr* 26: 47–62. http://dx.doi.org/10.1080/J006v26n04_04

Gan C, Campbell KA, Snider A, Cohen S, Hubbard J (2008) Giving Youth a Voice (GYV): a measure of youths' perceptions of the client-centredness of rehabilitation services. *Can J Occup Ther* 75: 96–104.

Gauffin H, Flensner G, Landtblom AM (2011) Living with epilepsy accompanied by cognitive difficulties: young adults' experiences. *Epilepsy Behav* 22: 750–758. http://dx.doi.org/10.1016/j.yebeh.2011.09.007

Gordon KE, Dooley JM, Sheppard KM, Macsween J, Esser MJ (2011) Impact of bisphosphonates on survival for patients with Duchenne muscular dystrophy. *Pediatrics* 127: e353–e358. http://dx.doi.org/10.1542/peds.2010-1666

Gorter JW (2009a) Rehabilitative therapies for the child with cerebral palsy: focus on family, function and fitness. *Minerva Pediatr* 4: 425–440.

Gorter JW (2009b) Transition to adult-oriented health care: perspectives of youth and adults with complex physical disabilities. *Phys Occup Ther Pediatr* 4: 362–366. http://dx.doi.org/10.3109/01942630903222100

Gorter JW (2012) Making links across the lifespan in neurology. *Can J Neurol Sci* 39: 1–2.

*Gorter JW, Stewart D, Woodbury-Smith M (2011) Youth in transition: care, health and development. *Child Care Health Dev* 37: 757–763. http://dx.doi.org/10.1111/j.1365-2214.2011.01336.x

Grant C, Pan J (2011) A comparison of five transition programmes for youth with chronic illness in Canada. *Child Care Health Dev* 37: 815–820. http://dx.doi.org/10.1111/j.1365-2214.2011.01322.x

Hilberink SR, Vos I, Roebroeck ME, Maathuis CGB (2013) Improving skills for growing up in youth with a physical disability. A feasibility and effectiveness study. Submitted for publication.

Huber M, Knottnerus JA, Green L, et al (2011) How should we define health? *BMJ* 343: d4163. http://dx.doi.org/10.1136/bmj.d4163

Kraus de Camargo O (2011) Systems of care: transition from the bio-psycho-social perspective of the International Classification of Functioning, Disability and Health. *Child Care Health Dev* 37: 792–799. http://dx.doi.org/10.1111/j.1365-2214.2011.01323.x

*Liptak GS (2008) Health and well being of adults with cerebral palsy. *Curr Opin Neurol* 21: 136–142. http://dx.doi.org/10.1097/WCO.0b013e3282f6a499

MacCulloch R (2012) *Interpreting the Myth of Independence 1: The Transition to Adulthood for Youth with Neurodevelopmental Disorders. Comprehensive Examination*. Montreal, QC: School of Social Work, McGill University.

Moola FJ, Norman ME (2011) 'Down the rabbit hole': enhancing the transition process for youth with cystic fibrosis and congenital heart disease by re-imagining the future and time. *Child Care Health Dev* 37: 841–851. http://dx.doi.org/10.1111/j.1365-2214.2011.01317.x

*Nieuwenhuijsen C, van der Laar Y, Donkervoort M, Nieuwstraten W, Roebroeck ME, Stam HJ (2008) Unmet needs and health care utilization in young adults with cerebral palsy. *Disabil Rehabil* 30: 1254–1262. http://dx.doi.org/10.1080/09638280701622929

*Nieuwenhuijsen C, Donkervoort M, Nieuwstraten W, Stam HJ, Roebroeck ME, the Transition research Group South West Netherlands (2009) Experienced problems of young adults with cerebral palsy: targets for rehabilitation care. *Arch Phys Med Rehabil* 90: 1891–1897. http://dx.doi.org/10.1016/j.apmr.2009.06.014

Oakeshott P, Hunt GM, Poulton A, Reid F (2010) Expectation of life and unexpected death in open spina bifida: a 40-year complete, non-selective, longitudinal cohort study. *Dev Med Child Neurol* 52: 749–753. http://dx.doi.org/10.1111/j.1469-8749.2009.03543.x

*Oskoui M (2012) Growing up with cerebral palsy: contemporary challenges of healthcare transition. *Can J Neurol Sci* 39: 23–25.

Palisano RJ, Shimmell LJ, Stewart D, Lawless JJ, Rosenbaum PL, Russell DJ (2009) Mobility experiences of adolescents with cerebral palsy. *Phys Occup Ther Pediatr* 29: 133–153. http://dx.doi.org/10.1080/01942630902784746

Priestly M (editor) (2001) *Disability and the Life Course. Global Perspectives*. Cambridge, UK: Cambridge University Press.

Punthakee Z, Gorter JW, for the TRACE Study Group (2011) TRansition to Adulthood with Cyber guide Evaluation (TRACE). Available at: www.canchild.ca/en/ourresearch/trace.asp (accessed 28 November 2012).

*Roebroeck ME, Jahnsen R, Carona C, Kent RM, Chamberlain MA (2009) Adult outcomes and lifespan issues for people with childhood-onset physical disability. *Dev Med Child Neurol* 51: 670–678.

Rotterdam Transition Profile (2010) Dutch en English versions. Available at: http://erasmusmc.nl/revalidatie/research/transition/ (accessed 28 November 2012).

Siebes RC, Wijnroks L, Ketelaar M, van Schie PE, Vermeer A, Gorter JW (2007) Validation of the Dutch Giving Youth a Voice Questionnaire (GYV-20): a measure of the client-centredness of rehabilitation services from an adolescent perspective. *Disabil Rehabil* 29: 373–380. http://dx.doi.org/10.1080/09638280600835218

*van Staa AL, Jedeloo S, van Meeteren J, Latour JM (2011) Crossing the transition chasm: experiences and recommendations for improving transitional care of young adults, parents and providers. *Child Care Health Dev* 37: 821–832. http://dx.doi.org/10.1111/j.1365-2214.2011.01261.x

Stewart D, Law M, Burke-Gaffney J, et al (2006) Keeping It Together: an information KIT for parents of children and youth with special needs. *Child Care Health Dev* 32: 493–500. http://dx.doi.org/10.1111/j.1365-2214.2006.00619.x

*Stewart D, Freeman M, Law M, et al (2009a) The Best Journey to Adult Life for Youth with Disabilities: An Evidence-based Model and Best Practice Guidelines for the Transition to Adulthood for Youth with Disabilities. Available at: http://transitions.canchild.ca/en/OurResearch/resources/BestPractices.pdf (accessed 28 November 2012).

Stewart D, Freeman M, Missiuna C, et al (2009b) *Keeping it Together: Youth Version.* Hamilton, ON: *CanChild* Centre for Childhood Disability Research, McMaster University.

Stewart DA, Lawless JJ, Shimmell LJ, et al (2012) Social participation of adolescents with cerebral palsy: trade-offs and choices. *Phys Occup Ther Pediatr* 32: 167–179. http://dx.doi.org/10.3109/01942638.2011.631100

Strauss DJ, Shavelle RM, Rosenbloom L, Brooks JC (2008) Life expectancy in cerebral palsy: an update. *Dev Med Child Neurol* 50: 487–493. http://dx.doi.org/10.1111/j.1469-8749.2008.03000.x

Verhoef JAC, Miedema HS, van Meeteren J, Stam HJ, Roebroeck ME (2013) A new intervention to improve work participation of young adults with physical disabilities: a feasibility study. Submitted for publication.

Verhoof E, Maurice-Stam H, Heymans H, Grootenhuis M (2012) Growing into disability benefits? Psychosocial course of life of young adults with a chronic somatic disease or disability. *Acta Paediatr* 101: e19–e26. http://dx.doi.org/10.1111/j.1651-2227

*Webb TS (2010) Optimizing health care for adults with spina bifida. *Dev Disabil Res Rev* 16: 76–81. http://dx.doi.org/10.1002/ddrr.99

Westbom L, Bergstrand L, Wagner P, Nordmark E (2011) Survival at 19 years of age in a total population of children and young people with cerebral palsy. *Dev Med Child Neurol* 53: 808–814. http://dx.doi.org/10.1111/j.1469-8749.2011.04027.x

World Health Organization (2001) *International Classification of Functioning, Disability and Health (ICF).* Geneva: WHO Press.

Young N, McCormick A, Mills W, et al (2006) The transition study: a look at youth and adults with cerebral palsy, spina bifida and acquired brain injury. *Phys Occup Ther Pediatr* 26: 25–45. http://dx.doi.org/10.1080/J006v26n04_03

*Young NL, Barden WS, Mills WA, Burke TA, Law M, Boydell K (2009) Transition to adult-oriented health care: perspectives of youth and adults with complex physical disabilities. *Phys Occup Ther Pediatr* 29: 345–361. http://dx.doi.org/10.3109/01942630903245994

*Young NL, Rochon TG, McCormick A, Law M, Wedge JH, Fehlings D (2010) The health and quality of life outcomes among youth and young adults with cerebral palsy. *Arch Phys Med Rehabil* 1: 143–148. http://dx.doi.org/10.1016/j.apmr.2009.08.152

Young NL, McCormick AM, Gilbert T, et al (2011) Reasons for hospital admissions among youth and young adults with cerebral palsy. *Arch Phys Med Rehabil* 1: 46–50. http://dx.doi.org/10.1016/j.apmr.2010.10.002

23
WHY WE NEED ADULT SPECIALISTS FOR PEOPLE WITH CHILDHOOD-ONSET NEURODEVELOPMENTAL CONDITIONS

Bernard Dan

Overview

The medical profession has become highly subspecialized. Children and young people with neurological and developmental conditions usually receive services from a variety of experts in child health, neurology, rehabilitation medicine, and so on. However, as these young people grow into adulthood there are few professionals in any of the health disciplines with experience and expertise in the needs of this group. This chapter presents the case in favour of training people to become adult specialists for the ever-growing population of people with 'developmental' conditions who are entering the 'adult' world with medical and social issues that currently are inadequately addressed. It is argued that such developments in health services will benefit both the young people who are 'graduating' from the child health arena into the world of adult health service and the adult-focused professionals who will expand their understanding of neurological and developmental issues as they concern people with these lifelong conditions.

Introduction

The notion of specialization in medical science and practice is probably as old as medicine itself, but formal systematization grossly similar to the current situation developed mostly over the course of the nineteenth century (Weisz 2003), with new additions up until recent years. It is obvious that the definition of self-contained medical specialties is to some extent arbitrary and has been occurring somewhat differently in different countries. Even within a country, there may be regional differences in the way practices are organized. The most competent available physician responsible for the care of a child with a neurodevelopmental condition might thus be a general practitioner or a specialist in paediatrics, developmental paediatrics, community paediatrics, paediatric neurology, neurology, psychiatry, or physical medicine. The title of the specialist does not necessarily equate to his or her level of expertise for this kind of clinical challenge.

To add to the complexity, medical specialties may be constructed along different axes. Whereas some are based on a particular organ or physiological system (e.g. cardiology or haematology), others deal exclusively with either surgical (e.g. neurosurgery) or internal medicine (e.g. neurology) aspects; yet others are concerned with diagnostic procedures (e.g. radiology or pathology) or therapeutic ones (e.g. radiotherapy); and some specialties are defined by the age of the patients (e.g. neonatology or gerontology). The last approach, which includes paediatrics and paediatric subspecialties, poses the specific challenge of transition between age groups if conditions persist or have a high risk of recurrence. This implies issues of knowledge transfer between specialists with regard to the specifics of the conditions but also to particular paradigms for approaching the clinical situations. Such knowledge transfer is central to the reasoning that should govern the care for individuals with childhood-onset neurodevelopmental conditions. Surprisingly, not only is knowledge transfer between practising specialists often poor in this area, but the very question of training professionals to care effectively for individuals with childhood-onset neurodevelopmental conditions who are now adults has been at best marginal in the vast majority of actual practices or training programmes. As a result, healthcare services for these adults lack the evidence-based grounding that exists for many adult-onset conditions, and practitioners are ill prepared to identify and meet their needs.

For want of more suitable options, a proportion of adults with childhood-onset neurodevelopmental conditions continue to be followed by their paediatrician under the assumption that paediatric care embraces 'all ages and stages of development from foetus to mature organism, to include the adult survivors of childhood disorders' (Johnson et al 2001, p. 1). But, paraphrasing the paediatric motto that 'children are not small adults', *adults with neurodevelopmental impairments are not big children with developmental impairments*. They have different needs and are confronted with different challenges. There have been attempts to train medical specialists in the care of individuals with developmental impairments across their lifespan with some remarkable local successes (Palmer et al 2003). Such a role was recognized by the American Board of Medical Subspecialties in 1999. The 4-year curriculum includes adult neurology, child neurology/developmental impairments, and related basic and clinical neuroscience. Dedicated multidisciplinary teams for young adults with conditions such as cerebral palsy, spina bifida, and muscular dystrophy have been developed in some places in the UK (Kent and Chamberlain 2004) and elsewhere. This approach, coupled with effective transition programmes, led to markedly increased participation in society among people with neurodisabilities at no additional financial cost compared with non-coordinated care (Bent et al 2002). Unfortunately, the availability of these specialists and settings is currently very limited. It may therefore be important to consider the inclusion of training on neurodevelopmental conditions in the curriculum of the medical specialties that are likely to provide healthcare service to adults with such impairments, although developmental impairment is not their primary focus.

Why train adult specialists on neurodevelopmental conditions?
There are many reasons why it has appeared relevant to promote sharing of information between professionals involved in the care of children and adults with neurodevelopmental conditions. The most obvious one is the recognition that chronic disorders that first manifest

in childhood persist in adulthood, where they pose particular challenges. It must also be recognized that abnormalities of neurological functions manifest differently if they occur early during development or result from the loss of established function as typical in adult neurology (see also Chapter 6). One of the most striking aspects is often the combination of disturbances that affect multiple neurological systems, resulting in motor, sensory, cognitive, and behavioural symptomatology. This has been conceptualized as comorbidity (Bax and Gillberg 2010). Furthermore, some of the manifestations that characterize neurodevelopmental conditions – for example, depression and epilepsy – may resolve to a large extent or not appear during childhood or adolescence but become problematic (again) in later life. Another reason is the fact that management has evolved to constitute a complex, coordinated approach involving multiple disciplines for addressing issues that arise in children. This approach differs considerably from the way in which services are commonly offered to adults with the same conditions. This evolution raises difficult questions when transition to adult care is considered, but it may also prove inspiring for optimizing the care of adults with impairments.

BECAUSE CHILDHOOD-ONSET NEUROLOGICAL CONDITIONS PERSIST IN ADULTHOOD
The persistence of childhood-onset neurological conditions is not due to defective management; on the contrary it is associated with increased longevity related to better handling of life-threatening complications. Individuals with conditions that used to be consistently lethal in childhood, such as spina bifida and Duchenne muscular dystrophy, may now survive well into adulthood. There have also been dramatic improvements in survival in relatively common neurological conditions, such as cerebral palsy (Stevenson et al 1997, Strauss et al 2007). Some authors have argued that 'the true extent of handicap from many childhood disorders can only be known in adulthood' (Johnson et al 2001). However, the consequences of such conditions in adulthood are often poorly understood (Rosenbaum 2003). Relative professional ignorance is even more marked in rarer conditions for which the natural history has been poorly or not at all documented, so that notions of clinical features in the adult are based on limited anecdotal reports, at best, or on misconceptions. For example, several reviews have stated lifespan to be normal in Angelman syndrome in reference to isolated mentions of patients in relatively good health in their seventies. This notion is not based on any systematic studies and would be inconsistent with the shortening of life expectancy commonly associated with the decreased mobility, severe scoliosis, dysphagia, aspiration, or severe epilepsy that concern a significant proportion of adults with this syndrome (Dan 2008, Roebroeck et al 2009). When data do exist, they may show that improved survival has not been linear, or has closely followed changes in identified factors (e.g. in Rett syndrome [Freilinger et al 2010]). It must be noted that, regardless of the prevalence of the individual conditions, collectively they represent significant numbers of patients that could potentially present to the adult medicine practitioners.

BECAUSE NEUROLOGICAL FEATURES ARE DIFFERENT IN CHILDHOOD-ONSET CONDITIONS
Some clinical manifestations of neurological insult may be different depending on whether the insult occurred during early development or in later life, probably owing to maturational factors, brain plasticity, and the influence of experiential factors. This is one of the main

justifications for defining cerebral palsy (Rosenbaum et al 2007). It has also called for some specific definitions of abnormal motor features in which the application of phenomenology from common adult neurology proved ineffective or confusing (Sanger et al 2003, 2006). The distinction between developmental and later-acquired dysfunction has been usefully entrenched in nosography in selected areas, e.g. dysphasia or dyspraxia (with the prefix dys-implying a developmental disorder) have different causes, features, and implications from aphasia or apraxia, respectively (with the prefix a- implying loss of previously acquired function). Many of the developmental conditions remain specific in affected adults. For example, adults with hemiplegic cerebral palsy show distinctive motor patterns compared with adults with stroke. Another important aspect in neurodevelopmental conditions is the fact that they may present with a dysfunction of multiple neurological circuits. These abnormalities may each reflect a 'primary' neurological lesion or disruption, or occur as a consequence of activity limitations that restrict learning and perceptual development experiences (Rosenbaum et al 2007).

Furthermore, while neurodevelopmental conditions persist in adulthood, there are varying emphases on symptoms that call for specific management. For example, fatigue and pain, which are rarely in the forefront in children with cerebral palsy, often become predominant complaints in adults (Turk et al 1997, Jahnsen et al 2004, Opheim et al 2009). On the contrary, some elements of the behavioural phenotype may be very disruptive in children (such as the exuberance and overactivity seen in fetal alcohol syndrome, Rett syndrome, or Angelman syndrome) and improve or disappear altogether after adolescence (Streissguth et al 1985, Pelc et al 2008a, Smeets et al 2012). In some conditions (e.g. Rett syndrome or Angelman syndrome) the seizure disorder may appear to resolve in adolescence (this used to be a common notion), but it often recurs in adults in whom it may be difficult to recognize (Clayton-Smith 2001, Pelc et al 2008b). The patients' needs also change with age in relation to natural history, personal, and societal factors. Self-perceived health-related quality of life has been found to be significantly lower in adolescents and adults with cerebral palsy, particularly with respect to the physical domain (Bjornson et al 2008, Gaskin et al 2008, van der Slot et al 2010).

BECAUSE OF THE NEED FOR TRANSITION FROM PAEDIATRIC CARE

The delivery of health care to children and adolescents who have neurodevelopmental conditions requires sharing of expertise among multiple disciplines (Patel et al 2008). In addition to the child and his or her family, there may be a host of specialists involved in this care, including a paediatrician, a paediatric neurologist, an orthopaedic surgeon, a physical therapist, a speech and communication therapist, an occupational therapist, a clinical psychologist, a neuropsychologist, an orthotist, an ear, nose, and throat specialist, an audiologist, an ophthalmologist, an orthoptist, a psychiatrist, a psychologist, a neurosurgeon, a social worker, a teacher, and more. In many settings, ways have been developed to favour interaction and coordination between the involved persons through the processes of evaluation, setting of objectives, intervention, and reappraisal. In spite of all this investment in childhood, many patients are lost to specialized follow-up when they become adults.

Several studies have found dramatically diminished contact with healthcare professionals after leaving school (Stevenson et al 1997, Ng et al 2003). Transition from paediatric to adult care is rarely organized. Many young adults with a neurodevelopmental condition lack the social skills to maintain services themselves (Cappelli et al 1999) and seek medical services only in an emergency (Viner 1999). As a result, adult healthcare professionals are usually unfamiliar with the conditions. There is abundant evidence that those lost to follow-up present later with treatable complications of their condition (Bax et al 1988). Therefore, there is a need for careful consideration of the issues relating to changeover in order to respond to the specific needs of adults with neurodevelopmental conditions. As with other chronic conditions, this transition should be an occasion for thorough reappraisal. The adult specialist might then note some long-overlooked aspect in the patient's history or clinical/paraclinical features that may lead people to question the diagnosis or prompt new management. The length of previous follow-up does not guarantee diagnostic accuracy. It carries implications for prognosis, genetic counselling, and management. As already mentioned, because many neurodevelopmental conditions have multisystem involvement and sequelae, multiprofessional care is often required. The existing paradigm that has been developed for child-focused services may serve as a model for optimizing adult care.

Who should be the focus of adult specialist training about neurodevelopmental conditions?

Many different healthcare professionals may be involved in the preventative (including secondary and tertiary prevention), curative (of some features that are part of the symptom complex), promotional, or rehabilitative services. All these professionals should have access to appropriate training in order to understand and meet the needs of adults with neurodevelopmental conditions. Furthermore, there is a case for systematically including more specific tuition in the curriculum for specialist training in medical (or paramedical) specialties that are directly concerned with those individuals' clinical presentation. These obviously include neurology, considering the primary problems and the orderly clinical method for approaching patients with disorders of the nervous system that characterize this specialty. Neurologists are best skilled in integrating clinical features with their neuroanatomical, neurophysiological, and neuropathological knowledge to propose adequate management, although most have little notion of or experience with neurodevelopmental conditions.

Another obvious discipline is physical medicine and rehabilitation, although the term 'habilitation' is more accurate in this context. It has been argued that specialists in rehabilitation medicine are particularly suitably placed as they have the diagnostic and management skills necessary to ensure the required coordination of health care (Chamberlain 2003). They liaise with other medical and surgical specialties. Their basic training allows them to identify and treat health problems such as musculoskeletal complications, pain, spasticity, and urological, as well as neurological, problems. They are used to analysing gait and posture and prescribing orthoses, adapted seating, and assistive technology. Orthopaedic surgeons are confronted with musculoskeletal problems that develop insidiously in a large proportion of individuals with neurodevelopmental conditions, most typically (but not exclusively) cerebral palsy.

Orthopaedic problems are very varied, including muscle/tendon contractures, bony torsion, hip displacement, and spinal deformity and are highly dependent on developmental factors that are completely absent from most conditions treated by orthopaedic surgeons. It has been stressed that they may not manifest fully until later life, when they can become the most dominant feature affecting mobility, physical well-being, and quality of life (Graham 2006). Patella alta, hip dysplasia, spondylolysis, and cervical stenosis are common progressive problems in adults with cerebral palsy (Murphy 2009). Recent data also indicate that comprehensive spasticity management, including botulinum toxin injections and orthopaedic surgery, provides meaningful improvement in self-performance and care delivery in activities of daily living in adults with intellectual impairment (Charles et al 2010). Similarly, psychiatrists would certainly be better equipped to treat the mood disorders, anxiety disorders, autistic spectrum disorder, and the host of behavioural problems that may be the most pervasive manifestations in adults with neurodevelopmental conditions.

The development of neurosurgical treatments for selected features that are common in adults with neurodevelopmental conditions, such as intrathecal baclofen therapy for severe spasticity, raises similar questions for neurosurgeons. Just as they need to be trained about adult-onset multiple sclerosis and stroke to optimize their eventual involvement with affected patients, they should know about cerebral palsy and neurodevelopmental conditions in the management of which they might play an important role. It has also been suggested that revision of ventricular shunts for hydrocephalus or posterior fossa decompression in spina bifida prompted by regular, careful monitoring of adolescents and adults with myelomeningocoele has decisive effects on the prevention of scoliosis (Rowe and Jadhav 2008). Urology and gynaecology should also be considered. In addition to these medical specialties, a number of allied professions should benefit from such basic training, including physical therapy, occupational therapy, speech and communication therapy (which also addresses feeding issues), orthotics, social care, etc. Such training could also be integrated into the training for organized interdisciplinary problem-based approaches in which fine understanding of underlying conditions is essential, such as pain clinics (see also Chapter 20).

What should be the focus of adult specialist training on neurodevelopmental conditions?

Historically, the field of neurodevelopmental impairments has evolved on a firm foundation of basic and clinical neurosciences (Palmer et al 2003). In order to optimize medical care of adults with neurodevelopmental conditions, involved professionals should be informed about the pathophysiology, clinical features, and management of these conditions and what is known of their repercussions in adulthood. They should also understand the developmental perspective that guides the paediatric approach to these conditions and its incidence on the lifelong scale (see also Chapter 6). In many situations, the very question of the definition of adulthood is essentially based (somewhat arbitrarily) on age rather than on the common psychological and societal connotations of autonomy. Indeed, the transition to adult services can be seen and stressed as a part of the rites of passage into adulthood (Schidlow and Fiel 1990). No less importantly, they should be aware of the conceptual and pragmatic framework in which this approach has developed, including reference to the International Classification of Functioning, Disability and Health (ICF), to quality of life issues, to the family-centred approach, and to the essentially team-based approach, also integrating education and social services. Professionals in training should acquire skills enabling them to plan appropriately and implement investigations and therapies, counsel patients and their relatives, follow them up, and develop a supportive role. They should become familiar with a number of ethical issues, including autonomy in decision making and end-of-life issues. They should also be encouraged to engage in societal advocacy for people with disabilities.

A recent categorization was proposed to address the adult outcome of selected paediatric neurological conditions (Camfield and Camfield 2011). Some of it might serve as a base for discussing neurodevelopmental conditions in a relevant way. In this categorization, Duchenne muscular dystrophy is suggested as the epitome of *disorders that were previously lethal in childhood and have (non-curative) treatments that allow survival into adulthood*. It illustrates a number of the points we have made in this chapter. Advances in therapy (Deconinck and Dan 2007) have indeed improved life expectancy so that about 85% of patients now live up to at least 35 years of age (Kohler et al 2009). As a result, some features, such as cardiomyopathy, become more apparent and must be recognized as being treatable. Expertise from multiple disciplines is required, including adult neurology, rehabilitation medicine, pulmonology, and cardiology, as well as various aspects of therapy and social services. Optimal management can probably be organized within an adult neuromuscular clinic.

There are also *disorders that are cured in childhood but have neurological sequelae that persist in adulthood*, such as brain tumours (Macedoni-Luksic et al 2003) and sickle cell anaemia (Ferster et al 1995). In these patients, neurological issues may be very complex and require special expertise. Another category concerns *disorders that are static in childhood but progress in adulthood*, with cerebral palsy as an illustration. The idea that cerebral palsy has a static course in childhood needs to be qualified. Although it must be distinguished from conditions that are due to pathophysiological mechanisms that remain active (Rosenbaum et al 2007), its clinical manifestations have long been noted to be 'persisting but not unchanging' (Mac Keith et al 1959), particularly in childhood. However, this category rightly stresses the risk for significant deterioration in adults (Dan 2007, Day et al 2007). Down syndrome would also belong to this tentative category, allowing emphasis on the possibilities for treatment of adult-onset Alzheimer disease (Costa 2012) and poorly recognized disorders such as senile myoclonic epilepsy (De Simone et al 2010).

Close to this category are *disorders diagnosed in childhood with their most serious manifestations in adulthood*, typified by neurofibromatosis type 1. Cerebrovascular disease, sarcomas, and renal failure are among the serious complications that begin in adult life in this condition. They contribute to restricting median survival to 59 years in the USA (Rasmussen et al 2001). This category would also include tuberous sclerosis complex in which, in addition to epilepsy, renal disease may become prominent in adulthood. Many childhood epilepsies would be included in *disorders that may or may not remit in childhood but have persistent effects on adult social function*. This categorization scheme also holds a special place for intellectual disability as part of *disorders that may be uncomfortable for adult care* because affected adults tend to be 'known well by no one' (Bigby 2008), an emblematic formulation that seems to substantiate the need to train adult specialists about neurodevelopmental conditions.

How should adult specialists be trained about neurodevelopmental conditions?

In order to improve healthcare management for people with neurodevelopmental impairments throughout their lifespan, we strongly suggest that specific programmes addressing childhood-onset neurological and developmental conditions should be designed and integrated into basic adult medicine training. These programmes should cover the domains described above. They should be primarily tailored to those engaging in general medicine and a number of medical specialties, including neurology, physical and rehabilitation medicine, orthopaedic surgery, neurosurgery, and psychiatry. In addition to a common core, each of these programmes should address speciality-specific issues. Setting up these programmes will imply hands-on clinical teaching with residency rotations in departments where children with neurodevelopmental disorders are cared for, thereby creating the necessary dynamic contacts between paediatric and adult medical specialities. This dynamic could be entertained through common meetings and also through the editorial policies of journals encouraging publication of articles relating to issues throughout the lifespan. In turn, paediatric specialists would learn much from their adult care colleagues. All this is also important for allied healthcare professions. As one of the key messages in these programmes is precisely interdisciplinarity, constant interaction should be promoted during the programmes (see also Chapter 20).

In addition to the inclusion of these programmes within the training curriculum of general practitioners and selected medical and surgical specialties, a more general programme should be designed to be of interest to any established practitioner who wishes to acquire skills to provide better health care to adults with neurodevelopmental conditions.

Given the advances in basic and clinical research, adult specialist training about neurodevelopmental conditions should also be proposed in the form of continuing education. This effort will undoubtedly create a context for documentation, audit, and research, which will also contribute to overall progress in the care for people with neurodevelopmental disabilities. Hopefully, improved competence in adult specialists will result in the empowerment of affected individuals.

Conclusion

In a not-so-distant past, rehabilitation was sometimes called the Cinderella of neurological research (Tesio et al 1995) by reference to the fairytale character who gets undeservedly neglected despite her merits and is forced into a wretched and obscure existence. Hopefully, this negative image has been dispelled following several decades of re-examination of needs, clinical practice, technological developments, sound scientific research, and training programmes. Active research into the rehabilitation of many neurological conditions such as stroke, multiple sclerosis, Parkinson disease, spinal injury, and amyotrophic lateral sclerosis, to name but a few, has dramatically improved functional outcomes, and both the underlying science and the pragmatic aspects of management are now part of neurologists' basic training. The Cinderella metaphor has also been discussed in relation to the habilitation of children with neurodevelopmental conditions (Soares Pinto et al 2005); again it can be hoped to have been largely dissipated following similar efforts that have led to strengthening a holistic approach to the child, integrating medical, social, and educational factors, tightly coupled with principles of evidence-based practice taking into account the complexity of these factors (Dan 2010).

The current challenge is to improve these patients' quality of life significantly throughout their lifespan. To achieve this goal, no intervention by a fairy godmother is expected, but rather the active implementation of adapted high-quality habilitation services for adults with neuro-developmental conditions in adult health care. To this end, medical and paramedical adult specialists should be trained in order to identify patients' needs and develop the appropriate expertise to meet them.

REFERENCES

Bax C, Gillberg M (2010) *Comorbidities in Developmental Disorders*. London: Mac Keith Press.

Bax MC, Smyth DP, Thomas AP (1988) Health care of physically handicapped young adults. *BMJ* 296: 1153–1155.

Bent N, Tennant A, Swift T, Posnett J, Scuffham P, Chamberlain MA (2002) Team approach versus ad hoc health services for young people with physical disabilities: a retrospective cohort study. *Lancet* 360: 1280–1286. http://dx.doi.org/10.1016/S0140-6736(02)11316-X

Bigby C (2008) Known well by no-one: trends in the informal social networks of middle-aged and older people with intellectual disability five years after moving to the community. *J Intellect Dev Disabil* 33: 148–157. http://dx.doi.org/10.1080/13668250802094141

Bjornson KF, Belza B, Kartin D, Logsdon RG, McLaughlin J (2008) Self-reported health status and quality of life in youth with cerebral palsy and typically developing youth. *Arch Phys Med Rehabil* 89: 121–127. http://dx.doi.org/10.1016/j.apmr.2007.09.016

Camfield P, Camfield C (2011) Transition to adult care for children with chronic neurological disorders. *Ann Neurol* 69: 437–444. http://dx.doi.org/10.1002/ana.22393

Cappelli M, MacDonald NE, McGrath PJ (1999) Assessment of readiness to transfer to adult care for adolescents with cystic fibrosis. *Child Health Care* 18: 218–224. http://dx.doi.org/10.1207/s15326888chc1804_4

Chamberlain MA (2003) Advances in rehabilitation: an overview and an odyssey. *Clin Med* 3: 62–67.

Charles PD, Gill CE, Taylor HM, et al (2010) Spasticity treatment facilitates direct care delivery for adults with profound intellectual disability. *Mov Disord* 25: 466–473. http://dx.doi.org/10.1002/mds.22995

Clayton-Smith J (2001) Angelman syndrome: evolution of the phenotype in adolescents and adults. *Dev Med Child Neurol* 43: 476–480. http://dx.doi.org/10.1017/S0012162201000871

Costa AC (2012) Alzheimer disease: treatment of Alzheimer disease in Down syndrome. *Nat Rev Neurol* 8: 182–184. http://dx.doi.org/10.1038/nrneurol.2012.40

Dan B (2007) Progressive course in cerebral palsy? *Dev Med Child Neurol* 49: 644. http://dx.doi.org/10.1111/j.1469-8749.2007.00644.x

Dan B (2008) *Angelman Syndrome*. London: Mac Keith Press.

Dan B (2010) Measuring outcomes: an ethical premise in management of childhood disability. *Dev Med Child Neurol* 52: 501. http://dx.doi.org/10.1111/j.1469-8749.2010.03688.x

Day SM, Wu YW, Strauss DJ, Shavelle RM, Reynolds RJ (2007) Change in ambulatory ability of adolescents and young adults with cerebral palsy. *Dev Med Child Neurol* 49: 647–653. http://dx.doi.org/10.1111/j.1469-8749.2007.00647.x

De Simone R, Puig XS, Gélisse P, Crespel A, Genton P (2010) Senile myoclonic epilepsy: delineation of a common condition associated with Alzheimer's disease in Down syndrome. *Seizure* 19: 383–389. http://dx.doi.org/10.1016/j.seizure.2010.04.008

Deconinck N, Dan B (2007) Pathophysiology of Duchenne muscular dystrophy: current hypotheses. *Pediatr Neurol* 36: 1–7. http://dx.doi.org/10.1016/j.pediatrneurol.2006.09.016

Ferster A, Christophe C, Dan B, Devalck C, Sariban E (1995) Neurological complications after bone marrow transplantation for sickle cell anaemia. *Blood* 86: 408–409.

Freilinger M, Bebbington A, Lanator I, et al (2010) Survival with Rett syndrome: comparing Rett's original sample with data from the Australian Rett Syndrome Database. *Dev Med Child Neurol* 52: 962–965. http://dx.doi.org/10.1111/j.1469-8749.2010.03716.x

Gaskin CJ, Morris T (2008) Physical activity, health-related quality of life, and psychosocial functioning of adults with cerebral palsy. *J Phys Act Health* 5: 146–157.

Graham HK (2006) Absence of reference to progressive musculoskeletal pathology in definition of cerebral palsy. *Dev Med Child Neurol* 48: 78–79. http://dx.doi.org/10.1017/S0012162206220164

Jahnsen R, Villien L, Stanghelle JK, Holm I (2003) Fatigue in adults with cerebral palsy in Norway compared with the general population. *Dev Med Child Neurol* 45: 296–303. http://dx.doi.org/10.1111/j.1469-8749.2003.tb00399.x

Johnson DA, Rivlin E, Stein DG (2001) Paediatric rehabilitation: improving recovery and outcome in childhood disorders. *Pediatr Rehabil* 4: 1–3.

Kent RM, Chamberlain MA (2004) Transition from paediatric to adult neurological services. *J Neurol Neurosurg Psychiatry* 75: 1208. http://dx.doi.org/10.1136/jnnp.2003.033076

Kohler M, Clarenbach CF, Bahler C, Brack T, Russi EW, Bloch KE (2009) Disability and survival in Duchenne muscular dystrophy. *J Neurol Neurosurg Psychiatry* 80: 320–325. http://dx.doi.org/10.1136/jnnp.2007.141721

Macedoni-Luksic M, Jereb B, Todorovski L (2003) Long-term sequelae in children treated for brain tumours: impairments, disability, and handicap. *Pediatr Hematol Oncol* 20: 89–101. http://dx.doi.org/10.1080/0880010390158595

MacKeith RC, MacKenzie ICK, Polani PE (1959) The Little Club Memorandum on terminology and classification of 'cerebral palsy'. *Cereb Palsy Bull* 1: 27–35.

Murphy KP (2009) Cerebral palsy lifetime care: four musculoskeletal conditions. *Dev Med Child Neurol* 51(Suppl. 4): 30–37. http://dx.doi.org/10.1111/j.1469-8749.2009.03431.x

Ng SY, Dinesh SK, Tay SK, Lee EH (2003) Decreased access to health care and social isolation among young adults with cerebral palsy after leaving school. *J Orthop Surg* 11: 80–89.

Opheim A, Jahnsen R, Olsson E, Stanghelle JK (2009) Walking function, pain, and fatigue in adults with cerebral palsy: a 7-year follow-up study. *Dev Med Child Neurol* 51: 381–388. http://dx.doi.org/10.1111/j.1469-8749.2008.03250.x

Palmer FB, Percy AK, Tivnan P, Juul D, Tunnessen WW, Scheiber SC (2003) Certification in neurodevelopmental disabilities: the development of a new subspecialty and results of the initial examinations. *Ment Retard Dev Disabil Res Rev* 9: 128–131. http://dx.doi.org/10.1002/mrdd.10069

Patel DR, Pratt HD, Patel ND (2008) Team processes and team care for children with developmental disabilities. *Pediatr Clin North Am* 55: 1375–1390. http://dx.doi.org/10.1016/j.pcl.2008.09.002

Pelc K, Cheron G, Dan B (2008a) Behaviour and neuropsychiatric manifestations in Angelman syndrome. *Neuropsychiatr Dis Treat* 4: 577–584.

Pelc K, Boyd SG, Cheron G, Dan B (2008b) Epilepsy in Angelman syndrome. *Seizure* 17: 211–217. http://dx.doi.org/10.1016/j.seizure.2007.08.004

Rasmussen SA, Yang Q, Friedman JM (2001) Mortality in neurofibromatosis 1: an analysis using U.S. death certificates. *Am J Hum Genet* 68: 1110–1118. http://dx.doi.org/10.1086/320121

Roebroeck ME, Jahnsen R, Carona C, Kent RM, Chamberlain MA (2009) Adult outcomes and lifespan issues for people with childhood-onset physical disability. *Dev Med Child Neurol* 51: 670–678. http://dx.doi.org/10.1111/j.1469-8749.2009.03322.x

Rosenbaum P (2003) Cerebral palsy: what parents and doctors want to know. *BMJ* 326: 970–974. http://dx.doi.org/10.1136/bmj.326.7396.970

Rosenbaum P, Paneth N, Leviton A, et al (2007) A report: the definition and classification of cerebral palsy April 2006. *Dev Med Child Neurol* 109(Suppl.): 8–14.

Rowe DE, Jadhav AL (2008) Care of the adolescent with spina bifida. *Pediatr Clin North Am* 55: 1359–1374. http://dx.doi.org/10.1016/j.pcl.2008.09.001

Sanger TD, Delgado MR, Gaebler-Spira D, Hallett M, Mink JW, Taskforce on Childhood Motor Disorders (2003) Classification and definition of disorders causing hypertonia in childhood. *Pediatrics* 111: e89–e97. http://dx.doi.org/10.1542/peds.111.1.e89

Sanger TD, Chen D, Delgado MR, et al (2006) Definition and classification of negative motor signs in childhood. *Pediatrics* 118: 2159–2167. http://dx.doi.org/10.1542/peds.2005-3016

Schidlow DV, Fiel SB (1990) Life beyond paediatrics. *Med Clin North Am* 74: 1113–1120.

van der Slot WMA, Nieuwenhuijsen C, van den Berg-Emons RJ, et al (2010) Participation and health-related quality of life in adults with spastic bilateral cerebral palsy and the role of self-efficacy. *J Rehabil Med* 42: 528–535. http://dx.doi.org/10.2340/16501977-0555

Smeets EE, Pelc K, Dan B (2012) Rett syndrome. *Mol Syndromol* 2: 113–117.

Soares Pinto K, Ponte Rocha A, Bonfim Coutinho AC, Mafra Gonçalves D, Siebra Beraldo PS (2005) Is rehabilitation the Cinderella of health, education and social services for children? *Dev Neurorehabil* 8: 33–43. http://dx.doi.org/10.1080/13638490400011173

Stevenson CJ, Pharoah PO, Stevenson R (1997) Cerebral palsy: the transition from youth to adulthood. *Dev Med Child Neurol* 39: 336–342. http://dx.doi.org/10.1111/j.1469-8749.1997.tb07441.x

Strauss D, Shavelle R, Reynolds R, Rosenbloom L, Day S (2007) Survival in cerebral palsy in the last 20 years: signs of improvement? *Dev Med Child Neurol* 49: 86–92. http://dx.doi.org/10.1111/j.1469-8749.2007.00086.x

Streissguth AP, Clarren SK, Jones KL (1985) Natural history of the fetal alcohol syndrome: a 10-year follow-up of eleven patients. *Lancet* 2: 85–91. http://dx.doi.org/10.1016/S0140-6736(85)90189-8

Tesio L, Gamba C, Capelli A, Franchignoni FP (1995) Rehabilitation: the Cinderella of neurological research? A bibliometric study. *Ital J Neurol Sci* 16: 473–477. http://dx.doi.org/10.1007/BF02229325

Turk MA, Geremski CA, Rosenbaum PF, Weber RJ (1997) The health status of women with cerebral palsy. *Arch Phys Med Rehabil* 78(Suppl. 5): 10–17. http://dx.doi.org/10.1016/S0003-9993(97)90216-1

Viner R (1999) Transition from paediatric to adult care. Bridging the gap or passing the buck? *Arch Dis Child* 81: 271–275. http://dx.doi.org/10.1136/adc.81.3.271

Weisz G (2003) The emergence of medical specialization in the nineteenth century. *Bull Hist Med* 77: 536–574. http://dx.doi.org/10.1353/bhm.2003.0150

24
LONGITUDINAL AND POPULATION-BASED APPROACHES TO STUDY THE LIFELONG TRAJECTORIES OF CHILDREN WITH NEURODEVELOPMENTAL CONDITIONS

Jenny Downs and Helen Leonard

Overview

In this chapter we discuss the use of population-based study designs, including those with a longitudinal component, to better understand trajectories and outcomes for children with developmental and childhood-onset neurological conditions. We argue that population-based studies are critical to overcome the selection bias seen in many clinical samples and to identify true variability within a condition. We discuss how longitudinal studies allow for monitoring of children's growth and development over time, both to look forward to accrue important prognostic information and to look back to assess the antecedents of outcomes. We advocate that longitudinal studies be continued into adulthood to work towards an understanding of the successful ageing of children with a developmental and childhood-onset neurological condition. Finally, we illustrate the arguments with the methodology and outcomes of the Australian Rett Syndrome Study, an example of research that combines population-based study methodology with a longitudinal follow-up component.

Introduction

Formative studies by pioneering investigators such as Jean Piaget (1927), Arnold Gesell (1928), and Ronald Illingworth (1963) laid the foundation for our modern understanding of child development, which throughout the latter half of the twentieth century began to view biological factors and the environment as complementary influences. This important principle has been applied to our understanding of the progress of children who are developing atypically (World Health Organization 2001). Continuing into the twenty-first century, there have been dramatic developments in the field of molecular biology, including understanding of the genome and the structure of specific genetic mutations, and their downstream effects on the biology of cellular and organ function. As a result a causative genetic mechanism has been identified in many intellectual impairment disorders of previous unknown aetiology. However, genetic pathways can also be modifiable by epigenetic influences, which include biological effects and developmental experiences in the social environment (Champagne 2010). A complex set of factors influences how our children, with or without an impairment, grow and develop, and both nature and nurture have key roles to play.

Concomitantly, research methodologies have become more sophisticated, enabling the study of diverse influences over time. One key methodology particularly relevant to child development is that of the longitudinal study, a design that essentially studies a large group of participants (a cohort) at multiple time points over many years (Last 2001). Longitudinal data are collected for multiple purposes. A longitudinal data set enables researchers and clinicians not only to look forward to predict future abilities and needs but also to look back at the antecedents of later outcomes. Looking forward, longitudinal studies can accrue important prognostic information for clinicians and guidance for families.

The parents of a young child with a newly diagnosed condition will have questions about what to expect for their child's future – whether their child will walk or talk, how current medical needs will progress with time, and what sort of treatments will result in the best outcomes. These questions will change as the child grows older – for example, what is the best way to support educational needs during school years, what can my child look forward to as an adult, and what are the important ingredients in order for my child to have and maintain a good quality of life? In contrast to cross-sectional studies, longitudinal studies can help to find answers to questions such as these. Looking back, one can compare specific outcomes of those who have received previous management strategies such as physiotherapy, medications, or surgery to those who did not receive these treatments, after adjusting for relevant confounders. Population-based studies are those in which cases are ascertained from a defined geographical population (Last 2001). Used in conjunction with modern statistical methods to model longitudinal data, a population-based study that includes a longitudinal component represents powerful design methodology.

This chapter will review the use of population-based and longitudinal studies of children with neurological and developmental conditions and illustrate the key theoretical principles using the example of the Australian Rett Syndrome Study.

Developmental and childhood-onset neurological conditions

Developmental and childhood-onset neurological conditions are those in which nervous system structure and function are adversely affected during growth and development in childhood. They are usually chronic in nature and are generally associated with varying degrees of intellectual as well as behavioural, motor, and/or sensory impairments. Their cause(s) is not always clear. However, many discrete disorders such as Rett syndrome, Down syndrome, and fragile X syndrome are now known to have a specific genetic aetiology. Less commonly the aetiology is environmental, e.g. fetal alcohol syndrome or congenital rubella syndrome. Other groups of disorders such as autism and cerebral palsy are defined according to their behavioural or motor characteristics and are heterogeneous in their aetiology (Bishop 2010). Finally, some children are exposed to factors that place them at a higher risk of poorer neurodevelopmental outcomes, e.g. preterm birth (Saigal and Doyle 2008).

Using the framework of the International Classification of Functioning, Disability and Health (ICF) (World Health Organization 2001), a neurological disorder may be associated with impairments such as altered muscle tone, dyspraxia, poor balance, and impaired coordination; limited functional abilities in relation to everyday activities such as mobility, communication, and learning; and restricted opportunities for educational, social, and recreational participation. There are additional influences from personal and contextual factors, e.g. those relating to the social, economic, and physical environment. These factors will have complex relationships within each child and family, and can change with time (Berkman and Kawachi 2000). Multivariable analyses are needed to determine associations among these factors and the very important outcomes of quality of life and well-being for both children and their families. (For more detailed information readers are directed to Chapters 2–5.)

At present there are no cures for most neurodevelopmental disorders. The needs of the child and family are complex, and careful planning is needed across the lifespan to assist management on a day-to-day basis and plan for future needs. A systematic review of the volume of research conducted on specific neurodevelopmental conditions, including those that are discrete and those associated with a more heterogeneous aetiology, found that the number of publications varies by condition and by the severity of the condition (Bishop 2010). For example, there has been a recent steep increase in published research about autism; a substantial body of research continues to be published for conditions such as cerebral palsy, epilepsy, and Down syndrome; but there is less research on fetal alcohol syndrome and intellectual impairments of unknown cause. The volume of genetic research has risen dramatically, although with less growth in clinical research; rather, studies are more frequently conducted in rare severe genetic conditions, although even this is patchy, with some conditions, e.g. Noonan syndrome, being less well researched (Bishop 2010). Thus far, research can provide some guidance in the management of neurological and developmental conditions but much more is needed to fully address family needs.

Population-based study for neurological and developmental conditions

Population studies are those in which cases are ascertained from a defined geographical population (Last 2001). They thus avoid the selection bias inherent in most clinical samples whereby those who are more severely affected are more likely to be included. There are two mechanisms for studying neurological and developmental conditions in a population framework. The first involves setting up a population-based register in which there is a mechanism for ascertaining all cases of the condition within a geographical area. In the absence of a population-based register, record linkage can also be used to define cases with specific criteria, e.g. children on medication for epilepsy. The second involves following a total birth cohort or a subsection thereof and identifying at what point the children develop the condition of interest. This can also be done using a variety of strategies including record linkage.

One example of a population-based register is the Australian Rett Syndrome Study in which there is ongoing ascertainment of the Australian population of girls and women with Rett syndrome as described in detail later in the chapter. There are surprisingly few other registers involving discrete disorders associated with intellectual impairment. However, the birth incidence, prevalence, and mortality of Prader–Willi syndrome in the UK have been estimated using population-based data. Multiple ascertainment strategies including contact with health, education, and social services professionals and the UK Prader–Willi Association were used to identify all known individuals with Prader–Willi syndrome who lived in a region of the UK comprising eight counties and approximately 5 million people (Whittington et al 2001).

Another example of a population-based register is the Intellectual Disability Exploring Answers (IDEA) database, which ascertains all individuals with intellectual impairments in Western Australia (WA) (Petterson et al 2005) and is one of the few databases of its kind in the world. Unique cases are identified from two overlapping administrative sources, the Disability Services Commission, the state government organization in Western Australia providing services for children and adults with intellectual disabilities, and/or the Western Australia Department of Education, which provides education services for children with special needs. A recent record linkage study using data from this and other sources compared maternal risk factors for children with intellectual impairment and autism. Mothers of children with mild to moderate intellectual impairment were likely to be younger, to be Aboriginal, and have greater social disadvantage than mothers of children with autism (Leonard et al 2011). The Victorian Cerebral Palsy Register is another population-based register that ascertains individuals born or accessing services in Victoria since 1970. The multiple sources for ascertainment include inpatient and outpatient attendance lists at the two tertiary children's hospitals for the state of Victoria, review of magnetic resonance imaging and gait laboratory assessment lists, and via referral from paediatricians and families. This register is now used as a sampling frame for a variety of research projects, e.g. has been used recently to investigate hearing loss in children with cerebral palsy (Reid et al 2011).

Record linkage can itself be used as a mechanism for identifying cases on a population basis. For example, national registry data in Finland for individuals using antiepileptic medications (registration contingent on a clinical diagnosis of epilepsy and additional information provided by the patient's neurologist) were linked to the whole population registry and to the hospital discharge databases to determine regional variations and trends over time in the incidence of epilepsy between 1986 and 2008. This registry is estimated to cover 97% of all persons with new-onset epilepsy, giving strength to the epidemiological findings (Sillanpaa et al 2011). This data source has provided population-based findings on the natural history of epilepsy followed over 37 years (Sillanpaa and Schmidt 2006) and on employment outcomes in children followed from childhood to a mean age of 23 years (Sillanpaa and Schmidt 2010).

The use of population-based registries illustrates the advantages for public health in examining a large number of participants with a cost-effective methodology and the provision of important epidemiological information. Research using such data can identify long-term outcomes with minimal selection bias. However, if registries are derived from administrative data initially collected for another purpose they may not always have the ability to collect information, such as that relating to function and participation, directly from the parents of affected children.

Prospective follow-up of a total birth cohort or a subsection of a birth cohort, identifying at what point the children develop the condition of interest, is another strategy that can be used. In the province of Alberta, Canada, all extremely low-birthweight infants are admitted to one of two regional neonatal intensive care units, and high ascertainment of the population of interest for follow-up has been achieved at the Northern regional centre (Robertson et al 2007). From follow-up of this group between 1974 and 2003, the prevalence of, and risk factors for, cerebral palsy in infants born at 20 to 29 weeks' gestational age has been estimated (Robertson et al 2007). This study draws strength from the long-term nature of the study and ascertainment of a high proportion of the population of interest (only 1% missing data).

In summary, although much of the neurological and developmental literature comprises clinic-based studies, only population-based studies can successfully reduce bias in relation to the selection and follow-up of participants. The use of population or birth cohort data can also inform our understanding of risk factors for neurodevelopmental impairment, although the clinical/functional detail available may be less than in studies in which there is direct contact with the participants. Population-based registries of specific disorders can help to identify the true variability associated with the condition, and an increasing number of studies have been reported in the literature over recent years. Encouraging the use of such methodology will bring benefits to both families and clinicians.

Longitudinal study for neurological and developmental conditions

DOCUMENTING GROWTH AND DEVELOPMENT

Longitudinal studies of children diagnosed with or at risk of a neurological or developmental condition provide opportunities for monitoring over time. To illustrate, this section identifies examples of longitudinal studies for specific discrete conditions (e.g. fragile X syndrome) and more heterogeneous groups (e.g. cerebral palsy) that may or may not have used population-based ascertainment. It also advocates for the continuation of longitudinal studies into adulthood to work toward understanding patterns of ageing in children with a childhood-onset neurological or developmental condition. Finally, it reviews selected literature relating to longitudinal studies of outcomes following preterm birth.

Longitudinal studies have been conducted in children with a discrete neurodevelopmental condition. For example, one study recruited 145 children with fragile X syndrome and an unaffected sibling through a national fragile X association and followed intellectual development over an average of 3 years and 11 months (Hall et al 2008); another recruited children with neurofibromatosis type 1, Williams–Beuren Syndrome, or fragile X syndrome from eight specialist centres and family associations and followed IQ and development over 2 years (Fisch et al 2010); and 11 children with Costello syndrome were recruited at an International Costello Syndrome Conference and functional outcomes were followed over 4 years (Axelrad et al 2009). These studies provide important information on the course of rare genetic disorders that have a large impact on families. However, these last studies are generally characterized by relatively short follow-up periods and modest sample sizes; analyses may not have controlled for confounding variables, and recruitment was not population based. There are also many other neurodevelopmental conditions about which less is known of their longitudinal course, especially those causing intellectual impairment (e.g. Cornelia de Lange syndrome).

More follow-up studies are available to indicate the course of conditions defined by their symptomatology (e.g. epilepsy, cerebral palsy) rather than their aetiology. The population-based study of children with epilepsy living in the geographic catchment of the Turku

University Hospital in Finland has a longitudinal component. Participants have now been followed to middle age, investigating the important outcomes of quality of life (Sillanpaa et al 2004) and employment (Sillanpaa and Schmidt 2010). For cerebral palsy, the Ontario Motor Growth Study followed the course of gross motor function in 657 children, many for over a 10-year period. Stratified by age and Gross Motor Function Classification System (GMFCS) level, the children were randomly selected from a sampling frame comprising 18 of 19 centres and one therapy-based centre in a community without a specialist centre. Up to 10 observations for more than 200 of the children over a 10-year period were collected to determine gross motor trajectories for each of the different GMFCS severity levels (Rosenbaum et al 2002, Hanna et al 2009). Examples of longitudinal assessment following specific treatments are also found in the field of cerebral palsy. Mobility outcomes were assessed 2 and 5 years after multilevel orthopaedic surgery in a consecutive clinic sample of 156 ambulant children with cerebral palsy (Harvey et al 2012). The effects of gastrostomy on growth outcomes after 6 months and 1 year were assessed in 57 children attending three specialist multidisciplinary feeding clinics in the UK (Sullivan et al 2005). These studies are building a picture that enables clinicians to predict the clinical course and to plan for appropriate services, although, overall, analyses have usually not taken account of confounding variables that may have affected trajectories.

Following preterm birth, children are often followed longitudinally, whether or not impairment is suspected. Longitudinal studies have identified a high prevalence of poorer neurodevelopmental outcomes and respiratory dysfunction during the early years, with learning and behavioural difficulties often becoming apparent during the school years at frequencies inversely proportional to gestational age at birth (Saigal and Doyle 2008). Further follow-up to adulthood has provided insight into additional downstream effects associated with preterm birth. For example, accelerated weight gain and crossing of body mass index centiles during adolescence in those who had been born with an extremely low birthweight are now being observed, and this could increase the risk of cardiovascular disease and type 2 diabetes when these children become adults (Saigal and Doyle 2008). For infants who survive the neonatal period, this body of longitudinal work has found that many infants are doing well in later life, information that is very important for counselling parents throughout the anxious time when their infant is acutely unwell, and for policy makers who are interested in outcomes following the implementation of expensive interventions such as neonatal intensive care.

An overall trend of longer life expectancy has been observed for persons with a neurodevelopmental condition (Janicki et al 2008), including Rett syndrome (Freilinger et al 2010) and Down syndrome (Yang et al 2002). The concept of 'successful ageing' is described in the gerontological literature (Doyle et al 2010), and there is a need for systematic studies to translate this concept for those with a neurodevelopmental condition. For example, there is evidence that persons with cerebral palsy experience musculoskeletal complications such as pain, deformity, and fatigue with age (Horsman et al 2010), but little is known of the influences of earlier management strategies (Haak et al 2009, Kembhavi et al 2011). Clinical practice guidelines for adolescents and young people with Down syndrome have been developed (Van Cleve et al 2006) and the authors advocate for seamless care as the children transition to adult services. Alzheimer disease develops earlier in people with Down syndrome than in the general population and other populations with intellectual impairment, with approximately 50%

affected in their fifties (Strydom et al 2010). Longitudinal studies have observed the evolution of symptoms during adulthood (Holland et al 2000, Ball et al 2006) but, as yet, no studies have tracked the antecedents of Alzheimer disease from childhood. Continued longitudinal studies across the lifespan can assist with the development of optimal care strategies during transition periods, and there is much work to be done.

As with any study, the validity of the findings depends on the quality of the study design. Longitudinal study designs depend particularly on assembling a complete population, or usually a representative cohort, maintaining high participation over the course of follow-up (e.g. the Australian Rett Syndrome Study has ongoing response fractions of >80% at each follow-up assessment), and using consistent measurement methods at each assessment with tools of established reliability and validity. Examples of consistent measurement methods in longitudinal studies include use of the same diagnostic criteria and classification of cerebral palsy over a 30-year follow-up period (Robertson et al 2007), and comprehensive initial training sessions followed by annual review for each of the physiotherapists who used the Gross Motor Function Measure to assess children with cerebral palsy over a 10-year period (Rosenbaum et al 2002, Hanna et al 2009).

There are also challenges in conducting longitudinal studies. It is a time consuming and expensive task to maintain the involvement of families as their child grows into adulthood, and this needs to be built into study budgets. Researchers need to recognize and address the burden of family participation. Careful design with efficiency of data collection for both family and budgetary reasons is an imperative. Researchers also need to provide timely and useful feedback on research findings to participating families. Finally, there is growing recognition that researchers should work with consumers to better direct research priorities, practice, and policies to the areas of greatest need (Telford et al 2004, Saunders et al 2007). Partnerships between researchers and consumers can optimize the relevance of the research to the community, the practicality of research methods, and the dissemination of research results.

IDENTIFYING CHANGING NEEDS THROUGH CHILDHOOD AND ADOLESCENCE AND INTO ADULTHOOD

At diagnosis, families have many questions that relate to their child's current problems and needs and, of course, concern for the future for their child. These questions will change with time as the developmental trajectory becomes clearer and different abilities and needs for supports are identified. This clarifies the foci of longitudinal studies: examples of questions on developmental issues and support needs at each of five broad life stages are shown in Table 24.1. Clinical care must respond to change as the child grows and develops, and a longitudinal model of research is optimally informative to understand evolving needs. There are often fewer services available as the individual with a neurodevelopmental condition ages, and longitudinal studies have an important role in continued advocacy for needs-based services.

An example: the Australian Rett Syndrome Study

DESCRIPTION OF RETT SYNDROME

Rett syndrome is a rare severe neurodevelopmental condition mainly seen in females. With an incidence of 1/9000 female births measured up to the age of 32 years (Fehr et al 2011a) Rett

TABLE 24.1

**Sample questions from families relevant to the needs of their child with a
neurological and/or developmental disorder at different life stages**

Life stage	Family questions
Newly diagnosed	What is this disorder?
	Does he or she need any more testing to check for likely complications?
	What is known about this disorder? Is there any written information?
	What is the cause?
	What do we do to look after our child? How do we feed him or her?
	What do we do now?
	Will he or she get worse or better?
	What is his or her future?
	How will this affect our planning for future children?
	Are there any other families in our neighbourhood who also have a child with this disorder?
	Is there a support group for parents?
Preschool years	What sort of therapy should our child get to help with the learning of developmental skills – movement and communication?
	Will he or she get epilepsy?
	How can we ensure that he or she grows optimally?
	Can he or she be toilet trained?
	What is the best way our family can work with others to provide good-quality treatment for our child? Which specialists should we see? Who are the best doctors?
	What do we tell our other children about our child's difficulties?
	What do we tell other people about our child's difficulties?
School years	What sort of school will best serve the needs of our child?
	What is the best system of communication for him or her? How can we be sure that he or she is able to communicate effectively with people outside our family?
	How can standing and walking practice be incorporated into daily life?
	How can we promote his or her participation in recreational activities?
	How can we support him or her in making friends?
	How can we manage the various health issues such as epilepsy and the development of deformity?
	How can we feel confident in the abilities of others to provide good-quality care for our child?
	Is there a respite facility suitable for our child?
Transition to adulthood	How can we support our teenager in developing friendships?
	How can we ensure that his or her goals of activity and participation can be supported when making the change from children's to adult services?
	How can we best help her to cope with her periods?
	How can we feel confident in the abilities of others to provide good quality-care for our teenager?
	Is there a respite facility suitable for our teenager?
	Who is going to be responsible for coordinating and providing medical care when our teenager is too old for children's services?
Adulthood	What are the ingredients for him or her to have a good quality of life?
	Now that he or she has left school, how will he or she spend the day?
	How can we ensure that access to therapy continues?
	How can we support his or her physical well-being throughout adulthood – the prevention of contracture, maintenance of mobility skills, and accessibility to good life experiences with different people and places?
	How can we support the maintenance of his or her social networks and skills?
	How can we support the maintenance of health and well-being throughout adulthood? How often should antiepileptic medications be reviewed now that he or she is an adult?
	How can we help him or her to live independently from us?
	How can we feel confident in the abilities of others to provide good-quality care for our son or daughter?

syndrome is one of the 8000 rare diseases that collectively affect up to 10% of the population (Zurynski et al 2008). It is typical of many rare diseases in that it begins in childhood, is difficult to diagnose, and continues throughout (and may shorten) life. It is associated with severe impairment and currently has no cure.

Clinical features of Rett syndrome were first described in the 1960s by Dr Andreas Rett from Austria. The latest criteria include a relatively normal prenatal and perinatal period with apparently normal development for the first 6 months of life, loss of hand and communication skills, acquisition of stereotypical hand movements, and evidence of impaired gait (Neul et al 2010). Comorbidities include scoliosis, poor growth, osteoporosis, epilepsy, breathing abnormalities, and sleep difficulties. In 1999, a causal association was identified between Rett syndrome and mutations in the methyl CpG-binding protein 2 (*MECP2*) gene (Amir et al 1999). More than 200 disease-causing *MECP2* mutations are now reported (Christodoulou et al 2003), with eight occurring more commonly. Current genetic testing uses a combined approach of mutation screening and sequencing of exons 3 and 4 for small sequence changes (Buyse et al 2000) and multiplex ligation-dependent probe amplification or quantitative polymerase chain reaction to screen for large deletions and duplications (Erlandson et al 2003).

THE AUSTRALIAN RETT SYNDROME DATABASE

Between 1993 and 1995, the Australian Rett Syndrome Database was established as a national population-based register of Rett syndrome. Ongoing ascertainment of cases is continuing through the Australian Paediatric Surveillance Unit (a unit of the Royal Australasian College of Physicians to facilitate research into rare paediatric disorders) (He et al 2010) and the Rett Syndrome Association of Australia. In January 2012, there were 382 females on the database with 58 (15.2%) having died since the initiation of the register. Multiple sources of case ascertainment contribute to the comprehensiveness of this data collection.

The Australian Rett Syndrome Study aims to describe the natural history of Rett syndrome, to investigate relationships between genotype and phenotype, and to understand the burden of Rett syndrome for those affected and their families. The database registers clinical and genetic data at the time of recruitment, and subsequently collects longitudinal data from families across Australia using questionnaires (since 1996) approximately biennially and videos (since 2004) at approximately 4-year intervals. Participation at each point of follow-up has been over 80%. Clinical data have also been collected including dual-energy X-ray absorptiometry scans on two occasions and objective measures of physical activity. As examples, the data have been used to investigate research questions relating to the time of diagnosis (Fehr et al 2011a), relationships between genotype and phenotype (Bebbington et al 2008), functional abilities (Downs et al 2008a, 2010), and, more recently, issues pertaining to when the girls transition from school to adult services. Importantly, the field of molecular biology is making inroads into the development of a cure for Rett syndrome, and the data and findings from the database can inform the structure of future clinical trials. Figure 24.1 illustrates the population-based recruitment and longitudinal structure of the Australian Rett Syndrome Study.

More specifically, study procedures include confirmation of the diagnosis of Rett syndrome for all referrals to the study, contact with families to seek consent to participate in the study, the collection of initial data describing early development, diagnosis, functional

337

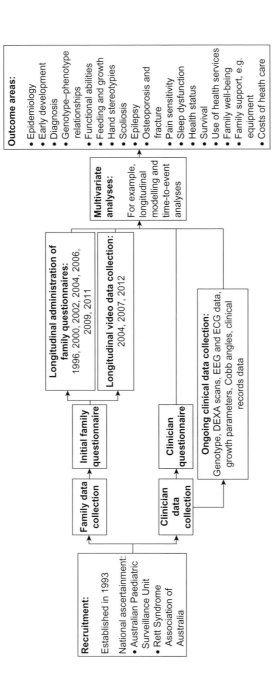

Fig. 24.1 Schematic diagram of the Australian Rett Syndrome Study showing national ascertainment, longitudinal data collection from multiple sources, and multivariate analyses of outcomes. DEXA, dual-energy X-ray absorptiometry; EEG, electroencephalography; ECG, electrocardiography.

abilities, and data about comorbidities and management. Follow-up questionnaires then track this clinical information and include additional questionnaires to measure family support, coping, and well-being. Importantly, consumers work with the study in the planning of methodology and provision of feedback. For example, a consumer reference group was formed in 2005 and comprises approximately 12 families from throughout Australia who meet quarterly via teleconference.

In summary, strengths include use of multiple sources of ascertainment and recruitment of the population of females with Rett syndrome in Australia, the comprehensive data collection, high participation at each point of follow-up, and the continuation of the study by a stable group of researchers. Up to 10 data points are now available for analysis on some females. Regular feedback is provided to families through biannual newsletters, study reports, and a website (www.aussierett.org.au), which includes lay summaries of papers resulting from the study. Studies arising from this database have already made a major contribution to our understanding of the epidemiology, natural history, comorbidities, and genetic and functional characteristics of Rett syndrome.

THE VALUE OF THE DATA COLLECTION

Studies have investigated the early development prior to diagnosis (Fehr et al 2011b) and factors associated with the age of diagnosis (Fehr et al 2010) to better understand early presentations. Many cross-sectional studies have been conducted to determine the extent that phenotype and clinical outcomes are associated with specific mutations. For example, it has been found that the p.R133C mutation has a milder phenotype (Leonard et al 2003) and the p.R270X and p.R255X mutations a more severe phenotype (Bebbington et al 2008). However, these genetic factors still need to be considered within the context of non-genetic factors that can influence functional outcomes. Consistent with the multiple body systems and functional domains affected by Rett syndrome, and the complexities of the contexts of the family, society, and the environment, many genotype–phenotype studies have used a variety of regression techniques including longitudinal modelling and time-to-event analysis. Examples include analyses investigating longitudinal trajectories of functional abilities (Downs et al 2011, Foley et al 2011), the occurrence of fractures over time (Downs et al 2008b), and the changing health status as the girls grow into women (Young et al 2011).

Clinicians are keen to use best practice but Rett syndrome is rare, and high-level evidence to support management is sparse or non-existent. Conducting clinical trials in conditions in which clinical practice is established and without an evidence base is ethically problematic. However, the longitudinal bank of information collected on the Australian population-based cohort over 16 years can be used to identify outcomes for some of the current management strategies using study designs alternative to randomized controlled trials (West et al 2008). We previously demonstrated the feasibility of this approach by using a longitudinal repeated measures design to compare change in function following scoliosis surgery with function in conservatively managed subjects (Downs et al 2009a). By constructing medication histories from successive questionnaires, we have shown that the risk of fracture is substantially increased in association with the use of sodium valproate to manage seizures (Leonard et al 2010). The database now makes possible the implementation of cohort studies to investigate the clinical effectiveness of treatments such as spinal fusion and gastrostomy that also cannot be tested with clinical trials. Finally, the Australian group directed the development of guidelines for the clinical management of scoliosis in Rett syndrome through systematic literature review and the Delphi technique, consulting with an expert panel of child neurologists, developmental paediatricians, orthopaedic surgeons, and physiotherapists (Downs et al 2009b). Currently available in English and Spanish, the guidelines have also been developed into booklet form for dissemination to clinicians and families.

Conclusion

In sum, longitudinal study designs provide greater confidence in defining trajectories and the effectiveness of treatment strategies than is possible with cross-sectional studies. By studying children with neurological or developmental conditions and their families throughout various life stages, we can work towards the identification of factors associated with improved trajectories. We can also try to understand mechanisms through which to facilitate the transition of vulnerable groups from poor to better health outcomes. The value of a longitudinal study is enhanced enormously by being population-based, an important strategy to avoid selection bias and ensure that the true variability of a condition is identified. Studies that combine population-based and longitudinal designs are rare but are urgently needed by children with neurological or developmental conditions and their families. The Australian Rett Syndrome Study is an example of one such study, and it has made a significant contribution to the understanding and management of Rett syndrome.

REFERENCES

Key references

Amir RE, Van den Veyver IB, Wan M, Tran CQ, Francke U, Zoghbi HY (1999) Rett syndrome is caused by mutations in X-linked MECP2, encoding methyl-cpg-binding protein 2. *Nat Genet* 23: 185–188. http://dx.doi.org/10.1038/13810

Axelrad ME, Schwartz DD, Fehlis JE, et al (2009) Longitudinal course of cognitive, adaptive, and behavioural characteristics in Costello syndrome. *Am J Med Genet A* 149A: 2666–2672. http://dx.doi.org/10.1002/ajmg.a.33126

Ball SL, Holland AJ, Hon J, Huppert FA, Treppner P, Watson PC (2006) Personality and behaviour changes mark the early stages of Alzheimer's disease in adults with Down's syndrome: findings from a prospective population-based study. *Int J Geriatr Psychiatry* 21: 661–673. http://dx.doi.org/10.1002/gps.1545

Bebbington A, Anderson A, Ravine D, et al (2008) Investigating genotype–phenotype relationships in Rett syndrome using an international data set. *Neurology* 70: 868–875. http://dx.doi.org/10.1212/01.wnl.0000304752.50773.ec

Berkman LF, Kawachi I (2000) *Social Epidemiology.* Oxford: Oxford University Press.

*Bishop DVM (2010) Which neurodevelopmental disorders get researched and why? *PLoS One* 5: e15112. http://dx.doi.org/10.1371/journal.pone.0015112

Buyse IM, Fang P, Hoon KT, Amir RE, Zoghbi HY, Roa BB (2000) Diagnostic testing for Rett syndrome by dhplc and direct sequencing analysis of the MECP2 gene: identification of several novel mutations and polymorphisms. *Am J Hum Genet* 67: 1428–1436. http://dx.doi.org/10.1086/316913

*Champagne F (2010) Epigenetic perspectives on development: evolving insights on the origins of variation. *Dev Psychobiol* 52: e1–e3. http://dx.doi.org/10.1002/dev.20443

Christodoulou J, Grimm A, Maher T, Bennetts B (2003) Rettbase: the IRSA mecp2 variation database – a new mutation database in evolution. *Hum Mutat* 21: 466–472. http://dx.doi.org/10.1002/humu.10194

Downs JA, Bebbington A, Jacoby P, et al (2008a) Gross motor profile in Rett syndrome as determined by video analysis. *Neuropediatrics* 39: 205–210. http://dx.doi.org/10.1055/s-0028-1104575

*Downs J, Bebbington A, Woodhead H, et al (2008b) Early determinants of fractures in Rett syndrome. *Pediatrics* 121: 540–546. http://dx.doi.org/10.1542/peds.2007-1641

Downs J, Young D, de Klerk N, Bebbington A, Baikie G, Leonard H (2009a) Impact of scoliosis surgery on activities of daily living in females with Rett syndrome. *J Pediatr Orthop* 29: 369–374. http://dx.doi.org/10.1097/BPO.0b013e3181a53b41

Downs J, Bergman A, Carter P, et al (2009b) Guidelines for management of scoliosis in Rett syndrome patients based on expert consensus and clinical evidence. *Spine* 34: e607–e617. http://dx.doi.org/10.1097/BRS.0b013e3181a95ca4

Downs J, Bebbington A, Jacoby P, et al (2010) Level of purposeful hand function as a marker of clinical severity in Rett syndrome. *Dev Med Child Neurol* 52: 817–823. http://dx.doi.org/10.1111/j.1469-8749.2010.03636.x

Downs J, Bebbington A, Kaufmann W, Leonard H (2011) Longitudinal hand function in Rett syndrome. *J Child Neurol* 26: 334–340. http://dx.doi.org/10.1177/0883073810381920

*Doyle YG, McKee M, Sheriff M (2010) A model of successful ageing in British populations. *Eur J Public Health* 22: 71–76. http://dx.doi.org/10.1093/eurpub/ckq132

Erlandson A, Samuelsson L, Hagberg B, Kyllerman M, Vujic M, Wahlstrm J (2003) Multiplex ligation-dependent probe amplification (MLPA) detects large deletions in the MECP2 gene of Swedish Rett syndrome patients. *Genet Test* 7: 329–332. http://dx.doi.org/10.1089/109065703322783707

Fehr S, Downs J, Bebbington A, Leonard H (2010) Atypical presentations and specific genotypes are associated with a delay in diagnosis in females with Rett syndrome. *Am J Med Genet A* 152A: 2535–2542. http://dx.doi.org/10.1002/ajmg.a.33640

Fehr S, Bebbington A, Nassar N, et al (2011a) Trends in the diagnosis of Rett syndrome in Australia. *Pediatr Res* 70: 313–319. http://dx.doi.org/10.1203/PDR.0b013e3182242461

Fehr S, Bebbington A, Ellaway C, Rowe P, Leonard H, Downs J (2011b) Altered attainment of developmental milestones influences the age of diagnosis of Rett syndrome. *J Child Neurol* 26: 980–987. http://dx.doi.org/10.1177/0883073811401396

Fisch GS, Carpenter N, Howard-Peebles PN, Holden JJ, Tarleton J, Simensen R (2010) The course of cognitive-behavioural development in children with the FMR1 mutation, Williams-Beuren syndrome, and neurofibromatosis type 1: the effect of gender. *Am J Med Genet A* 152A: 1498–1509.

Foley KR, Downs J, Bebbington A, et al (2011) Change in gross motor abilities of girls and women with Rett syndrome over a 3- to 4-year period. *J Child Neurol* 26: 1237–1245. http://dx.doi.org/10.1177/0883073811402688

*Freilinger M, Bebbington A, Lanator I, et al (2010) Survival with Rett syndrome: comparing Rett's original sample with data from the Australian Rett Syndrome Database. *Dev Med Child Neurol* 52: 962–965. http://dx.doi.org/10.1111/j.1469-8749.2010.03716.x

Gesell A (1928) *Infancy and Human Growth*. New York: Macmillan.

Haak P, Lenski M, Hidecker MJ, Li M, Paneth N (2009) Cerebral palsy and ageing. *Dev Med Child Neurol* 51(Suppl. 4): 16–23. http://dx.doi.org/10.1111/j.1469-8749.2009.03428.x

Hall SS, Burns DD, Lightbody AA, Reiss AL (2008) Longitudinal changes in intellectual development in children with Fragile X syndrome. *J Abnorm Child Psychol* 36: 927–939. http://dx.doi.org/10.1007/s10802-008-9223-y

*Hanna SE, Rosenbaum PL, Bartlett DJ, et al (2009) Stability and decline in gross motor function among children and youth with cerebral palsy aged 2 to 21 years. *Dev Med Child Neurol* 51: 295–302. http://dx.doi.org/10.1111/j.1469-8749.2008.03196.x

Harvey A, Rosenbaum P, Hanna S, Yousefi-Nooraie R, Graham HK (2012) Longitudinal changes in mobility following single-event multilevel surgery in ambulatory children with cerebral palsy. *J Rehabil Med* 44: 137–143. http://dx.doi.org/10.2340/16501977-0916

He S, Zurynski Y, Elliott E (2010) What do paediatricians think of the Australian Paediatric Surveillance Unit? *J Paediatr Child Health* 46: 412–418. http://dx.doi.org/10.1111/j.1440-1754.2010.01755.x

Holland AJ, Hon J, Huppert FA, Stevens F (2000) Incidence and course of dementia in people with Down's syndrome: findings from a population-based study. *J Intellect Disabil Res* 44: 138–146. http://dx.doi.org/10.1046/j.1365-2788.2000.00263.x

Horsman M, Suto M, Dudgeon B, Harris S (2010) Growing older with cerebral palsy: insiders' perspectives. *Paediatr Phys Ther* 22: 296–303. http://dx.doi.org/10.1097/PEP.0b013e3181eabc0f

Illingworth RS (1963) *The Development of the Infant and Young Child: Normal and Abnormal*. Edinburgh: E. & S. Livingstone.

Janicki M, Henderson CM, Rubin IL (2008) Neurodevelopmental conditions and ageing: report on the Atlanta Study Group charrette on neurodevelopmental conditions and ageing. *Disabil Health J* 1: 116–124. http://dx.doi.org/10.1016/j.dhjo.2008.02.004

Kembhavi G, Darrah J, Payne K, Plesuk D (2011) Adults with a diagnosis of cerebral palsy: a mapping review of long-term outcomes. *Dev Med Child Neurol* 53: 610–614. http://dx.doi.org/10.1111/j.1469-8749.2011.03914.x

Last JM (2001) *A Dictionary of Epidemiology*. Oxford: Oxford University Press.

Leonard H, Colvin L, Christodoulou J, et al (2003) Patients with the R133C mutation: is their phenotype different from patients with Rett syndrome with other mutations? *J Med Genet* 40: e52. http://dx.doi.org/10.1136/jmg.40.5.e52

*Leonard H, Downs J, Jian L, et al (2010) Valproate and risk of fracture in Rett syndrome. *Arch Dis Child* 95: 444–448. http://dx.doi.org/10.1136/adc.2008.148932

*Leonard H, Glasson E, Nassar N, et al (2011) Autism and intellectual disability are differentially related to sociodemographic background at birth. *PLoS One* 6: e17875. http://dx.doi.org/10.1371/journal.pone.0017875

Neul JL, Kaufmann WE, Glaze DG, et al, for the RettSearch Consortium (2010) Rett syndrome: revised diagnostic criteria and nomenclature. *Ann Neurol* 68: 944–950. http://dx.doi.org/10.1002/ana.22124

*Petterson B, Leonard H, Bourke J, et al (2005) IDEA (Intellectual Disability Exploring Answers): a population-based database for intellectual disability in western Australia. *Ann Hum Biol* 32: 237–243. http://dx.doi.org/10.1080/03014460500075035

Piaget J (1927) *The Language and Thought of the Child*. London: Kegan Paul, Trench & Trubner.

Reid SM, Modak MB, Berkowitz RG, Reddihough DS (2011) A population-based study and systematic review of hearing loss in children with cerebral palsy. *Dev Med Child Neurol* 53: 1038–1045. http://dx.doi.org/10.1111/j.1469-8749.2011.04069.x

*Robertson CMT, Watt M, Yasui Y (2007) Changes in the prevalence of cerebral palsy for children born very prematurely within a population-based program over 30 years. *JAMA* 297: 2733–2740.

*Rosenbaum PL, Walter SD, Hanna SE, et al (2002) Prognosis or gross motor function in cerebral palsy – creation of motor development curves. *JAMA* 288: 1357–1363. http://dx.doi.org/10.1001/jama.288.11.1357

*Saigal S, Doyle L (2008) An overview of mortality and sequelae of preterm birth from infancy to adulthood. *Lancet* 371: 261–269. http://dx.doi.org/10.1016/S0140-6736(08)60136-1

Saunders C, Crossing S, Girgis A, Butow P, Penman A (2007) Operationalizing a model framework for consumer and community participation in health and medical research. *Aust New Zealand Health Policy* 4: 13. http://dx.doi.org/10.1186/1743-8462-4-13

*Sillanpaa M, Schmidt D (2006) Natural history of treated childhood-onset epilepsy: prospective, long-term population-based study. *Brain* 129: 617–624. http://dx.doi.org/10.1093/brain/awh726

Sillanpaa M, Schmidt D (2010) Long-term employment of adults with childhood-onset epilepsy: a prospective population-based study. *Epilepsia* 51: 1053–1060. http://dx.doi.org/10.1111/j.1528-1167.2009.02505.x

Sillanpaa M, Haataja L, Shinnar J (2004) Perceived impact of childhood-onset epilepsy on quality of life as an adult. *Epilepsia* 45: 971–977. http://dx.doi.org/10.1111/j.0013-9580.2004.44203.x

Sillanpaa M, Lastunen S, Helenius H, Schmidt D (2011) Regional differences and secular trends in the incidence of epilepsy in Finland: a nationwide 23-year registry study. *Epilepsia* 52: 1857–1867. http://dx.doi.org/10.1111/j.1528-1167.2011.03186.x

*Strydom A, Shooshtari S, Lee L, et al (2010) Dementia in older adults with intellectual disabilities – epidemiology, presentation, and diagnosis. *J Policy Pract Intellect Disabil* 7: 96–110. http://dx.doi.org/10.1111/j.1741-1130.2010.00253.x

Sullivan PB, Juszczak E, Bachlet AME, et al (2005) Gastrostomy tube feeding in children with cerebral palsy: a prospective, longitudinal study. *Dev Med Child Neurol* 47: 77–85. http://dx.doi.org/10.1017/S0012162205000162

Telford R, Boote J, Cooper C (2004) What does it mean to involve consumers successfully in NHS research? A consensus study. *Health Expect* 7: 209–220. http://dx.doi.org/10.1111/j.1369-7625.2004.00278.x

Van Cleve SN, Cannon S, Cohen WI (2006) Part ii: Clinical practice guidelines for adolescents and young adults with Down syndrome: 12 to 21 years. *J Pediatr Health Care* 20: 198–205. http://dx.doi.org/10.1016/j.pedhc.2006.02.006

West S, Duan N, Pequegnat W, et al (2008) Alternatives to the randomized controlled trial. *Am J Public Health* 98: 1359–1366. http://dx.doi.org/10.2105/AJPH.2007.124446

*Whittington JE, Holland AJ, Webb T, Butler J, Clarke D, Boer H (2001) Population prevalence and estimated birth incidence and mortality rate for people with Prader-Willi syndrome in one UK health region. *J Med Genet* 38: 792–798. http://dx.doi.org/10.1136/jmg.38.11.792

World Health Organization (2001) *International Classification of Functioning, Disability and Health*. Geneva: WHO Press.

Yang Q, Rasmussen S, Friedman JM (2002) Mortality associated with Down's syndrome in the USA from 1983 to 1997: a population-based study. *Lancet* 359: 1019–1025. http://dx.doi.org/10.1016/S0140-6736(02)08092-3

Young D, Bebbington A, de Klerk N, Bower C, Nagarajan L, Leonard H (2011) The relationship between MECP2 mutation type and health status and service use trajectories over time in a Rett syndrome population. *Res Autism Spectr Disord* 5: 442–449. http://dx.doi.org/10.1016/j.rasd.2010.06.007

Zurynski Y, Frith K, Leonard H, Elliott E (2008) Rare childhood diseases: how should we respond? *Arch Dis Child* 93: 1071–1074. http://dx.doi.org/10.1136/adc.2007.134940

25
POLICIES, PROGRAMMES, AND PRACTICES: THE TENSIONS ABOUT LIFE QUALITY OUTCOMES

Gina Glidden and Rachel Birnbaum

Overview

This chapter explores policies, programmes, and practices that guide decision-making processes for children living with developmental impairments and their families and that may have important impacts on their life quality outcomes. Inherent tensions exist about who defines quality of life and the right to die or have access to assisted suicide. The authors conclude that it is incumbent on programme providers, policy makers, and governments to incorporate the children's experiences and their voices when targeting change to improve their quality of life and that of their families.

Introduction

There has been considerable focus on early intervention programmes for young children with developmental conditions (Blackman 2002). Research has been undertaken to explore the quality of life for children and young people with developmental conditions (Zekovic and Renwick 2003, Canty-Mitchell et al 2005, Wang and Brown 2009), to understand the economic costs of caring for children with developmental conditions (Anderson et al 2007, Burton and Phipps 2009), and, more recently, to identify the burdens and demands on the family as a result of caring for a child with a neurodevelopmental condition (Saposnek et al 2005, Birnbaum et al 2012, Mednick and Koocher 2012).

The Canadian Charter of Rights and Freedoms (1982) guarantees equal rights for everyone – including individuals with neurodevelopmental conditions.[a] However, policies, programmes, and practices for children with 'special needs' vary considerably from province to province in Canada, let alone from one country to another. Children experience diverse impairments, and each child is a unique individual. In the 2003 Update of Canada's Report to the UN Committee for the Rights of Children (Canadian Coalition for the Rights of Children, 2003), the authors

---

a   Section 15 enunciates rights for persons with disabilities and permits special programmes to advance disadvantaged groups in Canadian society.

report '… children with disabilities are not guaranteed free and appropriate early diagnosis, early intervention, and early childhood education in Canada' (p. 33).

This chapter will explore what policies, programmes, and practices exist that target change for improving the quality of life for children and young people who have developmental conditions and the impact of these policies on their families. Part I explores specific programmes and practices across the globe that highlight the tensions between policy implications and applications and how policies and programmes impact in particular on the needs of children and families. Part II explores targets for change to improve the quality of life for children and young people with developmental conditions. Part III concludes with the inherent tensions in the legislation across the globe that involves the right to die with dignity, in order to help us understand how policies respond positively or negatively in addressing the needs of disabled persons and their families. The authors argue that, although there are many policies and programmes in place to improve the quality of life for children and young people with developmental conditions, inherent tensions exist regarding quality of life. Additionally, the emphasis remains on deficit-based outcomes that focus on approaches directed at improving physical health rather than on policies, programmes, and practices that focus on the functioning abilities and quality of life of these populations.

Part I: Exploring programmes and practices

Disability legislation exists worldwide, sometimes within disability-specific laws and acts, at other times incorporated within existing national human rights legislation (Kovacs Burns and Gordon 2010, Kim and Fox 2011). Divergence in interpretations of the concepts of impairment and disability makes it such that it is measured and experienced differently around the world, resulting in significant global variation in the programmes and services that are created in support of people living with impairments and their families (Bedell et al 2011). This is important not only because definitions of impairment and disability help establish who is considered disabled in society and whether or not they are eligible for support services, but also because it reflects societal views which, in turn, influence the focus of policy. A universal understanding of disability and related concepts, including the environmental contextual factors of accommodation, equal access, and special needs such as those depicted in the International Classification of Functioning, Health and Disability (ICF) (World Health Organization 2001), may lead to a better ability to identify data that are comparable from one country to another. Comparable data may then help facilitate the identification of best practices and the creation of policies necessary to ensure their implementation (Bedell et al 2011).

Regardless of the variations in definition or structural location, disability legislation is met with differing views and arguments concerning necessity and efficacy. Those in support of disability legislation believe that it will be a good starting point for encouraging access: that it will (1) help to invigorate the disability movement and increase public awareness and alliances with disability groups, and (2) help to solidify a specific definition of disability using a social lens to promote understanding of the Canadian Charter of Human Rights and Freedoms and the provincial human rights codes (Prince 2010). Those who are sceptical about disability legislation believe that it is not essential and that it actually segregates the disability community and shifts the responsibility for issues of high priority away from governments and on to the shoulders of groups in the disability community. The main argument is that, once legislation is in place, the governing party will believe that it has properly addressed disability needs and concerns and thus simply move on to the needs of other groups (Prince 2010).

Despite these varying views and divergent understandings of disability worldwide, existing disability legislation reflects several important concepts. The first concerns *antidiscrimination* and refers to preventing the discrimination of people based on the existence of impairments, as well as repairing the harm done by discrimination and changing societal views concerning it (Kim and Fox 2011). The second concept, *strengths-based services*, reflects the importance of looking at abilities as well as needs. Services must address needs that are meaningful to each individual and must be based on accurate assessments that take into consideration each person's abilities and areas of interest (ICF concepts and their applicability are discussed in Chapter 4).

Services must also incorporate the evaluation of the professional who will provide the service (Turnbull et al 2001). These services encompass the evaluation of both the strengths and the available resources that will be used to enhance the improvement of the person's overall abilities. It is essential that the professional conducting the assessment be aware of the concept of disability, as the referral process towards services is contingent on the professional's knowledge of issues related both to impairment and to the services that would best meet the needs of the individual and the family (Bedell et al 2011). The emphasis on strengths and capacities promotes the concept of enhancing quality of life rather than only trying to repair the impairment (Turnbull et al 2001).

The third and fourth concepts that are important in the creation of disability legislation are *empowerment* and *autonomy*. Both help to ensure that services are offered in such a way that people living with a neurodevelopmental condition will gain control and mastery over their life, that they have a say in the direction of service provision, and that they will have the right to accept or refuse intervention and to change their mind (Turnbull et al 2001).

Other concepts are also considered in the creation and implementation of disability legislation, including: (1) *privacy and confidentiality*, meant to ensure that the private information gathered by and discussed with professionals is kept private; (2) *integration*, meant to ensure that, rather than being segregated and institutionalized, people living with neurodevelopmental conditions are included and can participate in all domains of life with typically developing people; (3) *production and contribution*, to ensure that persons living with impairments have the necessary accommodations to allow them to work and contribute to society; (4) *family integrity and unity*, which pushes for the necessary supports that will allow families to raise their children with impairments, and for children with impairments to have the benefit of being raised within their family unit; (5) *family centredness*, in which provision of services for the whole family ensures that the services are available to the entire family of someone living with a neurodevelopmental condition and that they take culture and ethnicity into consideration; and (6) *accountability*, which holds both policy makers and those implementing policies accountable (Turnbull et al 2001).

In addition to sharing disability-related concepts, services and programmes that are implemented worldwide through various legislative forums share common themes and concerns. Accessibility and inclusion to these services are underlying features and, although they are not all specifically related to 'childhood disability', the supports are often provided to adults (parents and legal guardians) who are caring for children (Kovacs Burns and Gordon 2010, Kim and Fox 2011). Many of the services and programmes fall into the following categories: (1) financial assistance, for example governmental cost-shared programmes, tax incentives, and funding for direct service provision (Prince 2001); (2) health and education (Jongbloed 2003, De Wispelaere and Walsh 2007, Kim and Fox 2011); (3) employment and vocational training to increase the levels of employment participation (Jongbloed 2003, Prince 2010, Kim and Fox 2011); (4) access to public services such as buildings and parks as well as transport, housing, and telecommunication (Jongbloed 2003, Kovacs Burns and Gordon 2010, Prince 2010, Kim and Fox 2011); and (5) judicial rights supporting the filing of discrimination complaints (Kovacs Burns and Gordon 2010, Prince 2010, Kim and Fox 2011).

CONSIDERATIONS AND CAUTIONS

Disability-specific legislation exists as a means of ensuring equal rights for people living with developmental conditions (Kim and Fox 2011). However, experience also demonstrates that, although laws can provide a framework, they are not enough to promote any access, let alone equal access (Prince 2010), and their existence alone does not ensure the implementation of the legislation (Kim and Fox 2011) (see also Chapter 13 on advancing the rights of children with neurodevelopmental conditions). Furthermore, when disability legislation is implemented, it does not and cannot fully ensure antidiscrimination (Kim and Fox 2011).

Prince (2004) argues that one major reason for this reality resides in a lack of coordinated management, harmonization, and teamwork between different levels of government responsible for elaborating and implementing the legislation. In addition, there is little accountability, resulting in great efforts on paper but little follow-up (Kovacs Burns and Gordon 2010). Disability issues are often lost or forgotten as they are shuffled through intergovernmental layers and within various departmental bureaucracies. Thus, great initiatives that require interdepartmental support and cooperation never come to fruition (Prince 2004). Prince (2004) concludes that, although government departments are able to join forces to meet disability-related goals, it is also important to establish clear lines of accountability at the federal level.

Part II: Creating targets for change

It was not until the late 1990s that the policy rights of people with impairments were even being acknowledged, let alone visible. In part, this can be attributed to the pervasive nature of the medical model when it comes to children and young adults with neurodevelopmental conditions (Campbell 2001). Whether it is about their rights to freedom of expression, thought, and association (Articles 13, 14, and 15), child protection and child welfare (Article 19), their right to be heard and represented (Articles 12 and 13), or about children with impairments (Article 23 of the United Nations Convention on the Rights of the Child), the voices of children are still heard through an adult perspective. This in turn leads to policies and programmes being formulated exclusively from an adult perspective and with little or no input from the population of interest. This is also true for children with impairments and their families (Hanvey 2002) and more so for aboriginal children (Valentine 2001) (see Chapter 13). For example,

There is no national standard of services and treatment programs provided to children with autism. After a cut-off age that varies between provinces, parents are often left to cover the costs—a situation which results in children being denied therapy.

(Standing Senate Committee on Human Rights 2005: 109)

Doctors are quick to diagnose Attention Deficit Hyperactivity Disorder and prescribe drugs to agitated children rather than looking into alternatives to medical diagnosis of such behavior.

(Standing Senate Committee on Human Rights 2005: 109)

Consequently, in Canada, there is wide variation in accountability across provinces and territories when it comes to services for children living with developmental conditions and the supports available to their families (Prince 2004). August (2009) argues that disability policy continues to borrow tools from the medical world. While a medical diagnosis can sometimes be an accurate way of describing and treating specific impairments, it cannot capture and measure the level of impairment or the social and economic costs that are associated with the developmentally impaired child and his or her family. Gannoni and Shute (2009) emphasize the importance of including children in the clinical process while shifting focus beyond the medical components of impairment towards social and environmental factors (Gibson et al 2009).

The ICF (World Health Organization 2001) defines disability in terms of the negative relationship between the physiological aspects of one's specific health condition and the environment (physical, attitudinal, structural) in which one lives (see Chapter 2 for more on the concept of 'disability' and Chapter 4 on the ICF). Despite this accepted definition, disability studies and current policy reflect the existing societal ideas regarding how disability and its related issues are viewed, accepted, and prioritized (Prince 2010). Society's image of what is considered 'normal' isolates and excludes people living with impairments (Prince 2004). Altering this view requires more education and sensitization, not only for the public but also for professionals in health, government, and community settings (Kovacs Burns and Gordon 2010). In addition to the need to modify society's view of disability is the need to review the continuing idea that children are the sole responsibility of their families, a notion that further promotes the idea that disability is not a societal responsibility but an individual family's problem that should be dealt with in the home (Kim and Fox 2011).

Society also tends to judge quality of life in terms of levels of functionality, and healthcare systems tend to be organized with this concept in mind. It is assumed that the more independence one has, the higher is one's quality of life (Gibson et al 2009). However, studies identify other important determinants. In a study of quality of life of children with cerebral palsy who required moderate to great levels of assistance in their daily activities, Young et al (2007) found that children identified family relationships and friendships with peers, as well as participation in leisure activities, as major elements that gave them high levels of enjoyment. Similarly, Rosenbaum et al (2007) determined that children's functional abilities did not directly correspond to the perception they had regarding their health and contentment with life.

Moreover, not all impairments impact in the same way on every child. A neurodevelopmental condition, be it cerebral palsy, attention deficit disorder, or autism, can have vastly different impacts on the emotional, medical, and physical well-being of children in both the short and long term (Birnbaum et al 2012). Additionally, there are problems with treating a developmental condition as a discrete concept because treatment methods can overlap. For example, having autism not only impacts on the child's processes of social communication but also interacts with the emotional aspects of the child and his or her family's circumstances. Moreover, the impact of a potentially disabling condition varies according to individual and economic circumstances and the personal characteristics of the child. People with neurodevelopmental conditions do not fit into one homogeneous group that shares the same needs, and even within disability communities themselves there exist hierarchies in which certain conditions are more greatly stigmatized than others (Campbell 1994).

These are not the only criticisms of the current state of disability policy. Currently, very little information is available regarding the extent to which support resources are utilized to address the needs of persons with neurodevelopmental conditions. In addition, Leonardi (2010) suggests there is a lack of comparable data worldwide regarding functioning and disability as a whole. Policy development is based on gathering data and ultimately how the government uses those data. Prince (2004) suggests that there is little room for policy makers to create informed disability-specific policy. In other words, policy is often reactionary. As we saw earlier, a possible explanation for the lack of data is that differences exist in the understanding of disability worldwide, and any data collected nationally are not universally comparable (Leonardi 2010, World Health Organization 2011). In some countries disability is defined in terms of performance levels in employment or in other social activities; in other countries it is defined in terms of medical or rehabilitation concepts, resulting in the existence of several different words for the same thing (Leonardi 2010). This often results in individuals falling between the cracks and missing out on support services that may be beneficial to them.

Part III: Disability policy and the tensions of life or death

Quality of life is an important outcome in the lives of all children; promoting it in the lives of those with neurodevelopmental conditions is crucial to disability policy. Considering the best interest of the child, policy can help determine which children receive the medically assisted technologies that may improve their quality of life; it can also guide which children are removed from life-saving technologies or simply not offered them at all. Policy also helps shape the types of support services that are made available to children who live with impairments and their families.

For example, the availability of assistive devices, sophisticated communication aids, and medical advances has made it easier for some individuals to live more comfortably and to improve their quality of life. However, for other individuals with degenerative or incurable diseases, medical technology has not provided relief but rather at times has prolonged their suffering (for more on suffering see Chapter 2, p. 16). These individuals have often sought the right to die. The question is: at what point has the quality of life deteriorated to the point at which it is acceptable to cease living, and who makes that decision?

In Canada, a number of provisions of the Criminal Code (RSC, 1985, c. C-46) are in place to protect individuals from euthanasia and cease their medical treatments. For example, in s.14 of the Criminal Code

> No person is entitled to consent to have death inflicted on him, and such consent does not affect the criminal responsibility of any person by whom death may be inflicted on the person by whom consent is given.

Additionally, in s.241 of the Criminal Code:

> Every one who: a. counsels a person to commit suicide, or: b. aids or abets a person to commit suicide, whether suicide ensues or not, is guilty of an indictable offence and liable to imprisonment for a term not exceeding fourteen years.[b]

Legislation permitting assisted suicide is very limited worldwide (Hwang 2005). In the European Union only the Netherlands,[c] Belgium,[d] and Luxembourg[e] have legislation that makes euthanasia legal. Voluntary euthanasia and assisted suicide were also legalized in Australia for 9 months until that law was repealed in 1997.

In the Netherlands the law officially changed in 2002 with the Termination of Life on Request and Assisted Suicide Act, making the Netherlands together with Switzerland the only countries in which foreigners can be patients. The Netherlands is also the only country that has provisions for children between the ages of 12 and 18 years (Fadem et al 2003). In Belgium, the Belgian Act of Euthanasia was passed in September 2002 and permits euthanasia but does not describe a method or procedure to follow.

The State of Oregon was the first state in the USA to legalize physician-assisted suicide. To be eligible under the Death with Dignity Act, 1994, residents must be 18 years of age or older and must have a terminal condition with a life expectancy of 6 months or less. They must also be assessed as being not depressed and must be able to administer the prescribed medication independently (Fadem et al 2003). The State of Washington mirrored this Act in 2008.

In Oregon, the legislation has been highly contested by disability organizations that fear that legalizing assisted suicide will devalue the lives of people with impairments by focusing

---

b s.749: Royal prerogative: Nothing in this Act in any manner limits or affects Her Majesty's royal prerogative of mercy. Applied in exceptional cases in which considerations of justice, humanity, and compassion override the natural administration of justice. Other provisions that may be relevant: s.45 – surgical operations; s.215 – duty of person to provide necessities of life; s.216 – duty of persons undertaking acts dangerous to life; s.217 – duty of persons undertaking acts; s.219 – criminal negligence; s.220 – death by criminal negligence; s.221 – causing bodily harm by criminal negligence; s.222 – homicide; s.229 – murder; s.231 – classification of murder; s.234 – manslaughter; s.245 – administering noxious things.

c Euthanasia is technically illegal for children under the age of 12.

d Belgium refers to the *Belgium Act on Euthanasia.*

e Bill passed on 19 March 2009 that requires the approval of two doctors and a panel of experts.

on the promotion of life-ending measures rather than structures that promote and facilitate living. In addition, fears have been raised that assisted suicide may encourage people who would otherwise strive for life to give up. Those who oppose such legislation also question who makes the rules and on what criteria the rules are based. Discussion about physician-assisted suicide most often takes place within the world of medicine, and seldom are disabled people included (Fadem et al 2003).

What do people with impairments say about Oregon's legislation? In a study using qualitative interviews with 45 people living with severe impairment, conducted by researchers who themselves lived with impairments, 30% of participants were in favour of the legislation, although they stressed the importance of not assuming that people with impairments simply do not want to live (Fadem et al 2003). Autonomy and end-of-life choices were important to the participants, who felt the decision to live or die should not be in anyone else's hands but their own. Two-thirds of the sample identified themselves as being a member of a disability community and, of those, almost half felt strongly guarded about the legislation, expressing the following concerns: a fear that disabled people would be encouraged to choose assisted suicide because their lives are devalued by society; a general lack of trust towards government and health industries; and a sense that no legislation should exist to control areas of life that are as personal as deciding to end one's life. Others felt that, if more community-based support services were available to disabled people, they would be able to live their lives to the fullest (Fadem et al 2003).

Common themes within the discussion of barriers that affect the quality of life of people living with neurodevelopmental conditions are negative societal views about the abilities and productivity levels of people living with impairments, as well as the lack of available and accessible support services to facilitate their inclusion and participation in education, employment, health care, and social outlets (World Health Organization 2011). Support services permit people living with impairments to live as independently as possible; this has a tremendous impact on their satisfaction with life, thus lowering their potential for depression and their subsequent desire to end their life (Batavia 2001). Loss of autonomy (91%), a lessened ability to engage in enjoyable activities (88.1%), and feeling like a burden on family members (35.3%) are some of the main reasons given by the 525 people who accessed assisted-suicide services in Oregon between its legalization in 1994 and January 2011 and who subsequently died (Oregon Public Health Division 2012). In addition, the World Health Report states that approximately 200 million people worldwide who reported living with an impairment encounter functional difficulties that lead, in part, to an increase in dependency on others and on constrained participation abilities (World Health Organization 2011). This emphasizes the significant place that inclusive supports should have within policy making and the tremendous impact that they could have on perhaps saving the lives of people living with impairments. We require the influence and involvement of players at all levels – government, private services, and disabled people and their families, as well as the general population – to push for and implement change (World Health Organization 2011).

The right to die with dignity when impaired by a degenerative or incurable disease has sparked many court challenges and has polarized debates on the rights of the those who wish to die with dignity versus those who believe that legislation will be misused and may lead to unintended consequences. Numerous cases in Canada have challenged the law for the right to die with dignity and, in turn, have raised the question of whether individuals have a right over their own bodies and ultimately over their time of death (Tiedmann and Valiquet 2008).

For example, in *Carter* v. *Canada* (2012) in the Supreme Court of British Columbia, the lawyer for Ms Taylor argued that the law makes it a criminal offence to help those who are impaired and who want to end their life (*The Huffington Post* 2011). Ms Taylor has amyotrophic lateral sclerosis (Lou Gehrig disease, also known as motor neurone disease), which will ultimately take her life, and she wanted the dignity to be able to choose when her life should end.

In another well-known Canadian case, *Rodriguez* v. *British Columbia* (1993), Ms Rodriguez had amyotrophic lateral sclerosis and went to court to challenge s.241 of the Canadian Charter of Rights and Freedoms as being unconstitutional. She argued that s.7 (the right 'to life, liberty and security of the person'), s.12 ('cruel and unusual punishment'), and s.15 ('equality') violated her rights under the Canadian Charter of Rights and Freedoms. The Supreme Court of British Columbia found that the provisions did not affect her freedom of choice. The court found that the disease, not the law, deprived her of her right to carry out her wishes to die with dignity. The decision was appealed to the British Columbia Court of Appeal and then to the Supreme Court of Canada, where it was dismissed on both occasions. In a five to four majority decision of the Supreme Court of Canada, Justice Sopinka wrote that the law accorded with the principles of fundamental justice. He stressed that it was necessary because: (1) it protects vulnerable people who may be persuaded to commit suicide; (2) it protects the sanctity of human life; (c) the court does not want to suggest that the state condones suicide; and (d) it would be difficult to establish safeguards to prevent abuse. (These issues are more fully discussed in Chapter 13.)

Although few countries have legalized assisted suicide, the practice of limiting life-sustaining interventions, even when this decision may lead to death, is widely accepted (Hwang 2003). Society today places greater value on the able-bodied person than on people living with impairments who are stigmatized and whose need for assistance is associated with a loss of dignity. Disability rights groups disagree with the notion that needing assistance equates to a loss of dignity and state that little has been done to address this prevalent societal view or to help the public learn about the actual autonomy and dignified lives of people with impairments (Coleman 2010). Negative attitudes in society and on the part of healthcare providers impact on the feeling of self-worth of children. For example, Lariviere-Bastine and Racine (2011) suggest that, as a result of their communication difficulties, children with cerebral palsy are often treated as though they are unable to provide an opinion about the direction of their care and, as such, treating the child as a complete person is compromised, which in turn compromises their sense of dignity (Hwang 2003, Lariviere-Bastien and Racine 2011). The following case example about the rights of the child highlights this tension.

The Supreme Court of Canada took the following position concerning a young person's desire to determine the outcome of her own health: although the young person had no impairment, she held strong religious views that would ultimately put her life at risk if she did not receive a blood transfusion. In *A.C.* v. *Manitoba* (2009), the Supreme Court of Canada held that courts must consider the opinions of 'mature adolescents' (those younger than 16 years of age) in medical decision making. While legislation, in this case the Manitoba Child and Family Services Act, gives a court the authority to authorize medical treatment that it finds to be in the 'best interests of the child', the Supreme Court ruled that the views of a child younger than 16 should be taken into consideration when determining the child's best interests. Justice Abella prescribed 'a sliding scale of scrutiny' that accords increasing respect to the adolescent's decisions depending on his or her degree of maturity, as well as taking into account the independence of those views and the gravity of the medical decision.

It goes against the caring nature of both parents and healthcare practitioners to have to make decisions that will directly or indirectly lead to the death of a child. Such decisions are highly difficult and are not taken lightly, but opting to keep alive a child who has a life-threatening illness or a terminal impairment to avoid the pain of deciding that they should die is equally hard (Carnevale 2007). In North America it is largely understood that parents play the ultimate role in deciding the outcome for their child. Using a framework of what is best for the child, parents decide what treatment or non-treatment would be the most beneficial to their child. In France, in contrast, the focus is that parents need to be protected from the enormity of making life or death decisions about their children; therefore, the responsibility falls on to the treating physicians, usually within team consultations. Parents are to be informed of the condition their child is in and the reasons why certain treatment options are or are not being offered, but it is the physician who makes the final decision as a means of alleviating any guilt a parent may feel (Carnevale et al 2006).

Resuscitation and other intensive medical involvements are typically not offered unless the physician believes them to be in the best interest of the child. In these cases, the physician will accede to parents' wishes when they have asked for life-saving measures not to be applied (Laventhal et al 2011). The reverse is also held to be true: if the physician determines that it is in the child's best interest to implement life-saving interventions, they will overrule the wishes of parents who wanted such measures not to be implemented. But how does a physician actually make this decision? The decision to resuscitate patients seems to be based more on individual circumstances than on the person's prognosis or on the consideration of what is best for the person (Laventhal et al 2011)

In a study conducted with 587 neonatologists and 108 high-risk obstetricians in the USA to assess their views on resuscitation in difficult ethical circumstances, Laventhal et al (2011) found that taking measures that ultimately result in the death of a child is usually based on what is considered to be in the best interest of the child, but at times the best interest of the family as a unit outweighs the best interest of the individual child (see also Chapter 13).

Conclusion

In this chapter we have explored the tensions and challenges in disability legislation that inform programmes and practices; the targets for change to improve the quality of life of children living with impairments that focus on functioning and abilities rather than deficits; and the tensions in the legislation regarding the right to die with dignity; the importance that support services may have on quality of life and decisions about ending life; and the unintended consequences that may result. What becomes apparent are the inherent inequities of applying legal statutes and/or diagnoses to support children in or prevent them from attaining their maximum potential, irrespective of their unique impairment. Regardless of impairment, geographic location, parental income, and cultural beliefs and values, children must be part of the discussion when it comes to programmes, policies, and practices designed to help them achieve their optimal quality of life.

REFERENCES

Key references

Anderson D, Dumont S, Jacobs P, Azzaria L (2007) The personal costs of caring for a child with a disability: a review of the literature. *Public Health Rep* 122: 3–16.

*August R (2009) Paved with good intentions: the failure of passive disability policy in Canada. Caledon Institute of Social Policy, Toronto, Ontario: 1–27.

Batavia A (2001) The ethics of PAS: morally relevant relationships between personal assistance services and physician-assisted suicide. *Arch Phys Med and Rehabil* 82: S25–S31.

Bedell GM, Khetani MA, Cousins MA, Coster WJ, Law MC (2011) Parent perspectives to inform development of measures of children's participation and environment. *Arch Phys Med Rehabil* 92: 765–773. http://dx.doi.org/10.1016/j.apmr.2010.12.029

*Birnbaum R, Lach L, Saposnek D, MacCulloch R (2012) Co-parenting children with neurodevelopmental disorders. In: Kuehnle K, Drozd L, editors. *Parenting Plan Evaluations: Applied Research for the Family Court*. Oxford: Oxford University Press, pp. 270–329.

Blackman J (2002) Early intervention: a global perspective. *Infants Young Child* 15: 11–19. http://dx.doi.org/10.1097/00001163-200210000-00004

*Burton P, Phipps S (2009) Economic costs of caring for children with disabilities in Canada. *Can Public Policy* 35: 269–290. http://dx.doi.org/10.3138/cpp.35.3.269

Campbell J (1994) Unintentional consequences in public policy: persons with psychiatric disabilities and the Americans with disabilities act. *Policy Studies Journal* 22: 133–145. http://dx.doi.org/10.1111/j.1541-0072.1994.tb02186.x

Campbell L (2001) Rights and disabled children. In: Franklin B, editor. *The New Handbook of Children's Rights: Comparative Policy and Practice*. London: Routledge, pp. 196–207.

*Canadian Coalition for the Rights of Children (2003) 2003 Update to Canada's Report to the UN Committee for the Rights of Children. Available at: http://rightsofchildren.ca/wp-content/uploads/2009/05/03update.pdf (accessed 13 March 2012).

Canty-Mitchell J, Austin JK, Perkins SM, Qi A, Swigonski N (2005) Health-related quality of life in Children with Special Health Care Needs (CSHCN). *Child Health Care* 34: 1–18. http://dx.doi.org/10.1207/s15326888chc3401_1

*Carnevale FA (2007) The birth of tragedy in pediatrics: a phronetic conception of bioethics. *Nurs Ethics* 14: 571–582. http://dx.doi.org/10.1177/0969733007080203

*Carnevale FA, Canou P, Hubert P, et al (2006) The moral experience of parents regarding life-support decisions for their critically-ill children: a preliminary study in France. *J Child Health Care* 10: 69–82. http://dx.doi.org/10.1177/1367493506060209

*Coleman D (2010) Assisted suicide laws create discriminatory double standard for who gets suicide prevention and who gets suicide assistance: Not Dead Yet responds to Autonomy, Inc. *Disabil Health J* 3: 39–50. http://dx.doi.org/10.1016/j.dhjo.2009.09.004

De Wispelaere J, Walsh J (2007) Disability rights in Ireland: chronicle of a missed opportunity. *Irish Political Stud* 22: 517–534. http://dx.doi.org/10.1080/07907180701699265

*Fadem P, Minkler M, Perry M, et al (2003) Attitudes of people with disabilities towards physician-assisted suicide legislation: broadening the dialogue. *J Health Polit Policy Law* 28: 977–1001. http://dx.doi.org/10.1215/03616878-28-6-977

Gannoni A, Shute RH (2009) Parental and child perspectives on adaptation to childhood chronic illness: a qualitative study. *Clin Child Psychol Psychiatry* 15: 39–53. http://dx.doi.org/10.1177/1359104509338432

Gibson BE, Darrah J, Cameron D, et al (2009) Revisiting therapy assumptions in children's rehabilitation: clinical and research implications. *Disabil Rehabil* 31: 1446–1453. http://dx.doi.org/10.1080/09638280802621390

*Hanvey L (2002) Children with disabilities and their families in Canada: a discussion paper. Commissioned by the National Children's Alliance for the First National Roundtable on Children with disabilities. Available at: http://www.nationalchildrensalliance.com/nca/pubs/2002/hanvey02.pdf

The Huffington Post (2011) Assisted suicide in Canada: dying woman challenges laws 20 years after last attempt. Available at: www.huffingtonpost.ca/2011/11/13/assisted-suicide-canada-law_n_1090820.html http//www.thecourt.ca/2012/01/18/canadas-assisted-suicide-debate-alive-and-well/ (accessed 12 February 2013).

*Hwang K (2005) Attitudes of persons with physical disabilities towards physician-assisted death. *J Disabil Policy Stud* 16: 16–21. http://dx.doi.org/10.1177/10442073050160010301

Jongbloed L (2003) Disability policy in Canada. *J Disabil Policy Stud* 13: 203–209. http://dx.doi.org/10.1177/104420730301300402

*Kim MK, Fox MH (2011) Disability and society: a comparative examination of disability anti-discrimination legislation in the United States and Korea. *Disabil Soc* 26: 269–283. http://dx.doi.org/10.1080/09687599.2011.560371

*Kovacs Burns K, Gordon GL (2010) Analysing the impact of disability legislation in Canada and the United States. *J Disabil Policy Stud* 20: 205–218. http://dx.doi.org/10.1177/1044207309344562

*Lariviere-Bastien D, Racine E (2011) Ethics in health care services for young persons with neurodevelopmental disabilities: a focus on cerebral palsy. *J Child Neurol* 26: 1221–1229. http://dx.doi.org/10.1177/0883073811402074

*Laventhal N, Larkin LK, Spelke MB, Andrews B, Meadow W, Janvier A (2011) Ethics of resuscitation at different stages of life: a survey of perinatal physicians. *Pediatrics* 127: e1221–e1229. http://dx.doi.org/10.1542/peds.2010-1031

*Leonardi M (2010) Measuring health and disability: supporting policy development: the European MHADIE project. *Disabil Rehabil* 32: S1–S8. http://dx.doi.org/10.3109/09638288.2010.520806

Mednick L, Koocher G (2012) Co-parenting children with chronic medical conditions. In: Kuehnle K, Drozd L, editors. *Parenting Plan Evaluations: Applied Research for the Family Court*. Oxford: Oxford University Press, pp. 235–270.

Oregon Public Health Division (2012) Characteristics and end-of-life care. Available at: http://public.health.oregon.gov/ProviderPartnerResources/EvaluationResearch/DeathwithDignityAct/Pages/index.aspx (accessed 22 February 2012).

*Prince MJ (2001) Canadian federalism and disability policy making. *Can J Polit Sci* 34: 791–817. http://dx.doi.org/10.1017/S0008423901778092

*Prince MJ (2004) Canadian disability policy: still a hit-and-miss affair. *Can J Socio* 29: 59–82. http://dx.doi.org/10.2307/3341945

*Prince MJ (2010) What about a disability rights act for Canada? Practices and lessons from America, Australia, and the United Kingdom. *Can Public Policy* 36: 199–214. http://dx.doi.org/10.3138/cpp.36.2.199

Rosenbaum P, Livingston MH, Palisano RJ, Galuppi BE, Russel DJ (2007) Quality of life and health-related quality of life of adolescents with cerebral palsy. *Dev Med Child Neurol* 49: 516–521. http://dx.doi.org/10.1111/j.1469-8749.2007.00516.x

Saposnek D, Perryman H, Berkow J, Ellsworth S (2005) Special needs children in family court. *Fam Court Rev* 43: 566–581. http://dx.doi.org/10.1111/j.1744-1617.2005.00056.x

Standing Senate Committee on Human Rights (2005) Who's in charge here? Effective implementation of Canada's international obligations with respect to the rights of children. Available at: http://publications.gc.ca/collections/collection_2011/sen/yc32-0/YC32-0-381-19-eng.pdf (accessed 13 March 2012).

*Tiedemann M, Valiquet D (2008) Euthanasia and assisted suicide in Canada. Available at: http://www.parl.gc.ca/Content/LOP/researchpublications/919-e.htm (accessed 13 March 2012).

*Turnbull RH III, Beegle G, Stowe MJ (2001) The core concepts of disability policy affecting families who have children with disabilities. *J Disabil Policy Stud* 12: 133–143. http://dx.doi.org/10.1177/104420730101200302

*Valentine F (2001) Enabling citizenship: full inclusion of children with disabilities and their parents. Canadian Policy Research Networks. Available at: http://cprn.org/documents/ACFZwv9Kd.PDF (accessed 13 March 2012).

Wang M, Brown R (2009) Family quality of life: a framework for policy and social service provisions to support families of children with disabilities. *J Fam Social Work* 12: 144–167. http://dx.doi.org/10.1080/10522150902874842

World Health Organization (2001) *International Classification of Functioning, Disability and Health*. Geneva: WHO.

*World Health Organization (2011) *World Health Report*. Available at: http://www.who.int/disabilities/world_report/2011/report/en/index.html (accessed 7 July 2012).

Young B, Rice H, Dixon-Woods M, Clover AF, Parkinson KN (2007) A qualitative study of the health-related quality of life of disabled children. *Dev Med Child Neurol* 49: 660–665. http://dx.doi.org/10.1111/j.1469-8749.2007.00660.x

Zekovic B, Renwick R (2003) Quality of life for children and adolescents with developmental disabilities: review of conceptual and methodological issues relevant to public policy. *Disabil Soc* 18: 19–34. http://dx.doi.org/10.1080/713662199

Cases and law

A.C. v. *Manitoba (Director of Child and Family Services)* [2009] SCC 30.

Canada Charter of Rights and Freedoms (1982) Enacted by the Canada Act 1982 [UK] c.11; proclaimed in force 17 April 1982. Amended by the Constitution Amendment Proclamation, 1983, SI/84-102, effective 21 June 1984. Amended by the Constitution Amendment, 1993 [New Brunswick], SI/93-54, *Can. Gaz. Part II*, 7 April 1993, effective 12 March 1993.

Carter v. *Canada (Attorney General)* [2012] BCSC 886.

Rodriguez v. *British Columbia* [1993] SCC.

26

THE ROLE OF PARENT AND COMMUNITY ORGANIZATIONS IN CHILD HEALTH PROMOTION

Christopher Morris and Val Shilling

Overview

This chapter will first consider the concept of 'health promotion' with reference to the World Health Organization's (WHO's) concepts. Second, examples of relevant parent and community organizations will be described, and the various ways in which they seek to promote the health and well-being of children with impairments and their families are discussed. Finally, the challenges that parent-led organizations face in achieving their goals will be identified and opportunities to further embed meaningful partnerships proposed. Many of the examples of organizations and policies are from the UK, reflecting the authors' location and experience. However, it is hoped that readers will recognize principles that are applicable to their own settings and will be able to identify examples of these parent-led initiatives, or opportunities, in their own countries.

Introduction

This chapter considers the roles that various parent and community organizations play in promoting the health and well-being of young people with neurological and developmental conditions and their families. Some organizations have been around for a long time. The oldest such non-medical organizations are probably philanthropic ventures set up in the nineteenth century for children with sensory impairments, such as schools specifically for deaf or blind children. The National Society for Crippled Children, founded in the USA in 1921 (later renamed as the Easter Seals) is often credited with being the oldest parent-led group. Since then, there has been a considerable increase in the number of parent and community organizations, particularly to support children with specific conditions. Enabling access to appropriate education has been a predominant theme. For instance, the National Spastics Society (the original name of Scope) was founded in the UK in 1952 by three parents and a social worker who wanted children with impairments to have equal rights to an education.

The various roles that these organizations play have evolved, and they continue to adapt their roles in different countries and settings. A consistent theme of this chapter is to call for more meaningful and productive partnerships between healthcare and social care profession-als and parent and community organizations. The various contributions of families should be sought and valued by professionals as being complementary and essential to their own work, with the aim of improving the health and well-being of children with impairments.

What do we mean by health promotion?

In other chapters in this book critical distinctions are made between concepts such as health status (Chapters 2 and 4), participation (Chapter 5), and variations on the theme of quality of life (Chapters 2 and 3). In promoting health, the WHO seeks broadly to foster the prin-ciples of social justice and equity of health outcomes across all these domains. In 1986 the WHO defined 'health promotion' as part of its landmark Ottawa Charter as: '…the process of enabling people to increase control over, and to improve, their health. To reach a state of complete physical, mental and social well-being, an individual or group must be able to iden-tify and to realize aspirations, to satisfy needs, and to change or cope with the environment. Health is, therefore, seen as a resource for everyday life, not the objective of living. Health is a positive concept emphasizing social and personal resources, as well as physical capacities. Therefore, health promotion is not just the responsibility of the health sector, but goes beyond healthy life-styles to well-being.' (World Health Organization 2009)

The Ottawa Charter and subsequent reports of WHO health promotion conferences make clear the statutory responsibility governments have to promote health through thoughtful policy making. 'Health promotion policy combines diverse but complementary approaches including legislation, fiscal measures, taxation and organizational change. It is coordinated action that leads to health, income and social policies that foster greater equity.' (World Health Organization 2009). However the WHO also emphasizes the need to empower communities to promote health 'through concrete and effective community action in setting priorities, making decisions, planning strategies and implementing them to achieve better health' (World Health Organization 2009). To encourage public involvement in decision making there is recognition of the need for access to information, learning opportunities, and funding.

Many of the WHO's efforts in health promotion have targeted adults' behaviours related to consumption of tobacco and alcohol, minimizing obesity, and improving women's health. However, in more recent documents, such as the 2005 Bangkok Charter, there is explicit recognition of the challenges faced by children and disabled people, highlighting their vulner-ability to exclusion (World Health Organization 2009). To overcome the challenges the WHO proposes coordinated actions: 'Partnerships, alliances, networks and collaborations provide exciting and rewarding ways of bringing people and organizations together around common goals and joint actions to improve the health of populations. Each sector – intergovernmental, government, civil society and private – has a unique role and responsibility' (World Health Organization 2009).

So how are we doing? A recent review of children's services in the UK National Health Service (NHS) showed that many of the ideals espoused in the WHO Charters are not being met owing to structural and cultural barriers in the NHS (Kennedy 2010). Sir Ian Kennedy's review catalogued a range of cultural barriers operating at national, regional, local, and indi-vidual care levels: (1) lack of priority for investment in children's services; (2) poor coordi-nation of health services particularly for children with complex needs; (3) poor coordination between health services and education and social care; and (4) poor sharing and access to information (Kennedy 2010). A principal recommendation from Kennedy was the need for everyone involved to agree on what we are trying to achieve for children and then to work together to achieve those goals: 'All the relevant agencies and professionals in a given area that are involved in commissioning and providing services must, with the active participation of children and young people, agree a common vision for the healthcare, health and well-being of children and young people, and collaborate in achieving it' (Kennedy 2010). This is a more strongly stated reprisal of the goals espoused in previous policies in the UK (e.g. Department of Health 2004, Department for Education and Skills 2005, Department of Health and Department for Children, Schools and Families 2009).

Therefore, a key role for parent and community organizations representing children with impairments is to engage with health service policy makers and providers to seek to agree on a common vision for the health outcomes we want to achieve. Equally important is for professionals in health and social care to value parent-led organizations and to work with them in a meaningful collaboration. Davies and Hall (2005) identified that health professionals may harbour reservations and/or negative beliefs about parent-led groups, including fearing that the parent-to-parent contact may undermine their expertise. Nevertheless, Davies and Hall (2005) argue in favour of the benefits of 'empowering' families, and fostering genuine partnerships between health professionals and parent-led organizations.

Parent and community organizations

At this point it would seem helpful to list some examples of the types of parent and community organizations that play a part in promoting the health of children with impairments and their families.

Charities and Voluntary Groups

A wide range of charitable and voluntary groups has been established to promote the health and well-being of children with impairments. Some organizations are condition specific (e.g. for autism, muscular dystrophy, etc.), while others support families of children with any impairment and take a non-categorical approach to childhood disability. Some organizations support children and/or families generally and support families of children with impairments as a subgroup. Most of the organizations focus their activities in one country or region; however, there are also international aid agencies that take a global perspective of children and/or impairment.

The typically stated mission is to enable or support children and families affected by frequently disabling conditions 'to live ordinary lives' or 'to live the lives they choose'. Some charities provide equipment or subsidize therapies; and some charities fund or engage with research into cures or to evaluate the effectiveness of treatments, or to explore other issues and experiences faced by families. It is perhaps a quirk of the UK system, but many organizations are registered as charities but provide, for a fee, education or mainstream, complementary, or alternative therapies.

In addition to structured organizations there are also informal local groups of parents and families that meet regularly. Groups may be supported in their activities through public sector funding and/or may be dependent on voluntary contributions.

STATUTORY AGENCIES

Local authorities and other publicly funded services may convene 'service user groups' to seek consultation on how they can improve the way they deliver their services. These provide children with impairments and their parents with the opportunity to come together and engage with service providers to have their say. For example, local authorities in England and Wales provide funding for Parent Partnerships, and central funding by the Department of Education supports the National Parent Partnership Network (www.parentpartnership.org.uk).

SCHOOLS

Education is a human right and a recognized determinant of health and well-being (World Health Organization 2009). Children with neurodevelopmental conditions may attend 'inclusive' mainstream or 'segregated' special schools or colleges depending on availability, national and local educational policies, their cognitive abilities, and children's and parents' preferences. Schools and colleges provide formal and informal opportunities for teachers, children, and parents to collaborate in finding ways to help children with additional needs to reach their potential, and also to support families.

PROVIDERS OF RECREATION AND LEISURE ACTIVITIES

Public sector, private, and community organizations provide a range of recreation and leisure opportunities for children and families. Among these are inclusive 'integrated' opportunities for all children and specialist 'segregated' opportunities designed specifically for children with impairments; families value both (Beresford et al 2010). Children's participation in positive and inclusive activities is associated with better health and well-being (Beresford et al 2010).

Roles

These kinds of parent and community organizations work in a number of ways to promote the health and well-being of children with impairments and their families. Some of the activities are undertaken jointly with professionals, while other activities are parent-led initiatives without the involvement of health professionals.

PEER SUPPORT

It is broadly acknowledged that the parents of children with impairments are at increased risk of relationship problems, stress, depression, and lack of sleep (Contact a Family 2003). Family relationships may suffer through exhaustion and stress, and parents report feeling isolated, lonely, and unsupported (Davies and Hall 2005). Parents have reported adverse physical and mental health effects, which they attribute to both the actual demands of caring and anxiety about their child's health and future (Murphy et al 2006). Parents often say they would like more contact with other parents of children with impairments to share information, advice, and social support (Schreiber et al 2011). Even the opportunity to talk to other parents in the waiting room can be a valued means of support for some parents (Cohn 2001). Parents do not always have enough knowledge or information to access the services and benefits that are available, and sometimes relationships with professionals are strained. The provision of peer support has the potential to mitigate some of the problems faced by families of children with impairments and to have a significant positive impact on later outcomes.

The defining characteristic of peer support is that it is support offered by people who have, or have had, similar experiences (Dennis 2003), i.e. parents of children with impairments supporting other parents of children with other impairments. A peer is 'an individual who shares common characteristics with the "targeted" group or individual, allowing her/him to relate to, and empathise with, that individual on a level that a non-peer would not be able to' (Doull et al 2008). The reason that this type of support is presumed to be important is because of the 'shared experience', a sense that another person understands what you are going through because he or she has been there. Meeting other parents can reduce isolation and help parents feel that they belong, and parents can share coping strategies and information (King et al 2000). Being able to share their own expertise and knowledge can also help parents feel valued and more self-confident (Davies and Hall 2005). Peer support can help parents understand what information and services are available to them as well as offering emotional support and a sense of shared experience and purpose (Koroloff et al 1999).

A number of psychological theories are thought to underlie peer support including social support, experiential knowledge, helper therapy principles, social learning theory, and social comparison theory. However, the nature of peer support has made it difficult to use traditional research methods to test these theories (Solomon 2004). Indeed, it is unusual for peer support for parents of children with impairments to be evaluated in research studies at all; as Law and colleagues (2001) reported, systematic, rigorous evaluations have seldom been conducted.

Peer support can differ in the type of interaction (e.g. one-to-one sessions, Internet forum), the setting (home, hospital, school), the aims (providing information, providing emotional support), the provider (professionally led programmes or volunteer organizations), and the structure (formal vs informal). Some examples are

- informal contact, such as chance encounters in the waiting room or at meetings
- informal parent-led support groups that may support parents of children with similar diagnoses or who attend the same school
- online Internet forums are popular: these are informal and flexible as parents can access forums in their own time and they are accessible to families with limited time or inclination to meet face to face – the fact that participants are anonymous may enable parents to raise issues that they might otherwise find it difficult to discuss face to face
- one-to-one telephone or email support by trained counsellors is offered by some organizations
- parent-led support groups are coordinated by some organizations, typically on a regional level – in some cases, training may be offered to group leaders
- one-to-one support in person from another parent: for example, Face 2 Face (a charitable national network in the UK) trains volunteer parents in counselling to become 'befrienders' who then support other parents supervised by a paid local coordinator.

PROVIDING INFORMATION

Another key role is in the provision of information. This is a role that parent-led and specialty organizations can often fulfil more expertly and comprehensively than professionals for several reasons. They usually have a regional or national perspective on the issues and the resources; and, frequently, they have a clear idea of the kinds of issues and questions that are most important to parents and young people with impairments.

Information is disseminated by parent-led organizations for various audiences, not just for other parents. For example, the Council for Disabled Children, part of the National Children's Bureau in the UK, offers different kinds of information for (1) young people, (2) parents, (3) public sector professionals, and (4) the voluntary sector. Their information and resources are relevant to promoting the health and well-being of children with any chronic health condition. Condition-specific charities, such as the National Autistic Society, the Epilepsy Foundation (in the USA), or Scope, provide a similar range of resources and also information about the conditions on which they focus. Many health professionals would find it informative and possibly enlightening to access information presented by parent-led organizations. This information aims to present the families' perspective in order to encourage professionals to take a holistic approach in their professional role, by making them aware of the range of issues with which families are coping.

Some of the key stages at which families seek information are to find out more about their child's condition, to find out about treatments and therapies, and to find out what other services and support might be available. Information about a health condition is often a valuable resource for families around the time of diagnosis (Davies and Hall 2005). The parent-led organization Contact a Family in the UK provides an A to Z listing of around 440 conditions. For each condition there is 'medical' information written in lay terms, brief information about treatment, and suggestions of organizations providing support to families of children with that condition (www.cafamily.org.uk/medicalinformation/conditions/azlistings/a.html).

Many organizations offer information about therapies and treatments. Such information varies in quality depending on who writes the articles and their motivation and any biases. There are numerous websites that promote unproven interventions and therapies; and many of these have a vested interest in actually selling treatments. However, some information is written by more reliable sources. The information provided by Contact a Family, for example, was written by members of the Royal College of Paediatrics and Child Health. However, there are many less reliable sources, some of which are websites for 'charities' that are in the business of selling unproven treatments. Our research group has recently made available some guidance for families to help them appraise the reliability of information they find on the Internet (www.pencru.org/evidence_searching.php). Parent-led organizations offer families information about what benefits and support they might be entitled to, depending on where they live. This is picked up in the next section on advocacy.

ADVOCACY AND OBTAINING RIGHTS

Parent and community organizations frequently advocate for individuals and/or lobby for the groups they represent to ensure that they obtain the support and services to which they are entitled. As mentioned above, this may involve providing information about the benefits and entitlements that are or may be available for individuals or families, and advice about how to claim those entitlements. There are a number of forms that are required to be completed to claim the different benefits to which families of children with impairments are fully entitled in the UK; however, even within the UK the entitlements and systems to claim vary by region.

Sadly, several parent-led agencies have found that completing the forms is complex and difficult, which makes it hard for families to claim their entitlement. Several organizations provide general guidance (e.g. www.cafamily.org.uk/families/rightsandentitlements/benefit-staxcredits) but these organizations also strongly recommend parents seek personal assistance to ensure that they provide all the appropriate information.

In the UK one of the leading campaign groups specifically for families of children with impairments is Every Disabled Child Matters (EDCM). The EDCM campaign lobbies the UK government to create legislation that will improve the health and well-being of children with impairments and also to ensure that the necessary resources are invested to bring those rights to reality (www.ncb.org.uk/edcm). An example of their activities is a recent campaign, conducted with the Internet-based parent organization Mumsnet, which lobbied for provision of adequate nappies for incontinent children with impairments. The campaign won a high-level response from the Department of Health to the effect that 'Pads (nappies) should be provided in quantities appropriate to the individual's continence needs. Arbitrary ceilings are inappropriate' (www.ncb.org.uk/edcm/campaigns/health.aspx).

Some of the most well-established social policy-oriented charities in the UK, such as the Joseph Rowntree Foundation and Barnardo's, include research about the life circumstances of children with impairments and their families in their work programmes. They then use, and encourage others to use, their findings to lobby government to improve support for children with impairments. While many of the lobbying issues are generic, the condition-specific charities also lobby on behalf of families of children affected by the conditions on which they are focused.

INVOLVEMENT IN POLICY MAKING

The potential benefits from involving 'service users' or 'consumers' in policy making and planning of services in health and social care are well recognized (World Health Organization 1978). Indeed, the right for children with impairments to be involved is enshrined in both the United Nations Conventions on the Rights of the Child (1989) and Persons with Disabilities (2006). Arnstein's 'ladder of citizen participation' is often cited as a model for involving service users; involvement ranges in the 'ladder' from tokenistic consultation to citizen control (Arnstein 1969). Although involving service users in policy making is being widely implemented (World Health Organization 2006), effective methods of implementing and achieving involvement are not well established (Nilsen et al 2006). There are also difficulties in defining and then measuring the impacts of involving service users (Fudge et al 2008).

The rationale for involving service users in policy making is based on democratic values and principles, but the extent to which pre-existing parent or community organizations are representative, rather than lobbyist, is debatable. Nevertheless such organizations are an obvious resource for national and local agencies responsible for health and social care to engage and recruit active and interested personnel to collaborate with developing better systems and programmes. Involving service users in UK health and social care policy making has been around for 30 years; the most recent system established is local involvement networks. The networks provide a forum for individuals to play a role in how services are designed and delivered (www.nhs.uk/NHSEngland/links/yourrights/Pages/whylink.aspx). There are many initiatives and opportunities for service users, i.e. families of children with impairments in the context of this chapter, to become involved in policy making. Nevertheless, at present it is not clear to what extent the input of service users really does impact on the organization and delivery of health and social care in practice (Craig 2008).

INVOLVEMENT IN RESEARCH

Alongside the growth of involving service users in policy making has been the emergence of involving patients and members of the public in research. Rosenbaum (2011) proposed the term 'family-centred research' to describe engaging families as partners in research. As we responded, there are three key established premises for involving families of children with impairments in childhood disability research (Morris et al 2011). From a philosophical perspective, families should be involved in deciding the research agenda as the research concerns them and those with similar life circumstances. Therefore families are uniquely placed to consider which lines of research enquiry are most relevant and likely to have salience to their lives. Second, there are pragmatic advantages to involving families in deciding which research questions will be addressed and how studies are designed. Families are more likely to want to take part in studies that address their own priorities and to do so using research procedures that are designed to be acceptable to them. The third premise is not universal, but in the UK involving patients and members of the public is mandatory when applying for government agency health services research funding. The rationale for involving members of the public in deciding the research agenda is predicated on the fact that, in a publicly funded system, it is their taxes that are used to subsidize the research, so they have a democratic right to have an influence on what is supported (Morris et al 2011).

Our definition of 'involvement' in this context encompasses all stages of research, including generating and developing ideas, prioritizing, refining research questions, designing studies, finding funding, carrying out the research, and disseminating results. INVOLVE is a UK advisory group which supports greater public involvement in NHS, public health, and social care research. INVOLVE defines three levels of involvement as consultation, collaboration, and user control (Hanley et al 2003), based broadly on Arnstein's 'ladder of citizen participation' (Arnstein 1969).

A key stage in research is deciding which topics are the most important to be addressed. The James Lind Alliance (JLA) advocates methods for bringing patients and clinicians together to identify the most important gaps in knowledge about the effects of treatments. These 'priority-setting partnerships' seek to identify, prioritize, and agree the 'top 10' most important research questions in relation to a particular condition (James Lind Alliance 2010). The JLA also supports broader initiatives to gather the views of patients; for example, they used a survey to identify patients' priorities for research into epilepsy (PatientView on behalf of DUETS and the James Lind Alliance 2008). In one of the few peer-reviewed studies of priority setting in childhood disability, an Australian group described a Delphi survey with three rounds to identify and prioritize consumer- and clinician-selected topics for cerebral palsy research (McIntyre et al 2009). Their results identified considerable overlap between each group's ideas, but they also found that some topics that families suggested were important were neglected by clinicians. Some of these were social issues such as 'cerebral palsy and poverty' or 'access in the community', which may not stimulate 'medically oriented' clinicians. Similarly, clinicians may not find 'effectiveness of alternative therapies' an important research topic. Nevertheless, many families seek out and use alternative therapies when conventional health care does not offer any help, or hope. It is therefore essential that the process for prioritizing topics for research needs to take account of all those the research is intended to inform (Morris et al 2011).

PROMOTING INCLUSION

Impairments are more prevalent in lower-income than in high-income countries and more likely to affect children from poorer households generally (World Health Organization and World Bank 2011). Children with impairments in the UK are reported to experience higher levels of poverty and personal and social disadvantage than typically developing children (Blackburn et al 2010), their housing is often inadequate (Beresford and Rhodes 2008), and, while household costs are greater, there are fewer opportunities for families to earn (Emerson et al 2005). Thus, many disabled children and young people face disadvantages in life chances and opportunities and are at risk of participation restrictions and social exclusion.

The World Report on Disability recommends a series of actions that 'disabled people's organizations' can take to promote inclusive and enabling opportunities for persons with impairments (Table 26.1). While some of the activities have already been described, e.g. advocacy, campaigning, and involvement in policy making, organizations carry out a number of other roles to promote inclusion. These activities target broad societal barriers such as improving public and professional attitudes towards disability and/or enabling and supporting individuals to live independently and develop skills.

Mass media campaigns are one way in which organizations seek to challenge and improve prevailing public attitudes towards impairments. Such campaigns have been conducted by a range of national and international organizations, e.g. that by UNICEF (2010) and the award-winning 'Creature Discomforts' campaign hosted by Leonard Cheshire Disability, which

TABLE 26.1

**Recommendations from the World Report on Disability for action that
'disabled people's organizations' can take to promote inclusion**

Disabled people's organizations can:

- Support people with disabilities to become aware of their rights, to live independently, and to develop their skills

- Support children with disabilities and their families to ensure inclusion in education

- Represent the views of their constituency to international, national, and local decision makers and service providers, and advocate for their rights

- Contribute to the evaluation and monitoring of services, and collaborate with researchers to support applied research that can contribute to service development

- Promote public awareness and understanding by professionals about the rights of persons with disabilities – for example through campaigning, advocacy, and disability equality training

Source: World Health Organization (2011).

provides a series of light-hearted animations with a serious message based on people's real experiences (www.creaturediscomforts.org).

On the individual level, many organizations seek to support young people in their quest to access positive and inclusive opportunities. These activities are typically oriented towards recreation and leisure activities for children and employment and enabling independent living for young adults. Often organizations seek to work with private and/or public sector employers to match young people to appropriate work, for example Scope (in the UK) and Easter Seals (in the USA) both operate schemes.

Challenges for the future

In a 'call for international action' in 1986, the WHO Ottawa Charter on Health Promotion concluded: 'The Conference is firmly convinced that if people in all walks of life, nongovernmental and voluntary organizations, governments, the World Health Organization and all other bodies concerned join forces in introducing strategies for health promotion, in line with the moral and social values that form the basis of this Charter, Health For All by the year 2000 will become a reality' (WHO 2009).

Despite progress, more than 25 years on, there remain significant inequities in health outcomes, particularly for young people affected by neurodevelopmental conditions and their parents/carers. The WHO notes the implementation gap: although many countries sign resolutions making commitments, the required actions are not always carried out in practice (World Health Organization 2009). The World Report on Disability echoes many of the same themes and continues the call for all agencies to work together to improve participation and inclusion (World Health Organization and World Bank 2011). It seems that we know what needs to be done but still find it difficult to deliver on the necessary deeds.

The recommendations of the World Report on Disability are targeted at the various stakeholders who can promote the health and well-being of children and young people affected by impairments and their families (World Health Organization and World Bank 2011). It has to be hoped that the necessary investments will be made, both in terms of the top-down finance and resources to make services work and in terms of the bottom-up change in the attitudes of individuals and communities to enable them to modernize and embrace variability.

Conclusion

It is hoped that this chapter will increase people's appreciation of the contribution that parent and community organizations can, and should be encouraged to, play in improving the health and well-being of children and families affected by impairments.

REFERENCES

Key references

Arnstein S (1969) A ladder of participation. *J Am Inst Planners* 35: 216–224. http://dx.doi.org/10.1080/01944366908977225

Beresford B, Clarke S, Borthwick, R (2010) *Improving the Wellbeing of Disabled Children and Young People through Improving Access to Positive and Inclusive Activities. Disability Knowledge Review 2*. London:

Centre for Excellence and Outcomes in Children and Young People's Services (C4EO). Available at: www.c4eo.org.uk/themes/disabledchildren/positiveactivities/files/c4eo_improving_the_wellbeing_improving_access_full_knowledge_review.pdf (accessed 31 July 2011).

Beresford B, Rhodes D (2008) *Housing and Disabled Children. Round-up: Reviewing the Evidence*. York, UK: Joseph Rowntree Foundation. Available at: www.jrf.org.uk/sites/files/jrf/2208.pdf (accessed 5 September 2011).

Blackburn CM, Spencer NJ, Read JM (2010) Prevalence of childhood disability and the characteristics and circumstances of disabled children in the UK: secondary analysis of the Family Resources Survey. *BMC Pediatrics* 10: 21.

Cohn ES (2001) From waiting to relating: parents' experiences in the waiting room of an occupational therapy clinic. *Am J Occup Ther* 55: 167–174. http://dx.doi.org/10.5014/ajot.55.2.167

Contact a Family (2003) *No Time for Us: Relationships Between Parents who Have a Disabled Child*. Available at: www.cafamily.org.uk/media/446233/no_time_for_us_report_2003final.pdf (accessed 27 November 2012).

Craig GM (2008) Involving users in developing health services. *BMJ* 336: 286–287. http://dx.doi.org/10.1136/bmj.39462.598750.80

*Davies S, Hall D (2005) 'Contact a Family': professionals and parents in partnership. *Arch Dis Child* 90: 1053–1057. http://dx.doi.org/10.1136/adc.2004.070706

Dennis CL (2003) Peer support within a health care context: a concept analysis. *Int J Nurs Stud* 40: 321–332. http://dx.doi.org/10.1016/S0020–7489(02)00092-5

Department for Education and Skills (2005) Statutory Guidance on Inter-agency Cooperation to Improve the Wellbeing of Children: Children's Trusts. London: Department for Education and Skills.

Department of Health (2004) National Service Framework for Children, Young People and Maternity Services. London: Department of Health.

Department of Health and Department for Children, Schools and Families (2009) Healthy Lives, Brighter Futures – The Strategy for Children and Young People's Health. London: Department of Health.

Doull M, O'Connor A, Welch V, Tugwell P, Wells G (2008) Peer support strategies for improving the health and well-being of individuals with chronic diseases. *Cochrane Library* 4.

Emerson E, Graham H, Hatton C (2005) Household income and health status in children and adolescents in Britain. *Eur J Publ Health* 16: 354–360. http://dx.doi.org/10.1093/eurpub/cki200

Fudge N, Wolfe CDA, McKevitt C (2008) Assessing the promise of user involvement in health service development: ethnographic study. *BMJ* 336(7639): 313–317. http://dx.doi.org/10.1136/bmj.39456.552257.BE

Hanley B, Bradburn J, Barnes M, et al (2003) Involving the Public in NHS, Public Health and Social Care Research: Briefing Notes for Researchers, 2nd edn. INVOLVE, pp. 8–12. Available at: www.invo.org.uk/pdfs/Briefing%20Note%20Final.dat.pdf (accessed 31 July 2011).

James Lind Alliance (2010) Guidebook. Available at: www.JLAguidebook.org (accessed 1 February 2011).

Kennedy I (2010) Getting it right for children and young people. Overcoming cultural barriers in the NHS so as to meet their needs. London: Department of Health. Available at: www.dh.gov.uk/prod_consum_dh/groups/dh_digitalassets/@dh/@en/@ps/documents/digitalasset/dh_119446.pdf (accessed 31 July 2011).

*King G, Stewart D, King S, Law M (2000) Organizational characteristics and issues affecting the longevity of self-help groups for parents of children with special needs. *Qual Health Res* 10: 225–241. http://dx.doi.org/10.1177/104973200129118381

Koroloff NM, Friesen BJ (1991) Support groups for parents of children with emotional disorders: a comparison of members and non-members. *Commun Ment Health J* 27: 265–279. http://dx.doi.org/10.1007/BF00757261

*Law M, King S, Stewart D, King G (2001) The perceived effects of parent-led support groups for parents of children with disabilities. *Phys Occup Ther Pediatr* 21: 29–48. http://dx.doi.org/10.1080/J006v21n02_03

Macaulay AC, Commanda LE, Freeman WL, et al (1999) Participatory research maximizes community and lay involvement. *BMJ* 319: 774–778. http://dx.doi.org/10.1136/bmj.319.7212.774

McIntyre S, Novak I, Cusick A (2009). Consensus research priorities for cerebral palsy: a Delphi survey of consumers, researchers and clinicians. *Dev Med Child Neurol* 52: 270–275. http://dx.doi.org/10.1111/j.1469–8749.2009.03358.x

*Morris C, Shilling V, McHugh C, Wyatt K (2011) Why it is crucial to involve families in all stages of childhood disability research. *Dev Med Child Neurol* 53: 769–771. http://dx.doi.org/10.1111/j.1469–8749.2011.03984.x

Murphy NA, Christian B, Caplin DA, Young PC (2006) The health of caregivers for children with disabilities: caregiver perspectives. *Child Care Health Dev* 33: 180–187. http://dx.doi.org/10.1111/j.1365–2214.2006.00644.x

Nilsen ES, Myrhaug HT, Johansen M, Oliver S, Oxman AD (2006) Methods of consumer involvement in developing healthcare policy and research, clinical practice guidelines and patient information material. *Cochrane Database Syst Rev* 3: CD004563. http://dx.doi.org/10.1002/14651858.CD004563.pub2

PatientView on behalf of DUETS and James Lind Alliance (2008) Patients' priorities for research into epilepsy: a survey of patient groups. Available at: www.lindalliance.org/pdfs/Epilepsy/Patients'%20Priorities%20for%20Epilepsy%20Research%20JLA%20%20DUETs.pdf (accessed 1 February 2011).

Rosenbaum PL (2011). Family-centred research: what does it mean and can we do it? Editorial. *Dev Med Child Neurol* 53: 99–100.

Schreiber J, Benger J, Salls J, Marchetti G, Reed L (2011) Parent perspectives on rehabilitation services for their children with disabilities: a mixed methods approach. *Phys Occup Ther Pediatr* 31: 225–238.

Solomon P (2004) Peer support/peer provided services underlying processes, benefits, and critical ingredients. *Psychiatr Rehabil J* 27: 392–401. http://dx.doi.org/10.2975/27.2004.392.401

UNICEF (2010) 'It's about ability.' Available at: www.unicef.org/montenegro/Its_About_Ability(1).pdf (accessed 5 September 2011).

United Nations (1989) Convention on the Rights of the Child. Available at: www.unicef.org/crc (accessed 31 July 2011).

United Nations (2006) Convention on the Rights of Persons with Disabilities. Available at: www.un.org/disabilities/index.asp (accessed 31 July 2011).

World Health Organization (1978) Declaration of Alma Ata: Report of the International Conference on Primary Health Care. Available at: www.who.int/hpr/NPH/docs/declaration_almaata.pdf (accessed 5 September 2011).

World Health Organization (2006) Ninth futures forum on health systems governance and public participation. Available at: www.euro.who.int/document/e89766.pdf (accessed 31 July 2011).

*World Health Organization (2009) Milestones in Health Promotion: Statements from Global Conferences. Available at: www.who.int/healthpromotion/Milestones_Health_Promotion_05022010.pdf (accessed 31 July 2011).

World Health Organization and World Bank (2011) World Report on Disability 2011. Available at: http://whqlibdoc.who.int/publications/2011/9789240685215_eng.pdf (accessed 5 September 2011).

Afterword

27
THE ICF AND LIFE QUALITY OUTCOMES

Peter L. Rosenbaum and Gabriel M. Ronen

Introduction

'Life quality' is a relatively new emphasis in clinical discussions and health services research. The topic moves us beyond the traditional primary focus on the biomedical dimensions of diseases, impairments, and conditions towards a broader consideration of the lives of people who experience these conditions, and, in the case of children and young people, the lives of their parents and families. While in no way minimizing the value of the best of current biomedicine, the purpose of this book is to explore 'life quality' as a focus for developments in the clinical, research, and policy arenas. We believe that there is an important responsibility to recognize that biomedicine provides at most a necessary but not sufficient contribution to the well-being and wholeness of people living with neurological and developmental impairments, and to the developmental trajectories of children and young people with these conditions and their families. This book has tried to provide perspectives on these ideas.

This book is dedicated equally to service providers, programme managers, researchers in the field of disability, and policy makers – all of whose actions may have potentially great impacts on children and young people with neurological and developmental impairments. In planning this book and engaging authors (all of whom responded enthusiastically to the invitation to contribute their perspectives) the editors drew on the concepts of the International Classification of Functioning, Disability and Health (ICF; World Health Organization 2001). We see these interrelated ideas as an important way of looking holistically at the life experiences of people with impairments that probably impinge on their neurological and developmental well-being. Thus, in drawing the book together here we have used ICF language once again both to highlight key ideas and to indicate where the ICF ends and additional perspectives are needed. We hope to challenge all our readers to recognize and seize opportunities to move the field forward with new research, advocacy initiatives, and policy developments that enrich the lives of all citizens – including those with impaired development or neurological function.

Grounding the issues within ICF concepts

It may help readers to revisit the relative emphases of ICF concepts as these have been discussed in this book. This final chapter reviews these ideas briefly.

BODY STRUCTURE AND FUNCTION

Readers will know that the body structure and function components of the ICF have been the traditional focus of 'disability' research in children and young people's health. Many traditional interventions have targeted 'impairments', applying biomedical thinking and 'treatments' as well as physical (re)habilitation in an effort to change the underlying biological differences that are thought to be associated with functional limitations. It has often been assumed that it was the impairments – and the manifestations thereof – that limited people's function, and that remediation of these problems would lead to better function and hence to a better life.

It will be apparent that virtually none of this book is about the biomedical aspects of impairment. The authors and editors take as a given that there is a biological basis to all the conditions in which we are interested and that a categorical approach will be needed for some aspects of intervention. There are myriad excellent texts that both provide an understanding of the biomedical underpinnings of neurological and developmental impairments and offer insights into the best available therapies and treatments. What we have tried to do in this book is to encourage readers to look at the many non-categorical *implications* of impairments in body structure and function on people's lives – implications for children's development, their families' well-being, and their life quality; implications for services, training of professionals, and professionals' behaviour; and implications for the social issues and life-course dimensions of these many and varied impairments.

ACTIVITY

Here as well there is more implied than written in this book about activity. At the same time there is considerable effort made throughout the book to encourage people to recognize that *what people do* should to a large extent be related to *what they want to do* (as discussed below regarding 'participation' and 'quality of life') and that whether something is done 'normally' is – to our way of thinking – far less significant than the capacity to achieve those activities that are important to the individual.

PARTICIPATION

This ICF theme is a major element of what this book is about. It can be argued that participation should be the target of all our clinical intervention efforts. We believe that we have a responsibility to encourage parents to empower their children to 'be, belong, and become' to the best of their ability and within the range of their personal interests. This means that we always need to ask 'So what?' questions about the therapeutic advice we offer in order to be certain that interventions are likely to enhance children and young people's participation (their engagement in aspects of their lives that are meaningful to them).

Implications of participation include providing opportunities for children's social inclusion that are free of stigma, that enable social engagement and play, that encourage families to recognize participation as a worthy goal and take a 'developmental' and 'positive psychology' view of their child's impairments, and that see sexuality as an important part of growing up 'even' when a young person has an impairment.

PERSONAL FACTORS

One of the major emphases throughout this book has been on the 'personhood' of children and young adults growing up with developmental impairments. We have stressed the importance of recognizing their individuality, their voices, their aspirations, their wholeness – and how all of these dimensions can potentially be challenged or altered (for better or worse) by forces outside of their immediate control. Thus, it is essential to identify and take advantage of each individual's personal factors – the child's (and family's) strengths, values, preferences, capacities, and capabilities – and to build on this constellation of elements to support the realization of the best 'life quality' for that individual.

ENVIRONMENTAL FACTORS

Another emphasis in this book involves recognizing the environmental and ecological forces that are essential determinants of the lives of children and emerging adults with developmental impairments, and those of their families. These include, first and foremost, the family itself, and much is offered in this book about them and their needs. We have argued here and elsewhere that, for people who work in the child health arena, the well-being of family is absolutely key to the developmental well-being of children – including (perhaps especially) for children with neurological and developmental impairments. This broader ecological perspective of child-in-family is gaining currency, but there is a long way to go before this truism is reflected in policies that see the family (rather than the impaired child) as the unit of interest. We also believe that inherent in a 'family-centred' approach to our relationships with all families is respect for their uniqueness and individuality. Adopting and practicing such an approach enables service providers to learn about and accommodate the sociocultural factors that are such an important component of the multicultural and multiracial communities in which we live and work.

For these reasons the social–ecological environment of laws, policies, social structures, and attitudes is highlighted. This has been done in part to remind readers that there are important and often formative forces on children and families that are well outside the province of the health systems, the improvement of which would have a considerable impact on all children and families, including those about whose lives this book is written.

Our authors have also talked about issues such as knowledge translation (KT) and exchange, training, and inter-professional education as important 'environmental' elements that support professionals to be as well informed and equipped as possible to serve young people with neurological and developmental conditions and their families. Much of what is necessary in KT concerns conceptual shifts and developments (such as embracing ICF language and ideas and abandoning older notions that have been shown not to work). These challenges are, we believe, best addressed in environments that value and reward transdisciplinary learning, research, and service delivery, and move people beyond our traditional disciplinary boundaries. This in turn reminds us of the need for effective training of adult specialists who should be comfortable providing services to 'adults with children's conditions'. In addition, there is the need for interaction with and support of parent and advocacy groups, provision of evidence-based guidance to the courts and public policy makers, monitoring the quality of the ever-growing but often uncritical medical news stories, and interacting in a constructive and accountable engagement with journalists and news media to ensure objective communications (Wilson 2010, Macilwain 2010, Ronen and Dan 2013).

What does the ICF NOT do?

It is important to comment on the possible limitations of the ICF as the sole lens through which to consider all the issues discussed in this book. First, although the ICF as presently constituted makes it possible to describe a moment-in-time snapshot, it is in effect static. The ICF provides what we like to think of as a template that encourages us to identify and 'rule in' (include) current aspects of people's lives across the several elements of the framework. By so doing, both people's strengths and challenges can be included within a single two-dimensional picture of the ICF model, helping us to recognize where there are potential 'points of entry' to work with this child or young person and his or her family, and how these elements may be connected. Thus at a clinical (individual) level the ICF can provide a transdimensional picture of the status of a person, while at the policy level it becomes possible to identify those aspects of people's predicaments that cannot be resolved with better 'medical treatment' alone but need complementary political, social, or environmental interventions.

To this moment-in-time perspective we need to add the dimensions of *time and space*, to try to identify where the specific configuration of elements of a specific person with an impairment might be heading. These additional elements may include an awareness of the dynamic processes of development and life, such as early preparation for transition to adult care. Other contemporaneous factors lie within the community and society in which a person with a neurological or developmental condition is growing up and later grows older – factors such as attitudes towards disability, educational or social policies of inclusion, family support mechanisms, and so on that can all impact significantly on the life quality of the individual with an impairment and that of the family. It is here that one can identify opportunities to make changes – in any aspect of the ICF picture – and assess the impact of those changes on relevant targets over the added dimensions of time and space. This way of thinking and acting then provides the expanded longitudinal perspective that is not part of the ICF but is inherent in the dynamic concept of 'outcomes' across the lifespan.

Second, the ICF can provide an *objective* descriptive account of the elements of a person's life, but *does not include the essential subjective dimension of quality of life!* Although the 'personal factors' component of the ICF allows people to identify their individual likes and dislikes, strengths and weaknesses, it does not seek people's self-reported values or judgements about their lives (patient-reported outcomes). As has been highlighted in many places in this book, the 'disability paradox' identified by Albrecht and Devlieger (1999) brings home clearly the importance of knowing the 'subjective' perceptions of people about their lives, because often the personal and the 'objective' are vastly different. Thus, knowing about people's self-assessed 'quality of life' must be seen to be as important as, and complementary to, the picture provided by the ICF.

A final thought …

The ICF is not meant to be prescriptive. We believe that at best it provides opportunities to identify – with the people who are the focus of our work – what aspects of *their* lives are important to *them* and might be the targets of our resources, advice, and experience. It is our hope that the ideas articulated in this book will have provoked thought and possibly action to enrich the lives (and life quality) of children and young adults with neurological and developmental conditions and their families. We particularly hope that academics and research colleagues will recognize the myriad opportunities to explore the challenges to our field identified by our authors. Any single thought or study can and should be used as a point of entry to move the fields forward. If this goal is realized, the next edition of this book will be even richer and more useful than we have striven to make this version!

REFERENCES

Albrecht GL, Devlieger PJ (1999) The disability paradox: high quality of life against all odds. *Soc Sci Med* 48: 977–988. http://dx.doi.org/10.1016/S0277-9536(98)00411-0

Macilwain C (2010) Calling science to account. *Nature* 463: 875. http://dx.doi.org/10.1038/463875a

Ronen GM, Dan B (2013) Ethical considerations in pediatric neurology. In Dulac O, Lassonde M, Sarnat HB, editors. *Handbook of Clinical Neurology Vol. 111, Pediatric Neurology, Part I*. Chennai: Elsevier.

Wilson PM (2001) A policy analysis of the expert patient in the United Kingdom: self-care as an expression of pastoral power? *Health Soc Care Commun* 9: 134–142. http://dx.doi.org/10.1046/j.1365–2524.2001.00289.x

World Health Organization (2001) *International Classification of Functioning, Disability and Health*. Geneva: WHO Press.

INDEX

Notes

Page numbers in *italics* refer to material in figures, whilst numbers in **bold** refers to material in tables. Abbreviations used: CP, cerebral palsy; ICF, International Classification of Functioning, Disability and Health; KTA, knowledge to action; QoL, quality of life.

Other titles from Mac Keith Press www.mackeith.co.uk

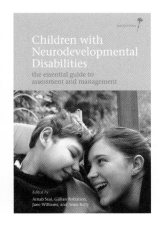

Children with Neurodevelopmental Disabilities: the essential guide to assessment and management
Arnab Seal, Gillian Robinson, Anne M. Kelly and Jane Williams (Eds)

2013 ▪ 744pp ▪ softback ▪ 978-1-908316-62-2
£65.00 / € tbc / $ tbc

A comprehensive textbook on the practice of paediatric neurodisability, written by practitioners and experts in the field. Using a problem-oriented approach, the authors give best-practice guidance, and centre on the needs of the child and family, working in partnership with multi-disciplinary, multi-agency teams. Drawing on evidence-based practice, the authors provide a ready reference for managing common problems encountered in the paediatric clinic.

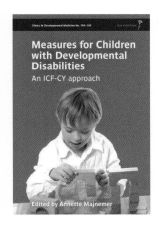

Measures for Children with Developmental Disabilities
An ICF-CY approach
Annette Majnemer (Ed)

Clinics in Developmental Medicine No 194-195
2012 ▪ 552pp ▪ hardback ▪ 978-1-908316-45-5
£150.00 / €186.00 / $235.00

This title presents and reviews outcome measures across a wide range of attributes that are applicable to children and adolescents with developmental disabilities. It uses the children and youth version of the International Classification of Functioning, Disability and Health (ICF-CY) as a framework for organizing the various measures into sections and chapters. Each chapter coincides with domains within the WHO framework of Body Functions, Activities and Participation, and Personal and Environmental Factors.

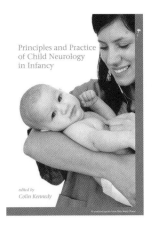

Principles and Practice of Child Neurology in Infancy
Colin Kennedy (Ed)

A practical guide from Mac Keith Press
2012 ▪ 384pp ▪ softback ▪ 978-1-908316-35-6
£29.95 / €38.10 / $49.50

This handbook of neurological practice in infants is designed to be of practical use to all clinicians, but particularly those in under-resourced locations. Seventy per cent of children with disabilities live in resource-poor countries and most of these children have neurological impairments. This book presents recommendations for investigations and treatments based on internationally accepted good practice that can be implemented in most settings.

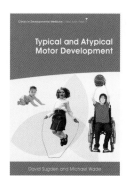

Typical and Atypical Motor Development
David Sugden and Michael Wade

Clinics in Developmental Medicine
2013 ▪ 400pp ▪ hardback ▪ 978-1-908316-55-4
£145.00 / €180.00 / $234.95

Sugden and Wade, leading authors in this area, comprehensively cover motor development and motor impairment, drawing on sources in medicine and health-related studies, motor learning and developmental psychology. A theme that runs through the book is that movement outcomes are a complex transaction of child resources, the context in which movement takes place, and the manner in which tasks are presented.

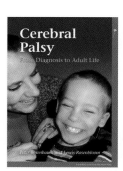

Understanding Cerebral Palsy: From Diagnosis to Adult Life
Peter Rosenbaum and Lewis Rosenbloom

A practical guide from Mac Keith Press
June 2012 ▪ 224pp ▪ softback ▪ 978-1-908316-50-9
£29.95 / €36.10 / $50.00

This book has been designed to provide readers with an understanding of cerebral palsy as a developmental as well as a neurological condition. It details the nature of cerebral palsy, its causes and its clinical manifestations. Using clear, accessible language (supported by an extensive glossary) the authors have blended current science with metaphor to explain the biomedical underpinnings of cerebral palsy.

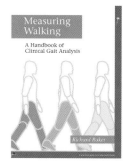

Measuring Walking: A Handbook of Clinical Gait Analysis
Richard Baker

A practical guide from Mac Keith Press
2013 ▪ 248pp ▪ softback ▪ 978-1-908316-66-0
£49.95 / €60.00 / $199.95

This book is a practical guide to instrumented clinical gait analysis covering all aspects of routine service provision. It reinforces what is coming to be regarded as the conventional approach to clinical gait analysis. Data capture, processing and biomechanical interpretation are all described with an emphasis on ensuring high quality results. There are also chapters on how to set up and maintain clinical gait analysis services and laboratories.

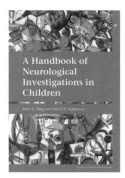

A Handbook of Neurological Investigations in Children
Mary D. King and John B. P. Stephenson

A practical guide from Mac Keith Press
2009 ▪ 400pp ▪ softback ▪ 978-1-898683-69-8
£39.95 / €48.00 / $73.95

This book sets out the investigations that are really needed to establish the cause of neurological disorders. Its problem-oriented approach starts with the patient's presentation, not the diagnosis. It includes more than 60 case vignettes to illustrate clinical scenarios.

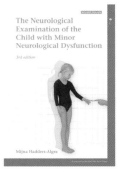

The Neurological Examination of the Child with Minor Neurological Dysfunction, 3rd edition
Mijna Hadders-Algra

A practical guide from Mac Keith Press
2010 ▪ 160pp ▪ softback ▪ 978-1-898683-98-8
£49.95 / €60.00 / $76.00

Bert Touwen's classic handbook has been updated to reflect contemporary clinical practice. This refined, sensitive and age-appropriate technique is designed to take into account the developmental aspects of the child's rapidly changing nervous system. The accompanying DVD contains videos illustrating typical and atypical performance and also provides an electronic assessment form.

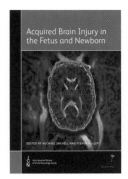

Acquired Brain Injury in the Fetus and Newborn
Michael Shevell and Steven Miller (Eds)

International Review of Child Neurology Series
2012 ▪ 330pp ▪ hardback ▪ 978-1-907655-02-9
£125.00 / €155.00 / $195.00

Given the tremendous advances in the understanding of acquired neonatal brain injury, this book provides a timely review for the practising neurologist, neonatologist and paediatrician. The editors take a pragmatic approach, focusing on specific populations encountered regularly by the clinician. They offer a "bench to bedside" approach to acquired brain injury in the preterm and term newborn infant. The contributors, all internationally recognized neurologists and scientists, provide reader with a state-of-the art review in their area of expertise.